Medical and Psychiatric Comorbidity Over the Course of Life

Medical and Psychiatric Comorbidity Over the Course of Life

Edited by

William W. Eaton, Ph.D.

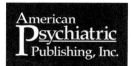

American Psychiatric Publishing, Inc.

Washington, DC
London, England

Manufactured in the United States of America on acid-free paper
09   08   07   06   05   5   4   3   2   1
First Edition

Typeset in Adobe's Janson Text and The Mix.

American Psychiatric Publishing, Inc.
1000 Wilson Boulevard
Arlington, VA 22209–3901
www.appi.org

Library of Congress Cataloging-in-Publication Data
Medical and psychiatric comorbidity over the course of life / edited by William W. Eaton. — 1st ed.
　　　p. ; cm.
　　Includes bibliographical references and index.
　　ISBN 1-58562-231-1 (pbk. : alk. paper)
　　1. Psychiatric epidemiology. 2. Mental illness—Etiology. 3. Mental illness—Longitudinal studies. 4. Comorbidity.
　　　[DNLM: 1. Mental Disorders—epidemiology. 2. Mental Disorders—etiology.
　3. Comorbidity.   WM 140 M489 2005]   I. Eaton, William W.
　　RC455.2.E64M43 2005
　　362.2′0422—dc22
　　　　　　　　　　　　　　　　　　　　　　　　　2005008199

British Library Cataloguing in Publication Data
A CIP record is available from the British Library.

Contents

PART IV

- -

Emotions and Health

PART V

- -

Schizophrenia

Contributors

George S. Alexopoulos, M.D.
Professor, Department of Psychiatry, Weill Medical College of Cornell University; Director, Weill-Cornell Institute of Geriatric Psychiatry, White Plains, New York

Adrian Angold, M.R.C.Psych.
Associate Professor, Department of Psychiatry and Behavioral Sciences, Center for Developmental Epidemiology, Duke University Medical School, Durham, North Carolina

Haroutune K. Armenian, M.D., Dr.P.H., M.P.H.
Professor, Department of Epidemiology, Johns Hopkins Bloomberg School of Public Health, Baltimore, Maryland

Michaeline A. Bresnahan, Ph.D., M.P.H.
Associate Professor, Department of Epidemiology, Mailman School of Public Health, Columbia University, New York, New York

Joseph R. Carbone, M.D.
Assistant Professor, Departments of Psychiatry and Neurology, Mount Sinai School of Medicine, New York, New York

Giovanni Cizza, M.D., Ph.D., MH.Sc.
Principal Investigator, Clinical Endocrinology Branch, National Institute of Diabetes, Digestive, and Kidney Disease, National Institutes of Health, Bethesda, Maryland

E. Jane Costello, Ph.D.
Professor, Department of Psychiatry and Behavioral Sciences, Duke University Medical School, Durham, North Carolina

George Davey Smith, D.Sc.
Professor of Clinical Epidemiology and Head, Epidemiology Division, Department of Social Medicine, University of Bristol, United Kingdom

William W. Eaton, Ph.D.
Professor and Chair, Department of Mental Health, Johns Hopkins Bloomberg School of Public Health, Baltimore, Maryland

Helen Link Egger, M.D.
Assistant Professor, Department of Psychiatry and Behavioral Sciences, Center for Developmental Epidemiology, Duke University Medical School, Durham, North Carolina

Joshua Fogel, Ph.D.
Assistant Professor, Department of Economics, Brooklyn College of the City University of New York (CUNY), Brooklyn, New York

Jeanne Goodman
Department of Psychiatry, Mount Sinai School of Medicine, New York, New York

Jack M. Gorman, M.D.
Esther and Joseph Klingenstein Professor and Chair, Department of Psychiatry; Professor, Department of Neuroscience, Mount Sinai School of Medicine, New York, New York

Tara L. Gruenewald, Ph.D.
Assistant Professor, Department of Medicine, University of California–Los Angeles School of Medicine, Los Angeles, California

Dan W. Haupt, M.D.
Associate Professor, Department of Psychiatry, Washington University School of Medicine, St. Louis, Missouri

Matthew Hotopf, Ph.D.
Professor of General Hospital Psychiatry, Department of Psychological Medicine, Institute of Psychiatry, King's College London, United Kingdom

Laura D. Kubzansky, Ph.D.
Assistant Professor, Department of Society, Human Development, and Health, Harvard School of Public Health, Boston, Massachusetts

Bruce G. Link, Ph.D.
Professor of Epidemiology and Sociomedical Sciences, Columbia University; Research Scientist, New York State Psychiatric Institute, New York, New York

Preben Bo Mortensen, M.D., Dr.Med.Sci.
Professor and Head, National Centre for Register-Based Research, University of Aarhus, Denmark

Norbert Müller, M.D., Ph.D.
Professor and Vice-Chair, Department of Psychiatry, Ludwig-Maximilians University, Munich, Germany

John W. Newcomer, M.D.
Associate Professor, Department of Psychiatry, Washington University School of Medicine, St. Louis, Missouri

Mark G. A. Opler, Ph.D., M.P.H.
Associate Research Scientist, Department of Epidemiology, Mailman School of Public Health, Columbia University, New York, New York

Jo C. Phelan, Ph.D.
Associate Professor of Sociomedical Sciences, Columbia University, Sleepy Hollow, New York

Michael Riedel, M.D.
Department of Psychiatry, Ludwig-Maximilians University, Munich, Germany

Markus J. Schwarz, M.D.
Department of Psychiatry, Ludwig-Maximilians University, Munich, Germany

Teresa E. Seeman, Ph.D.
Assistant Professor, Department of Medicine, University of California– Los Angeles School of Medicine, Los Angeles, California

Ezra S. Susser, M.D., Dr.P.H.
Gelman Professor and Chair, Department of Epidemiology, Mailman School of Public Health, Columbia University, New York, New York

Myrna M. Weissman, Ph.D.
Professor of Psychiatry and Epidemiology, College of Physicians and Surgeons of Columbia University; Chief, Division of Clinical Genetic Epidemiology, New York State Psychiatric Institute, New York, New York

Simon Wessely, F.R.C.Psych.
Director, King's Centre for Military Health Research, Institute of Psychiatry, King's College London, United Kingdom

Megan B. Willems, M.D.
Department of Psychiatry, Mount Sinai School of Medicine, New York, New York

Preface

Life Course Epidemiology and Comorbidity

COMORBIDITY IS THE coexistence of two or more diseases, conditions, or "clinical entities" in the same individual (Feinstein 1967). When applied to the field of life course epidemiology (Kuh and Ben-Shlomo 1997), the relevant concept is lifetime comorbidity, a concept that does not require that the disorders exist simultaneously. When the focus is narrowed to medical and psychiatric comorbidity, there are myriad relevant subfields, such as psychosomatics, behavioral medicine, and health psychology. The American Psychopathological Association (APPA) has traditionally focused on etiological frameworks for understanding psychopathology, with a strong appreciation for the epidemiological method. The 2004 APPA annual meeting brought together specialists in these fields, and their presentations have been edited into chapters for this book.

Much of the interest in medical comorbidity originated in the drive for good clinical care, for improving the outcome of treatment, and for "prognostic portent" (Kaplan and Feinstein 1974). That interest continues today (Hall et al. 2002). For psychiatric disorders, comorbidity emerged as an important issue in classification as editions of the American Psychiatric Association's *Diagnostic and Statistical Manual of Mental Disorders* (American Psychiatric Association 1968, 1980, 1987, 1994, 2000) generated ever more narrow and numerous diagnoses, thus producing an increase in comorbidity among psychiatric conditions.

Supported by National Institute of Mental Health grants 47447 and 53188.

The study of lifetime comorbidity has the potential to suggest etiological clues, a principal use of epidemiology (Morris 1975). This aspect of comorbidity was appreciated early as a possibility but was relatively neglected compared with the focus on prognosis and clinical care. The concept of *etiologically relevant period* (Rothman 1981) or *incubation period* (Armenian and Lilienfeld 1983) helps to understand this potential. The punctuation marks for this period of time include the beginning of the causal action, which is usually probabilistic in nature. At some point in time, the causal action converts from risk to pathogenesis, making the disease process irreversible, so that it will inevitably present with signs and symptoms sufficient for diagnosis. The time between the point of irreversibility, which is not observable, and the observable clinical presentation is the latency period. The etiologically relevant period begins with the earliest causal action and ends with the diagnosis.

A principle of the life course approach to epidemiology is that the etiologically relevant period has certain characteristics. These aspects are important in the study of comorbidity. One aspect is that the etiologically relevant period can be long—for example, measures taken in childhood, such as the basic 11 tests, can predict onset of dementia six or seven decades later (Whalley et al. 2000); or temperament, a relatively enduring emotional predisposition, may situate the individual more or less permanently at high risk, culminating in irreversibility only after decades of induction (Kubzanksy, Chapter 10). In pleiotropy (Hodgkin 1998), the action of identical genes present since conception produces different disorders that may occur at different stages of the life, such as the comorbidity of panic disorder and cystitis (Weissman, Chapter 4). A second feature of the etiologically relevant period is that it may involve critical stages—that is, relatively narrow periods during development to which the action of a given cause is limited. The stage of most focus has been that of fetal growth (Opler et al., Chapter 3), or puberty (Costello et al., Chapter 1), but critical periods of varying durations may exist throughout the course of life (Cizza, Chapter 7). A third important feature of the etiologically relevant period for life course epidemiology is that it may have a cumulative quality to it, such that years, or even decades, of accumulation are required to reach the point of irreversibility. For example, it may take years of the burden of lower-class life (Link and Phelan, Chapter 5) or of increased allostatic burden (Seeman and Gruenewald, Chapter 9) for the causal nexus to reach sufficiency. A fourth aspect of the incubation period for the situation of life course epidemiology is that it may involve multiple causes, representing different disciplines and different spheres of action, that are spread throughout the life course.

These life course aspects of the etiologically relevant period make the causal picture complex but enhance the value of the study of comorbidity. The Figure shows models for comorbidity that illuminate these complexities and potential rewards. Part A shows two independent diseases, starting with risk factors on the left. The risk process progresses to pathogenesis. Eventually the disease begins, generating a variety of signs and symptoms distributed through time in a natural history. Part B shows one form of life course comorbidity involving primary and secondary conditions. A complexity is that the individual diseases are not always easy to recognize as such because the signs and symptoms overlap—indeed, our designation of them as separate diseases may be more an act of convention than of nature. Here one disease, and one subgroup of symptoms, tends to start earlier than the other. This may generate the reward, because when we understand the course and pathology of the primary disease we may shed light on the pathogenesis of the secondary disease. Relevant chapters in this volume include those of Alexopoulos (Chapter 8), Carbone et al. (Chapter 6), Cizza (Chapter 7), and Newcomer and Haupt (Chapter 14). The practical benefits are the possible primary prevention of secondary disorders (Kessler and Price 1993).

Part C of the figure shows another complex scenario, in which the risk structure and the pathogenesis overlap ("pathogenetic interplay" in the words of Alvan Feinstein [1970]). The reward here is that the overlap in pathogenesis may be enlightening in a manner similar to the ways in which animal models of diseases are enlightening: when we learn something about pathogenesis of disease A, we may be able to learn about disease B. Indeed, all the knowledge we acquire about one disease is possibly relevant to the other—hence the value of learning whether, for example, immune diseases (Müller et al., Chapter 13) or other medical illnesses are related to psychiatric disorders (Mortensen, Chapter 12). This aspect has the potential to accelerate the learning process considerably.

In summary, a principal reward from study of comorbidity for etiological understanding may arise from areas of overlapping pathogenesis. However, the figure described here is so extremely simplified as to be a caricature. Chronic medical and psychiatric disorders generally have complex patterns of risk factors and numerous multiple chains of pathogenesis—that is, the web of causation (Krieger 1994). The medical and psychiatric disorders have many overlapping signs and symptoms, with boundaries between well and ill that are difficult to distinguish. An area of mutual pathogenesis may link disparate realms of knowledge and provide a crucial clue to etiology and nosological distinctiveness of both disorders.

William W. Eaton, Ph.D.

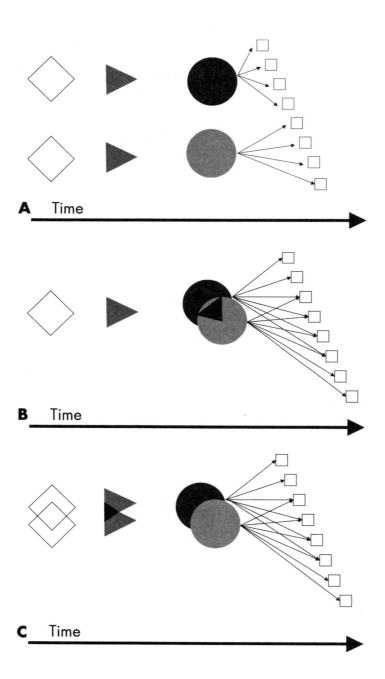

FIGURE 1.   Models for comorbidity.

(A) Two independent diseases. *Diamonds* represent risk factors, which progress to pathogenesis, represented by a *triangle*. Eventually the disease (*circles*) begins, generating a variety of signs and symptoms (*small squares*) distributed through time.

(B) Comorbidity: primary and secondary conditions. Individual diseases are not always easy to recognize as such, because the signs and symptoms overlap. One disease, and one subgroup of symptoms, tends to start earlier than the other. An understanding of the course and pathology of the primary disease may shed light on the pathogenesis of the secondary disease (represented by the *dark triangle inside overlapping circles*).

(C) Comorbidity: shared risk and pathogenesis. This shows another complex scenario in which the risk structure (*diamonds*) and the pathogenesis (*triangles*) overlap (*dark triangle*).

REFERENCES

American Psychiatric Association: Diagnostic and Statistical Manual of Mental Disorders, 2nd Edition. Washington, DC, American Psychiatric Association, 1968

American Psychiatric Association: Diagnostic and Statistical Manual of Mental Disorders, 3rd Edition. Washington, DC, American Psychiatric Association, 1980

American Psychiatric Association: Diagnostic and Statistical Manual of Mental Disorders, 3rd Edition, Revised. Washington, DC, American Psychiatric Association, 1987

American Psychiatric Association: Diagnostic and Statistical Manual of Mental Disorders, 4th Edition. Washington, DC, American Psychiatric Association, 1994

American Psychiatric Association: Diagnostic and Statistical Manual of Mental Disorders, 4th Edition, Text Revision. Washington, DC, American Psychiatric Association, 2000

Armenian HK, Lilienfeld AK: Incubation period of disease. Epidemiol Rev 5:1–15, 1983

Feinstein A: Clinical Judgment. Baltimore, MD, Williams & Wilkins, 1967

Feinstein AR: The pretherapeutic classification of comorbidity in chronic disease. J Chronic Dis 23:455–468, 1970

Hall SF, Rochon PA, Streiner DL, et al: Measuring comorbidity in patients with head and neck cancer. Laryngoscope 112:1988–1996, 2002

Hodgkin J: Seven types of pleiotropy. Int J Dev Biol 42:501–505, 1998

Kaplan MH, Feinstein A: The importance of classifying initial comorbidity in evaluating the outcome of diabetes mellitus. J Chronic Dis 27:387–404, 1974

Kessler RC, Price RH: Primary prevention of secondary disorders: a proposal and agenda. Am J Community Psychol 21:607–633, 1993

Krieger N: Epidemiology and the web of causation: has anyone seen the spider? Soc Sci Med 39:887–903, 1994

Kuh D, Ben-Shlomo Y: A Life Course Approach to Chronic Disease Epidemiology. Oxford, England, Oxford University Press, 1997

Morris JN: Uses of Epidemiology, 3rd Edition. Edinburgh, Churchill Livingstone, 1975

Rothman KJ: Induction and latent periods. Am J Epidemiol 114:253–259, 1981

Whalley LJ, Starr JM, Athawes R, et al: Childhood mental ability and dementia. Neurology 55:1455–1459, 2000

Epidemiology

Physical and Psychiatric Illness Across Adolescence

A Life Course Perspective

E. Jane Costello, Ph.D.

Helen Link Egger, M.D.

Adrian Angold, M.R.C.Psych.

ALTHOUGH THERE IS a considerable literature on the links between childhood psychiatric disorder and medical conditions such as headaches (Egger et al. 1998; Garvey et al. 1984; Pine et al. 1996; Stewart et al. 1989; Swartz et al. 2000), stomachaches (Garber et al. 1990; Jolly et al. 1994; Kaufman et al. 1997; Walker et al. 1993), accidents and injuries (Chadwick 1985; Rowe et al. 2004), and musculoskeletal pain (Egger et al. 1999), there is much less about what the temporal ordering of medical and psychiatric

This work was supported in part by grants from the National Institute of Mental Health (R01-MH063970, R01-MH01002, K02-MH01167), the National Institute on Drug Abuse (R01-DA011301, R01-DA016977), and the William T. Grant Foundation.

conditions across the life course can tell us about the direction of effect (Ben-Shlomo and Kuh 2002). In this chapter we follow the lives of some 1,400 children through adolescence to address some questions about the relative timing of medical and psychiatric conditions. Starting from a broad range of both types of disorder, we end with a highly specific story about girls whose early oppositional behavior predicted sexually risky behavior as they moved through adolescence, which in turn greatly increased the risk of infectious disease.

SUBJECTS AND METHODS

The Great Smoky Mountains Study (GSMS) is a longitudinal study of the development of psychiatric disorder and need for mental health services in rural and urban youth (Angold and Costello 1995; Angold et al. 1995, 1996; Burns et al. 1995; Costello et al. 1996, 1998). A representative sample of three cohorts of children ages 9, 11, and 13 years at intake was recruited from 11 counties in western North Carolina. Potential participants were selected from the population of some 20,000 children using a household equal-probability, accelerated cohort design (Schaie 1965). The accelerated cohort design means that over several years of data collection, each cohort reaches a given age in a different year, thus controlling for cohort effects (Kleinbaum et al. 1982). Youth with behavior problems were oversampled. A screening questionnaire was administered to a parent (usually the mother) of the first stage sample ($N=3,896$). The questionnaire consisted mainly of the externalizing (behavioral) problems scale of the Child Behavior Checklist (Achenbach and Edelbrock 1981) and was administered by telephone or in person. All children scoring above a predetermined cut-point (the top 25% of the total scores), plus a 1-in-10 random sample of the rest (i.e., the remaining 75% of the total scores), were recruited for detailed interviews. Ninety-five percent of families contacted completed the telephone screen.

About 8% of the area residents and the sample were African American, and fewer than 1% were Hispanic. American Indians made up only about 3% of the population of the study area, which was overwhelmingly white, but were oversampled from school records to constitute 25% of the study sample. This was done by using the same screening procedure but recruiting everyone irrespective of screen score. Of the 456 American Indian children identified, screens were obtained on 96%, and 81% of these ($n=350$) participated in the study. All subjects were given a weight inversely proportional to their probability of selection, so that the results presented are representative of the population from which the sample was drawn. Although race was included in all analyses, no conclusions are drawn in this paper about race/ethnic similarities or differences, which are reported elsewhere (Costello et al. 1997, 1999b; Federman et al. 1997). This chapter presents data on a total of 6,674 parent–child pairs of interviews carried out across the age range 9–16 years. Participants were interviewed as closely as possible to their birthday each year.

MEASURES

The Child and Adolescent Psychiatric Assessment (CAPA) is an interviewer-based interview (Angold and Fisher 1999). The goal of interviews using this format, such as the Present State Examination or the Schedules for Clinical Assessment in Neuropsychiatry (Wing 1976; Wing et al. 1992) designed for use with adults, is to combine the advantages of clinical interviews with those of highly structured "epidemiological" interview methods. A detailed glossary provides the operational rules for identifying clinically significant symptoms.

The CAPA interviews parent and child separately, using different interviewers. In this paper, we counted a symptom as present if reported by either parent or child or both, as is standard clinical practice. The time frame of the CAPA for determining the presence of most psychiatric symptoms is the previous 3 months. In the case of a few rare and severe acts, such as fire-setting or assault, a lifetime frame of reference is used as required by DSM-IV-TR (American Psychiatric Association 2000). Two-week test–retest reliability of CAPA diagnoses in children ages 10 through 18 is comparable with that of other highly structured child psychiatric interviews (Angold and Costello 1995; Angold and Fisher 1999).

Health information was collected with questions adapted from the 1993 version of the Questionnaire for Parents of Children Under 18, used in the National Health Interview Survey (NHIS). The NHIS is an ongoing survey of the health of the American population and the principal source of information on the health of the civilian noninstitutionalized population of the United States. It is one of the major data collection programs of the National Center for Health Statistics, a part of the Centers for Disease Control and Prevention. Questions were asked about two time periods: ever and the previous 12 months. The list of conditions can be found in Table 1–1. If a condition was reported during the previous 12 months, additional questions were asked about age at onset, number of bed days, nights in hospital, days of school missed, limitations on activities, medical consultations, med-

TABLE 1–1.   Medical conditions from National Health Interview Survey questionnaire

Accidents, injuries, poisonings, and resulting conditions
Missing body part
Impairment, stiffness, or deformity of back, foot, or leg
Impairment, stiffness, or deformity of fingers, hand, arm
Tonsillitis, adenoiditis
Repeated ear infection
Food or digestive allergy
Frequent diarrhea or colitis
Persistent bowel trouble
Diabetes
Sickle cell anemia
Asthma
Mononucleosis
Hepatitis
Meningitis
Bladder or urinary tract infection
Rheumatic fever
Pneumonia
Hay fever
Respiratory allergy
Deafness or trouble hearing
Blindness
Crossed eyes
Trouble seeing
Eczema
Epilepsy or seizures not associated with fever
Seizures associated with fever
Frequent or severe headaches or migraine
Cancer
Arthritis or joint disease or problem
Bone, cartilage, muscle, or tendon problem
Cerebral palsy
Congenital heart disease
Other heart disease or condition
Other condition requiring surgery
Other condition

ication, surgery, pain or discomfort, and how much the child was "bothered" by the condition. The parent was also asked whether the child had ever had a life-threatening illness.

PROCEDURE

Interviewers were residents of the area in which the study is taking place. All had at least bachelor's level degrees. They received 1 month of training and constant quality control. Interviewers were trained by Department of Social Services staff in the state's requirements for reporting abuse or neglect, and all suspected cases were referred to the appropriate agency. Families were visited by two interviewers, either at home or in a location convenient for them. Before the interviews began, parent and child signed informed consent forms. Each parent and child was paid $10 after the interview.

DATA MANAGEMENT AND ANALYSIS

Scoring programs for the CAPA, written with Statistical Analysis System (SAS) software (SAS Institute Inc, Cary, NC), combine information about the date of onset, duration, and intensity of each symptom to create diagnoses according to DSM-IV criteria (American Psychiatric Association 1994).

The medical history information was coded by two physicians into four clusters: 1) accidents, injuries, and poisonings (referred to for brevity as accidents); 2) atopies (allergies, eczema, asthma); 3) infections (diarrhea, bowel problems, urinary tract infections, pneumonia, tonsillitis, ear infections, mononucleosis, hepatitis, meningitis, rheumatic fever); and 4) serious chronic conditions (cancer, epilepsy, blindness, deafness, missing limb, diabetes, sickle cell anemia). The way the questionnaire was designed made it impossible to be sure whether, for example, a missing limb was the result of an accident or was a birth defect. However, in most cases the interviewer's notes helped to classify cases into these four groups.

Statistical models were tested using the SAS program GENMOD, defining the type of the correlation as unstructured, and using the Generalized Estimation Equation (GEE) option with a logistic link function. We also used the robust variance estimates (i.e., sandwich type estimates), together with sampling weights, to adjust the standard errors of the parameter estimates to account for the two-phase sampling design. GEE has the advantage of using the data available, so the casewise omission of cases with missing data is not necessary. The use of multiwave data with the appropriate sample weights thus capitalized on the multiple observation points over time while controlling for the effect on variance estimates of repeated measures.

Finally, lagged variables were created to address the order of effects. Logistic regressions were run using GENMOD as described earlier, with subjects' age and race (white vs. American Indian) entered as covariates.

RESULTS

Medical Conditions

Table 1–2 shows the 12-month prevalence of groups of medical conditions for the sample as a whole and separately by gender and for subjects when younger (9–12) and older (13–16). Table 1–3 shows the 3-month prevalence of key groups of psychiatric disorders: any depressive disorder, any anxiety disorder, any disruptive behavior disorder (DBD), attention-deficit/hyperactivity disorder, and drug abuse or dependence. The final column shows the results of testing for age group and gender simultaneously. Details for individual conditions can be obtained from the first author (Costello).

Two-fifths of the sample reported one or more medical conditions in any 12-month period. The most common conditions were atopic conditions. One third of the sample had at least one: eczema (7.7%), asthma (14.1%), hay fever (14.0), or allergies (5.3%). One child in seven had a condition reported by the parent as chronic, severe, or both. The most common of these were arthritic conditions (2.6%), problems with hearing (3.6%) and seeing (2.2%), and diabetes (1.5%). A similar number (14.5%) reported an accident, injury, or poisoning in the past year. Infections were also quite common (12%).

More children than adolescents had atopic conditions and infections. Adolescents had more accidents and injuries, so overall there was not a significant difference in the proportion of children and adolescents who had at least one condition. Nor was there a significant age difference in the average number of illnesses reported per year. Children reported somewhat more infectious conditions than adolescents, in particular adenoiditis and tonsillitis (6.7% vs. 2.5%, $P=0.002$), ear infections (7.7% vs. 2.9%, $P = 0.0004$), and persistent bowel trouble (2.9% vs. 0.5%, $P=0.0001$).

The only class of conditions that showed a gender difference was infections; 66% more girls than boys (15% vs. 9%, $P=0.001$) reported these. Among the infectious conditions, the biggest gender difference was in uri-

TABLE 1–2. Twelve-month prevalence of certain categories of medical illness, by age, gender, and ethnicity

Medical condition	Total (N=1,420)	Female (n=630)	Male (n=790)	Ages 9–12 years (41.3%)	Ages 13–16 years (58.7%)	White (n=983)	African American (n=88)	American Indian (n=349)	Tests of group differences
					No. (95% CI)				
Accident	16.0 (14.4, 18.1)	14.6 (12.2, 17.5)	17.8 (15.1 20.5)	14.5 (11.9, 17.7)	16.9 (14.7 19.3)	16.5 (14.5, 18.7)	11.2 (7.7, 16.1)	16.5 (14.3, 18.9)	Y<O, $P=0.008$ B>G, $P<0.05$
Atopia	22.4 (19.5, 25.6)	22.4 (18.5, 27.0)	22.3 (18.4, 27.0)	22.6 (18.4, 27.0)	22.4 (19.2, 26.0)	22.6 (19.4, 26.0)	22.7 (12.9, 36.7)	17.5 (14.5, 21.0)	Y=O B=G
Infection	8.7 (7.4, 10.1)	11.2 (9.2, 13.6)	6.3 (4.9, 8.1)	8.2 (6.3, 10.4)	9.0 (7.4, 10.9)	8.9 (7.3, 10.5)	5.8 (3.1, 10.7)	10.1 (8.1, 12.4)	Y>O, $P=0.08$ B<G, $P=0.0001$
Severe chronic condition	8.4 (6.9, 10.1)	8.5 (6.5, 11.0)	8.3 (6.3, 10.9)	8.2 (6.1, 11.0)	8.7 (6.9, 10.7)	8.4 (6.9, 10.2)	8.1 (3.4, 18.3)	8.1 (6.3, 10.5)	Y=O B=G
Any medical condition	58.5 (55.5, 61.5)	58.3 (54.2, 62.3)	58.8 (54.3, 63.2)	63.2 (59.1, 67.2)	56.6 (52.9, 60.3)	58.9 (55.6, 62.1)	54.5 (41.7, 66.7)	57.8 (54.3, 61.3)	Y>O, $P=0.004$ B=G

Note. CI=confidence interval; B=boys; G=girls; Y=young (ages 9–12 years); O=old (ages 13–16 years).

TABLE 1–3. Three-month prevalence of certain categories of psychiatric illness, by age, gender, and ethnicity

Medical condition	No. (95% CI)								Tests of group differences
	Total (N=1,420)	Female (n=630)	Male (n=790)	Ages 9–12 years (41.3%)	Ages 13–16 years (58.7%)	White (n=983)	African American (n=88)	American Indian (n=349)	
Depressive disorder	2.2 (1.6, 3.0)	2.9 (1.8, 4.4)	1.6 (1.0, 2.5)	0.9 (0.6, 1.4)	3.1 (2.1, 4.4)	2.3 (1.6, 3.3)	0.9 (0.4, 2.0)	2.2 (1.5, 3.3)	Y<O, P<0.0001 9–12: B=G 13–16:B<G, P=0.01
Anxiety disorder	2.4 (1.8, 3.1)	2.9 (2.0, 4.0)	1.9 (1.2, 2.9)	2.7 (1.9, 4.0)	2.0 (1.4, 3.0)	2.4 (1.8, 3.1)	2.4 (1.0, 5.5)	2.5 (1.7, 3.5)	Y=O G=B Y=O
Conduct disorder or oppositional defiant disorder	5.6 (4.7, 6.7)	3.5 (2.6, 4.6)	7.8 (6.3, 9.6)	5.5 (4.4, 6.9)	5.6 (4.5, 7.0)	5.3 (4.3, 6.4)	10.0 (5.3, 18.0)	7.0 (5.4, 9.1)	B>G, P<0.0001
Attention-deficit/hyperactivity disorder	0.9 (0.6, 1.2)	0.3 (0.2, 0.5)	1.5 (1.0, 2.2)	1.7 (1.1, 2.5)	0.3 (0.2, 0.5)	1.0 (0.7, 1.4)	0.4 (0.1, 1.1)	0.6 (0.3, 1.4)	Y>O, P<0.0001 B>G, P<0.0001
Drug abuse/dependence	2.4 (1.8, 3.1)	2.0 (1.4, 2.9)	2.9 (1.9, 4.0)	0.03 (0.01, 0.1)	4.0 (3.0, 5.3)	2.5 (1.8, 3.3)	0.9 (0.4, 2.0)	3.7 (2.7, 5.1)	O>Y, P<0.0001 B=G

Note. CI=confidence interval; B=boys; G=girls; Y=young (ages 9–12 years); O=old (ages 13–16 years).

nary tract infections (UTIs), reported by five times as many girls as boys (3.8% vs. 0.7%, *P*=0.0004). Girls also reported more pneumonia (3.5% vs. 1.5%, *P*<0.05) and mononucleosis (1.7% vs. 0.8%, *P*=0.08).

Psychiatric Conditions

Table 1–3 shows the mean 3-month prevalence of a group of psychiatric disorders across the 9–16 age range. Almost one child in eight had at least one disorder. A discussion of age, gender, and race differences and similarities can be found in other publications (Costello et al. 1996, 1997, 2001, 2003).

Comorbidity Among and Between Medical and Psychiatric Conditions

Tests of concurrent comorbidity among groups of medical conditions showed a moderate but significant degree of comorbidity, with odds ratios in the 2 to 3 range, among infectious diseases, atopic conditions, and chronic/serious conditions, but none with accidents/injuries/poisonings controlling for all the other types of comorbidity. Comorbidity among psychiatric disorders has been described in other papers (Angold et al. 1999; Costello et al. 1999a) and is not discussed further here. However, it is worth noting for the next set of analyses that disruptive behavior disorders (DBDs: attention-deficit/hyperactivity disorder, conduct disorder, oppositional defiant disorder [ODD]) were highly comorbid with depression in girls (bivariate odds ratio [OR]=21.1; 95% confidence interval [CI]=12.7, 34.9; *P*<0.0001).

The co-occurrence of medical and psychiatric conditions is summarized in Table 1–4, expressed as odds ratios. Table 1–4 shows each bivariate test uncontrolled for other comorbidities. Of the 210 possible tests of association, 52 (24.7%) were significant at *P*<0.05, 26 (12.3%) at *P*<0.01, and 6 (2.8%) at *P*<0.001, suggesting that there was a concurrent association between medical and psychiatric disorder that exceeded chance.

However, our interest in this chapter is in prediction over time. We therefore ran two sets of models similar to those whose results are shown in Table 1–4; first we predicted the medical conditions from the psychiatric ones, and then we predicted the psychiatric conditions from the medical ones. In each analysis, we controlled for current comorbidity. Details of all these analyses can be obtained from the first author (Costello). Here we concentrate on the strongest set of associations to emerge: those between DBDs (conduct disorder, ODD) and infectious diseases in girls.

TABLE 1–4.   Cross-sectional association between medical conditions and psychiatric disorders

Medical condition	Total	Female	Male	Ages 9–12	Ages 13–16
Any illness					
Any psychiatric disorder	1.4**	1.7*	1.1	1.9*	1.2
Depression	1.1	0.6	2.4	2.1	1.1
Anxiety	1.6	1.7	1.7	3.7**	1.1
ADHD	2.6**	6.7*	2.2*	3.6**	1.1
CD/ODD	1.4	2.4**	1.1	0.8	1.8*
Drug abuse	0.8	1.1	0.6	0.7	0.8
Accident					
Any psychiatric disorder	1.5*	1.3	1.6*	2.2	1.2
Depression	1.3	0.6	1.5	0.2	1.5
Anxiety	0.8	0.8	0.9	2.3	0.4
ADHD	1.8	4.5**	1.3	2.6	1.4
CD/ODD	1.6	1.2	1.7	0.8	2.1**
Drug abuse	1.0	1.0	1.0	—	0.9
Atopia					
Any psychiatric disorder	0.9	1.3	0.7	1.0	0.9
Depression	1.6	1.3	1.4	7.7***	1.0
Anxiety	1.0	1.3	1.8	1.9	0.8
ADHD	1.7	1.3*	2.2*	3.6**	1.1
CD/ODD	1.2	1.5	1.0	1.2	1.2
Drug abuse	0.7	0.9	0.6	4.9	0.8

TABLE 1–4. Cross-sectional association between medical conditions and psychiatric disorders *(continued)*

Medical condition	Total	Female	Male	Ages 9–12	Ages 13–16
Infection					
Any psychiatric disorder	1.7**	1.8**	1.8**	1.5	1.9**
Depression	1.7	1.1	2.3	2.2	1.75
Anxiety	1.6	1.7	1.1	1.8	1.5
ADHD	1.8*	3.0*	1.9	2.5**	0.6
CD/ODD	1.7*	3.1**	1.3	1.6	1.8
Drug abuse	1.3	1.8	0.9	—	1.3
Severe/chronic condition					
Any psychiatric disorder	1.5**	1.4	1.6	1.4	1.6*
Depression	0.5	0.5	0.4*	0.6	0.3
Anxiety	2.6	4.3*	0.7	1.0	4.3*
ADHD	1.3	1.9	1.5	0.7	1.1
CD/ODD	2.5**	2.4	2.6*	1.9	2.9**
Drug abuse	0.4	0.1***	0.7	—	0.4

Note. — =Numbers too small; model would not converge. ADHD=attention-deficit/hyperactivity disorder; CD/ODD=conduct disorder/oppositional defiant disorder.

*P<0.05; **P<0.01; ***P<0.001.

Predictive Analyses: Disruptive Behavior Disorders and Infectious Diseases in Girls Across Childhood and Adolescence

1. *Does past DBD increase the risk of infectious disease?*
   A history of DBDs increased the likelihood of an infectious disease three-fold (OR=3.0; 95% CI=1.7, 5.3; P=0.0003). Infectious diseases were even more likely in the year immediately after diagnosis of a DBD (OR=4.0; 95% CI=2.1, 7.9; P<0.0001). No such association was seen in boys.
2. *Does past infectious disease increase the risk of DBD?*
   DBDs were no more likely following an infectious disease than without one (OR=1.1, not significant). Thus it appears that the causal arrow, if there is one, must go from DBDs to infectious disease, not the other way.

Predictive Analyses: The Effect of Comorbid Depression on the Pathway From Disruptive Behavior Disorders to Infectious Diseases

As noted earlier, depression and DBDs were highly comorbid in girls. Although depression was not concurrently comorbid with infectious diseases, it seemed possible that girls with a history of depression might be at increased risk of medical conditions such as infectious diseases. However, depression predicted neither infectious diseases nor DBDs, nor did it increase the risk of infectious disease in girls with a history of DBDs. Thus, it appears that the increased risk of infectious conditions was specific to DBDs.

Disruptive Behavior Disorders

Conduct disorder and DBDs were entered separately as predictors of infectious disease. The only significant predictor was ODD. Current ODD was not significant. Thus, we concluded that girls with a history of ODD were at increased risk of infectious disease, irrespective of their current psychiatric status.

Infectious Conditions Predicted by Oppositional Defiant Disorder

Of the nine infectious conditions included in the NHIS questionnaire, bladder infections and UTIs were most significantly predicted by ODD. This suggested that girls with a history of ODD might be more likely to engage in behaviors, specifically sex without the use of condoms or sex with multiple partners, that would increase their risk of UTI. That is, we predicted that high-risk sexual activity would mediate the link between ODD and infectious disease.

TABLE 1–5. Results of final logistic model predicting urinary tract infection (Generalized Estimation Equation parameter estimates and empirical standard error estimates)

	Odds ratio	95% Confidence interval	P
Intercept	0.0004	0.0000, 0.007	<0.0001
Past oppositional defiant disorder	3.0	1.4, 6.4	0.0036
Sexual risk	2.8	1.2, 6.2	0.0131
Control variables			
Current oppositional defiant disorder	1.1	0.4, 2.9	NS
Past infectious disease	0.9	0.4, 2.3	NS
Age	1.2	1.0, 1.5	0.0415

Note. NS=not significant.

Sexual Risk

We created a scale of items from the CAPA that were consistent with the literature on risk for sexually transmitted diseases: multiple sexual partners, sex without a condom, and forced sex (sexual abuse, rape, sexual coercion). The occurrence of any one or more of these more than doubled the likelihood of UTI, from 8.4% to 22.0% (OR=2.9; 95% CI=1.5, 5.4; P=0.001). Girls with a history of ODD were three times as likely to report sexual risk (OR=3.2; 95% CI=1.7, 6.1; P=0.0003). However, when we tested the mediational model by entering both ODD history and sexual risk as predictors of infectious disease, both remained significant (ODD: OR=3.8; 95% CI=1.8, 7.8; P=0.0003 vs. sexual risk: OR=2.5; 95% CI=1.3, 4.5; P=0.003) (see Table 1–5). A test for interaction was not significant. Thus, it appears that both a history of ODD and a history of sexual risk contributed independently to an increased likelihood of UTIs.

Early Maturation

Finally, we tested the effect of age at sexual maturation, because previous research has linked early maturation to ODD and sexually risky behaviors (Ge et al. 2002; Magnusson et al. 1985; Moffitt et al. 1992; Stattin and Magnusson 1990). Girls were defined as early maturing if they reached Tanner stage 4 before age 12 years (18.2%). For the oldest cohort, who were 13 years at entry into the study, we selected the same percentage of the cohort with the earliest age at reported menarche. Early maturing girls were modestly, but not significantly, more likely to have a history of ODD (OR=2.4, not significant) and sexual risk (OR=1.4, not significant) but were somewhat less likely to report UTIs (OR=0.5, not significant). We therefore concluded that the link between ODD and UTI was not mediated by early sexual maturation.

SUMMARY AND CONCLUSION

We started with a broad question: is there a link between psychiatric and medical disorders over time in a representative population sample of children and adolescents? We used time-lagged analyses to test for the temporal ordering of any such associations, in a data set containing up to eight assessments of more than 1,400 participants. It quickly became clear that (apart from the obvious link between DBDs and accidents in both boys and girls) there was only one set of associations of interest: DBDs predicted infectious diseases in girls. Infectious diseases did not predict DBDs, and the concurrent association between DBDs and infectious diseases was not significant. It took time for the onset of a DBD to lead to infectious disease. Despite the strong concurrent association between depression and DBDs, depression had no effect on the likelihood of infectious disease.

At the next stage of the analysis, we narrowed down the global variables to the specific components that carried the weight of the findings. In the case of DBDs, the most important component was ODD, a condition marked by difficulty with impulse control (e.g., losing one's temper, arguing) and hypersensitivity to perceived slights (e.g., being resentful, touchy, spiteful). In the case of infectious disorders, UTIs were the most important component, and, to a lesser extent, diarrhea, colitis, and other kinds of bowel problems. (Although some of these may not have been infectious in origin, given the limited information from the NHIS, the medical experts on the study [authors Angold and Egger] independently decided to classify them in this category.)

This focus on ODD and UTI suggested that the link might have to do with sexually risky behaviors. Although there is a plentiful literature on the links between behavioral problems and sexual activity in adolescents (e.g., Bardone et al. 1998; Fergusson and Woodward 2000; Kessler et al. 1997; Lavan and Johnson 2002; Paul et al. 2000; Tubman et al. 2003), and on sexual activity as a risk factor for UTI in women (Foxman et al. 1995; Nguyen and Weir 2002), a literature search revealed no studies directly linking DBDs and UTI. It was indeed the case that UTIs were more common in girls who reported multiple sex partners and/or sex without condom use and that these girls also were more likely to have a history of ODD. However, the test of sexual risk as a mediator of the ODD–UTI link failed, because including it in the model did not reduce the odds ratio (Baron and Kenny 1986; Shrout and Bolger 2002). It appears that ODD and sexual risk, although both increasing the risk for UTI, did so somewhat independently.

Several researchers (Dufour et al. 1994; Frick et al. 1995; Robins and Price 1991) have noted developmental interrelationships among DBDs, depression, and somatization disorder, suggesting that we might be observing an increased likelihood of reporting illness by girls with DBDs, especially girls who were also vulnerable to depression. It should be noted, however, that 1) the information on medical illnesses was provided by the mother, not the girl, making this explanation perhaps less likely (although not impossible, given the intergenerational nature of somatization [Frick et al. 1995]); and 2) no link was observed between DBDs and other types of medical condition, such as atopias and chronic/serious conditions. This argues against a general tendency by girls with ODD to exaggerate any kind of physical complaint. The ODD–UTI link was strong in younger (9–12 years) as well as older (13–16 years) girls, which is another argument against its being mediated by sexual risk, because such risk was not seen below age 13 years in this sample.

Previous research has suggested that deviant behavior in girls is likely to predict somatic complaints in late adolescence and early adulthood (Robins and Price 1991; Zoccolillo 1993). The sample used here was too young to test this hypothesis beyond the link with UTI. On the basis of this work, however, we can predict that this group of vulnerable girls is at risk of further physical as well as psychiatric illness as they move into adulthood. The link between UTI and HIV (Greenblatt et al. 1999) makes this group an important focus for prevention.

REFERENCES

Achenbach TM, Edelbrock CS: Behavioral problems and competencies reported by parents of normal and disturbed children aged four through sixteen. Monogr Soc Res Child Dev 46:1–82, 1981

American Psychiatric Association: Diagnostic and Statistical Manual of Mental Disorders, 4th Edition. Washington, DC, American Psychiatric Association, 1994

American Psychiatric Association: Diagnostic and Statistical Manual of Mental Disorders, 4th Edition, Text Revision. Washington, DC, American Psychiatric Association, 2000

Angold A, Costello EJ: A test-retest reliability study of child-reported psychiatric symptoms and diagnoses using the Child and Adolescent Psychiatric Assessment (CAPA-C). Psychol Med 25:755–762, 1995

Angold A, Fisher PW: Interviewer-based interviews, in Diagnostic Assessment in Child and Adolescent Psychopathology. Edited by Shaffer D, Lucas C, Richters J. New York, Guilford, 1999, pp 34–64

Angold A, Prendergast M, Cox A, et al: The Child and Adolescent Psychiatric Assessment (CAPA). Psychol Med 25:739–753, 1995

Angold A, Erkanli A, Costello EJ, et al: Precision, reliability and accuracy in the dating of symptom onsets in child and adolescent psychopathology. J Child Psychol Psychiatry 37:657–664, 1996

Angold A, Costello EJ, Erkanli A: Comorbidity. J Child Psychol Psychiatry 40:57–87, 1999

Bardone A, Moffitt T, Caspi A, et al: Adult physical health outcomes of adolescent girls with conduct disorder, depression, and anxiety. J Am Acad Child Adolesc Psychiatry 37:594–601, 1998

Baron RM, Kenny DA: The moderator-mediator variable distinction in social psychological research: conceptual, strategic, and statistical considerations. J Pers Soc Psychol 51:1173–1182, 1986

Ben-Shlomo Y, Kuh D: A life course approach to chronic disease epidemiology: conceptual models, empirical challenges and interdisciplinary perspectives. Int J Epidemiol 31:285–293, 2002

Burns BJ, Costello EJ, Angold A, et al: Children's mental health service use across service sectors. Health Aff 14:147–159, 1995

Chadwick O: Psychological sequelae of head injury in children. Dev Med Child Neurol 27:72–75, 1985

Costello EJ, Angold A, Burns BJ, et al: The Great Smoky Mountains Study of Youth: goals, designs, methods, and the prevalence of DSM-III-R disorders. Arch Gen Psychiatry 53:1129–1136, 1996

Costello E, Farmer E, Angold A, et al: Psychiatric disorders among American Indian and white youth in Appalachia: The Great Smoky Mountains Study. Am J Public Health 87:827–832, 1997

Costello EJ, Angold A, March J, et al: Life events and post-traumatic stress: the development of a new measure for children and adolescents. Psychol Med 28:1275–1288, 1998

Costello EJ, Erkanli A, Federman E, et al: Development of psychiatric comorbidity with substance abuse in adolescents: effects of timing and sex. J Clin Child Psychol 28:298–311, 1999a

Costello EJ, Farmer EMZ, Angold A: Same place, different children: white and American Indian children in the Appalachian Mountains, in Where and When: Historical and Geographical Aspects of Psychopathology. Edited by Cohen P, Robins L, Slomkowski C. Mahwah, NJ, Lawrence Erlbaum, 1999b, pp 279–298

Costello EJ, Compton SN, Erkanli A, et al: Does preventing poverty prevent child psychopathology? Analysis of a natural experiment. Invited presentation for the World Psychiatric Association Section on Epidemiology and Public Health Scientific Meeting, Baltimore, MD, June 2001

Costello EJ, Mustillo S, Erkanli A, et al: Prevalence and development of psychiatric disorders in childhood and adolescence. Arch Gen Psychiatry 60:837–844, 2003

Dufour S, Tremblay R, Virtaro F: Prediction of somatization disorders in prepubertal girls. Can J Psychiatry 39:384–390, 1994

Egger HL, Angold A, Costello EJ: Headaches and psychopathology in children and adolescents. J Am Acad Child Adolesc Psychiatry 37:951–958, 1998

Egger HL, Angold A, Costello EJ: Somatic complaints and psychopathology in children and adolescents: stomach aches, musculoskeletal pains and headaches. J Am Acad Child Adolesc Psychiatry 38:852–860, 1999

Federman EB, Costello EJ, Angold A, et al: Development of substance use and psychiatric comorbidity in an epidemiologic study of white and American Indian young adolescents: The Great Smoky Mountains Study. Drug Alcohol Depend 44:69–78, 1997

Fergusson D, Woodward L: Educational, psychosocial, and sexual outcomes of girls with conduct problems in early adolescence. J Child Psychol Psychiatry 41:779–792, 2000

Foxman B, Geiger AM, Palin K, et al: First-time urinary tract infection and sexual behavior. Epidemiology 6:162–168, 1995

Frick PJ, Kuper K, Silverthorn P, et al: Antisocial behavior, somatization, and sensation-seeking behavior in mothers of clinic-referred children. J Am Acad Child Adolesc Psychiatry 34:805–812, 1995

Garber J, Zeman J, Walker LS: Recurrent abdominal pain in children: psychiatric diagnoses and parental psychopathology. J Am Acad Child Adolesc Psychiatry 29:648–656, 1990

Garvey MJ, Tollefson GD, Schaffer CB: Migraine headaches and depression. Am J Psychiatry 141:986–988, 1984

Ge X, Brody G, Conger R, et al: Contextual amplification of pubertal transition effects on deviant peer affiliation an externalizing among African American children. Dev Psychol 38:42–54, 2002

Greenblatt RM, Bacchetti P, Barkan S, et al: Lower genital tract infections among HIV-infected and high-risk uninfected women: findings of the Women's Interagency HIV Study (WIHS). Sex Transm Dis 26:143–151, 1999

Jolly JB, Wherry JN, Wiesner DC, et al: The mediating role of anxiety in self-reported somatic complaints of depressed adolescents. J Abnorm Child Psychol 22:691–702, 1994

Kaufman KL, Cromer B, Daleiden EL, et al: Recurrent abdominal pain in adolescents: psychosocial correlates of organic and nonorganic pain. Child Health Care 26:15–30, 1997

Kessler RC, Berglund PA, Foster CL, et al: Social consequences of psychiatric disorders, II: teenage parenthood. Am J Psychiatry 154:1405–1411, 1997

Kleinbaum DG, Kupper LL, Morgenstern H: Epidemiologic Research: Principles and Quantitative Methods. New York, Van Nostrand Reinhold, 1982

Lavan H, Johnson JG: The association between Axis I and II psychiatric symptoms and high-risk sexual behavior during adolescence. J Personal Disord 16:73–94, 2002

Magnusson D, Stattin H, Allen VL: Biological maturation and social development: a longitudinal study of some adjustment processes from mid-adolescence to adulthood. J Youth Adolesc 14:267–283, 1985

Moffitt TE, Caspi A, Belsky J, et al: Childhood experience and the onset of menarche: a test of a sociobiological model. Child Dev 63:47–58, 1992

Nguyen H, Weir M: Urinary tract infection as a possible marker for teenage sex. South Med J 95:867–869, 2002

Paul C, Fitzjohn J, Herbison P, et al: The determinants of sexual intercourse before age 16. J Adolesc Health 27:136–147, 2000

Pine DS, Cohen P, Brook J: The association between major depression and headache: results of a longitudinal epidemiologic study in youth. J Child Adolesc Psychopharmacol 6:153–164, 1996

Robins LN, Price RK: Adult disorders predicted by childhood conduct problems: results from the NIMH Epidemiologic Catchment Area project. Psychiatry 54:116–132, 1991

Rowe R, Maughan B, Goodman R: Childhood psychiatric disorder and unintentional injury: findings from a national cohort study. J Pediatr Psychol 29:119–13, 2004

Schaie KW: A general model for the study of developmental problems. Psychol Bull 64:92–107, 1965

Shrout PE, Bolger N: Mediation in experimental and nonexperimental studies: new procedures and recommendations. Psychol Methods 7:422–445, 2002

Stattin H, Magnusson D: Pubertal Maturation in Female Development. Mahwah, NJ, Lawrence Erlbaum, 1990

Stewart WF, Linet MS, Celentano DD: Migraine headaches and panic attacks. Psychosom Med 51:559–569, 1989

Swartz KL, Pratt LA, Armenian HK, et al: Mental disorders and the incidence of migraine headaches in a community sample. Arch Gen Psychiatry 57:945–950, 2000

Tubman JG, Gil AG, Wagner EF, et al: Patterns of sexual risk behaviors and psychiatric disorders in a community sample of young adults. J Behav Med 26:473–500, 2003

Walker LS, Garber J, Greene JW: Psychosocial correlates of recurrent childhood pain: a comparison of pediatric patients with recurrent abdominal pain, organic illness, and psychiatric disorders. J Abnorm Psychol 102:248–258, 1993

Wing JK: A technique for studying psychiatric morbidity in inpatient and outpatient series and in general population samples. Psychol Med 6:665–671, 1976

Wing JK, Babor T, Brugha T, et al: SCAN: Schedules for Clinical Assessment in Neuropsychiatry. Arch Gen Psychiatry 47:589–593, 1992

Zoccolillo M: Gender and the development of conduct disorder. Dev Psychopathol 5:65–78, 1993

The Consequences of Psychopathology in the Baltimore Epidemiologic Catchment Area Follow-Up

William W. Eaton, Ph.D.

Joshua Fogel, Ph.D.

Haroutune K. Armenian, M.D., Dr.P.H., M.P.H.

LIFE COURSE EPIDEMIOLOGY OF
MEDICAL AND PSYCHIATRIC COMORBIDITY

The life course approach to epidemiology (see Chapter 3; Kuh and Ben-Shlomo 1997) addresses two important pitfalls in the understanding of medical and psychiatric comorbidity. The first pitfall is the bias associated with a visit to a clinic or hospital—so-called Berkson's bias (Berkson 1946). Because each health condition is imperfectly associated with the tendency to visit the clinic or hospital, individuals who have two conditions are more likely to be in the clinic than those with one condition. In research samples

This work was supported by National Institute of Mental Health grants MH47447 and MH14592.

originating from clinics and hospitals, comorbidity is overestimated. The second pitfall is the tendency to assume that the etiologically relevant period (Rothman 1981, 1986) is short enough to be observed during one follow-up period, professional lifetime, or generation of research. The chronic diseases do not always fit this expectation, and even some infections (Torrey and Peterson 1973), injuries, behaviors (Whalley et al. 2000), and early growth patterns (Barker 1995) have catastrophic effects on health that do not appear until several decades have passed. This pitfall leads to underestimation of the relationship between diseases and health conditions. This bias is not quite the same as the so-called prevalence bias, or the "clinician's illusion," in which severity and chronicity are overestimated in samples drawn at a single point in time (Cohen and Cohen 1984). Here the problem is that the temporal and potentially causal connection between syndromes is missed because the period of observation is not long enough to include both syndromes, which may have occurred decades apart. For want of a better name, this bias is called "short incubation bias" (Armenian and Lilienfeld 1983).

THE NATIONAL INSTITUTE OF MENTAL HEALTH EPIDEMIOLOGIC CATCHMENT AREA PROGRAM

The National Institute of Mental Health (NIMH) Epidemiologic Catchment Area (ECA) Program had five important aspects of its design (Eaton and Kessler 1985; Eaton et al. 1981; Regier et al. 1984; Robins and Regier 1991):

1. Interest in specific mental disorders according to the operational diagnostic criteria of DSM-III (American Psychiatric Association 1980);
2. Surveys that combined data from community and institutional populations, thereby estimating "total true" prevalence rates;
3. A prospective aspect allowing estimation of incidence as well as prevalence;
4. Linkage with data on use of services; and
5. A multisite aspect that promoted insight into variation across research sites arising from both methodological and substantive differences between sites.

The first of these design aspects led to the study's characterization as the first of the "third generation" of psychiatric epidemiology (Dohrenwend and Dohrenwend 1982). Important early publications studied comorbidity, but because there had not been standardized collection of data on physical disorders across all five ECA sites, the results on comorbidity were limited to psychiatric disorders (Boyd et al. 1984). The second aspect was soon forgotten as it became clear that, due to changes in the structure of institutions, the population in group quarters had little effect on the total rates of prevalence. Although within any given institution there might be a very high rate of prevalence, the probabilities of selection ensured that the household population would dominate the rates (Leaf et al. 1985). Analyses connected to the third design aspect of estimating incidence showed that many psychiatric disorders had onset earlier than the youngest ECA respondent (18 years; Christie et al. 1988). Analyses also demonstrated how woefully short the 1-year follow-up period was, generating a limited number of new cases (Eaton et al. 1989). Finally, it became clear using quasi-prospective analyses that the prodromal periods for psychopathology were so long that a 1-year follow-up was of limited use (Eaton et al. 1995). Analyses on use of services suffered because the same subject reporting the psychopathology was also asked to report on use of services, leading to a recall bias in favor of high association between use of services and psychopathology. Yet because the evidence obtained showed unexpectedly low service use among those with disorders, the data were influential in this aspect (Regier et al. 1988; Shapiro et al. 1984).

The multisite aspect allowed some experimentation and variation between the five sites (Yale University, Johns Hopkins University, Washington University–St. Louis, Duke University, and University of California–Los Angeles [UCLA]). Researchers at Yale were interested in the elderly and in disability, for example; at UCLA there was interest in comparisons between white and Hispanic populations. In Baltimore (i.e., Johns Hopkins) there was interest in, among other things, the relationship between psychiatric disorders and physical illnesses.

A decade after the conclusion of the ECA multisite collaboration, a retrospective series of articles reviewed its successes and failures (Eaton 1994a, 1994b; Kessler 1994; Regier 1994; Shrout 1994).

THE BALTIMORE EPIDEMIOLOGIC CATCHMENT AREA FOLLOW-UP

The Baltimore site of the ECA study was one of three to follow its sample for more than the single year required in the overall design. At Yale, there was a mortality follow-up 9 years later (Bruce et al. 1994). At Washington University–St. Louis there was a follow-up of a portion of the sample

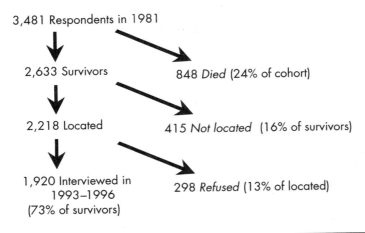

3,481 Respondents in 1981

2,633 Survivors

848 *Died* (24% of cohort)

2,218 Located

415 *Not located* (16% of survivors)

1,920 Interviewed in
1993–1996
(73% of survivors)

298 *Refused* (13% of located)

FIGURE 2–1. Attrition experienced in Baltimore Epidemiologic Catchment Area follow-up, 1981–1996.

(Bucholz et al. 1996). The Baltimore site is unusual in its follow-up of the entire household sample from 1981 (Badawi et al. 1999; Eaton et al. 1997). Following up the cohort involved attrition due to three broad sources: death, loss of contact among those known or conjectured to be alive, and refusal among those who are located and approached. The follow-up from 1981 to 1993 was successful, in part, because the field period of the follow-up was extended several additional years, with the final subject being located and interviewed in 1996. About a quarter of the sample had died, and more than 15% of those who survived could not be located even after extensive efforts (Figure 2–1). More than 10% of those located did not agree to participate in an interview. Nevertheless, more than 73% of the survivors were interviewed in the follow-up survey.

Psychopathology has the potential to be predictive of all three types of attrition. Attrition in the ECA has been studied from the baseline sample designation through to completion of the baseline interview (Cottler et al. 1987; Von Korff et al. 1985), from baseline interview to 1-year follow-up (Eaton et al. 1992), and at the Baltimore site, from baseline interview to 13-year follow-up (Badawi et al. 1999). Yet psychopathology was not as strong a predictor of attrition as many had predicted, as shown in Table 2–1, which compares results for nine disorders from the four-site follow-up after 1 year (Eaton et al. 1992) with the Baltimore 13-year follow-up (Badawi et al. 1999). There was not a single significant predictor of refusal to participate in the interview. The 1-year follow-up did not include death as an outcome

TABLE 2–1. Two analyses of psychopathology and attrition: Epidemiologic Catchment Area (ECA) surveys

Mental disorder	Four ECA sites* 1-year follow-up		Baltimore ECA site** 13-year follow-up		
	Lost	Refused	Lost	Refused	Died
Major depression	**1.4**	0.6	1.3	1.2	1.2
Obsessive-compulsive disorder	1.4	0.8	1.0	1.0	0.8
Phobic disorder	1.1	0.9	1.0	0.7	**1.3**
Panic disorder	**2.0**	0.9	1.1	0.9	1.4
Cognitive impairment	1.2	0.8	**2.5**	0.4	**1.8**
Schizophrenia	1.5	1.6	0.5	0.5	1.4
Drug abuse/dependence	**1.4**	0.9	1.1	1.0	**4.0**
Alcohol abuse/dependence	**1.3**	1.0	1.2	0.6	**1.8**
Antisocial personality	**1.7**	1.2	**2.5**	0.5	**3.0**

Note. **Bold font** indicates that 95% confidence interval does not include 1.0.

*Baseline *N* of 10,167; odds ratio adjusted for site, gender, age, race, education, marital status, and language of interview (Eaton et al. 1992).

**Baseline *N* of 3,481; odds ratio adjusted for gender, age, race, and education (Badawi et al. 1999).

because it was so rare after so short a time. In the 13-year follow-up, death was predicted by cognitive impairment, drug and alcohol disorders, and antisocial personality. The latter three variables also predicted loss of contact in the 1-year follow-up. The Baltimore 13-year follow-up field extended to 3.5 years, possibly allowing us to find persons with these characteristics that might not be located when the field period is limited to 1 year, as was the case for the overall 1-year follow-up in the ECA surveys. In our follow-up in Baltimore, only cognitive impairment and antisocial personality were predictive of failure to locate the individual. We presume this failure is related to entry into institutions: nursing homes for cognitively impaired subjects and prisons and jails for those with antisocial personality disorder.

MEDICAL AND PSYCHIATRIC COMORBIDITY

Inclusion of questions on physical illness in the baseline surveys, combined with the broad range of data on patterns of psychiatric symptoms and disorders, facilitated study of the consequences of psychopathology for medical conditions in the Baltimore ECA follow-up. Because the baseline ECA surveys had included a broad range of psychopathology according to the latest operational definitions, the stage was set for demonstrating and comparing the long-term consequences of the various psychiatric disorders. This aspect displays the advantages of the general cohort study, in which a variety of outcomes can be studied in relationship to a given exposure (Lilienfeld and Stolley 1994)—in this case, the "exposure" is the occurrence of a psychiatric disorder, and the outcomes included mortality (Kouzis and Eaton 1995, 1997, 2000; Kouzis et al. 1995), use of services (Cooper-Patrick et al. 1999; Eaton 1998), socioeconomic status (Eaton et al. 2001), and physical conditions, which are discussed in more detail in the following sections.

Diabetes

The earliest publication in this area for the Baltimore ECA follow-up showed the predictive relationship of depressive disorder to onset of type 2 diabetes (Eaton et al. 1996), with results shown in Table 2–2. There existed at that time a strong literature on the comorbidity of depression and diabetes, but there was little or no evidence about the direction of influence because the data were based on samples of persons with diabetes (Lustman et al. 1988) or cross-sectional samples of the general population (Gavard et al. 1993; Lustman et al. 1988). The cohort design with baseline and follow-up questions on diabetes allowed estimation of the incidence of diabetes, and

TABLE 2–2.   Psychopathology and the development of diabetes: Baltimore Epidemiologic Catchment Area follow-up, 1981–1993/1996

Psychiatric disorder	Odds ratio	95% Confidence interval
Dysphoric episode	1.02	0.61, 1.68
Depression syndrome	1.02	0.50, 2.07
Major depressive disorder (including grief reaction)	2.23	0.90, 5.55
Panic disorder	1.07	0.14, 8.33
Phobic disorder	0.84	0.48, 1.48
Alcohol disorder	0.66	0.28, 1.57
Obsessive-compulsive disorder	1.23	0.37, 1.18

Note.   Individual models each adjusted for age, gender, and body mass index.
Source.   Eaton et al. 1996.

the effect of a history of depressive disorder on that incidence, with a clear temporal ordering of measurement. The evidence in Table 2–2 shows that the association is moderately strong, that clinical depression is a more powerful predictor than episodes of depressed mood, and that other forms of psychopathology have much less impact. This result attracted some attention because there had not been a cohort study with this capability before, even though the results did not meet traditional levels of statistical significance and even though it was based on self-reported occurrence of diabetes. A study in Japan replicated the results using oral glucose tolerance tests instead of self-reported diabetes and found virtually the same relative odds, but with more convincing level of significance due to the larger sample size (Kawakami et al. 1999). There have been several replications since that time (Carnethon et al. 2003; Golden et al. 2004) and at least one failure to replicate (Saydah et al. 2003).

Heart Attack

Another analysis of the Baltimore ECA follow-up data, conducted in parallel with the work on diabetes, showed that a history of depression was a risk factor for a first heart attack (Pratt et al. 1996). The adjusted relative odds were 3.9, stronger than the predictive strength of standard risk factors for heart attack such as hypertension, high cholesterol, or family history of heart attack. Similar to the work on diabetes, depression was a stronger risk factor than other types of psychopathology; somewhat differently, the anal-

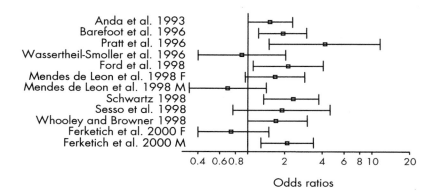

FIGURE 2–2.   Depression and coronary heart disease: prospective studies.
Source.   Rugulies 2002.

ysis showed that even milder forms of depression raised risk for a heart attack. Analyses of medications being taken suggested that the heart attack did not result from treatment for depression. A later meta-analytic review integrated this finding with literature through 2002 (Rugulies 2002), and it is redrawn here as Figure 2–2. Almost all the studies show the same effect of depression on risk of coronary heart disease.

Other Outcomes From Depression

The consequences of depression cut across a variety of physical conditions, but they are not general, as shown in Table 2–3. The results in Table 2–3 are a selection of topics from the published analyses of the Baltimore ECA follow-up focusing on five major medical conditions of middle age: diabetes (Eaton et al. 1996), heart attack (Pratt et al. 1996), cancer (Gallo et al. 2000), stroke (Larson et al. 2001), and arthritis (Armenian et al. 1996). Analyses about other physical conditions and depression that are omitted from Table 2–2 include work on migraine (Swartz et al. 2000), fatigue (Addington et al. 2001; Bogner et al. 2002), and back pain. Also omitted are publications on depression and cognitive impairment (Rosenblatt et al. 2003) and depression and substance use disorders (Bovasso 2001; Crum et al. 2001).

The data in Table 2–3 are a simplification of the information available from the individual publications and manuscripts. In general, the analyses took advantage of the broad range of measures of psychopathology; as in

TABLE 2–3.   Predictive relationship of depressive disorder to five medical conditions: Baltimore Epidemiologic Catchment Area follow-up, 1981–1993/1996

Condition	Predicting medical condition			Predicting depressive disorder		
	At risk	New cases	Odds ratio	At risk	New cases	Odds ratio
Type 2 diabetes	1,715	89	2.2	1,633	71	1.1
Heart attack	1,551	64	**4.5**	1,633	71	1.7
Cancer	2,017	203	1.0	1,633	71	0.6
Stroke	1,705	95	**2.7**	1,633	71	**8.4**
Arthritis	1,332	270	1.3	1,633	71	1.0

Note.   **Bold font** indicates that 95% confidence interval does not include 1.0.
Source.   Armenian et al. 1996; Eaton et al. 1996; Gallo et al. 2000; Larson et al. 2001; Pratt et al. 1996.

Table 2–2, it was usually depressive disorder that had the most impact. The questions used to determine the presence of physical conditions were drawn from the Health Interview Surveys of the National Center for Health Statistics; they are simple to understand but often not as precise as could be hoped. For example, the analyses on diabetes depended on the question: Have you ever had high sugar or diabetes? It must be assumed that the diabetes is of the adult-onset type, because all onsets occurred after age 30 years. (Yet this complicates the analysis of the consequences of diabetes for depression, described later.) At the baseline, the question about the heart was: Have you ever had heart problems? In the follow-up, a specific question on heart attacks was asked, but it is not perfectly clear that subjects know when they have had a heart attack. (Later analyses on heart attacks confirmed by medical records in this sample reveal considerable error, but the strength and direction of the findings remain stable even so.) The question at baseline on cancer was: Have you ever had cancer? At the follow-up there were detailed questions on the types of cancer, and there was a search of death certificates for causes of death that included cancer. One of the intriguing results, not shown in Table 2–3, is that depressive disorder raised the risk for breast cancer by a factor of 3.8 (25 new cases) and prostate cancer by 11.8 (10 new cases). Both these relative risks were barely significant in the statistical sense at the level of alpha = 0.05.

The pattern in Table 2–3 is that depressive disorder predicts onset of diabetes, heart attack, and stroke. These are all conditions associated with weakness or decline in the vasculature, obesity, and metabolic syndrome. The results do not seem to be a result of a low threshold for reporting illness in general, because the most likely candidate in that situation would be a relationship to arthritis, the most painful of the conditions shown.

Depression as the Outcome

What about the effects of the physical conditions on the incidence of depressive disorder? There were 71 new cases of depressive disorder over the 13 years of the follow-up (Eaton et al. 1997). The pattern here is even more striking in that there appears to be little or no effect of these physical conditions on risk for onset of depressive disorder, with the exception of stroke (see Table 2–3). The lack of strong effect on depression of many of these conditions is not consistent with some literature in the field of health psychology and is presumably due, in part, to the requirement of the full depressive episode as opposed to an episode of dysphoria in reaction to the physical condition. Another explanation is the length of the follow-up—after 13 years, individuals have had time to adjust to the existence of a physical condition. The relative risk for stroke is 8.4 (95% confidence interval=1.6, 42.6). This result is consistent with the documented effects of stroke and associated brain lesions on risk for depressive disorder in longitudinal studies in clinical settings (Robinson 1997; Robinson et al. 1983, 1984).

THE WEB OF CAUSATION

These findings illustrate the value of the life course approach and the value of general cohort studies. The life course approach emphasizes the importance of the languid temporal evolution of individual health over the entire course of life. Causal relations may exist that become apparent only when studied in decades rather than days, weeks, months, or years. The general cohort approach demonstrates how unexpected findings can emerge in a broad range of areas, which eventually can form a recognizable pattern.

The web of causation (Krieger 1994) is complex. It could be that a single diathesis—say, a genetic constellation, or an early insult, or a combination of the two—predisposes the individual to a series of later conditions. In this scenario, the temporal associations we see, as reported earlier, do not actually represent an ongoing causal process but rather the unfolding of a single disorder whose etiologically relevant period ended early in life, with symptomatic expression scheduled over the life course. This alternative is some-

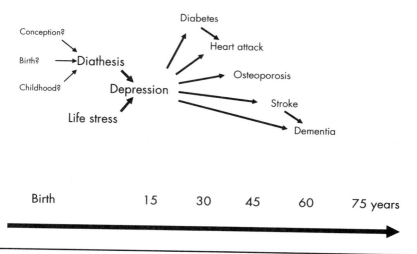

FIGURE 2–3.   Multiple-source diathesis: depression as mediator. Multiple chains of cause and multiple endpoints.

what pessimistic because prevention activities would have to begin before any of the disorders actually appeared. This first alternative includes depression as simply one among many syndromes expressing the diathesis. The other alternative is that the causal process itself is probabilistic and unfolds continuously over the life course (Figure 2–3). Here depression becomes somewhat more important because it influences the causal dynamics early and in many ways. For example, depression may affect the risk for stroke and heart attack because it raises risk for diabetes, or it may independently raise risk for diabetes, thereby raising risk for stroke and heart attack as well as independently raising risk for the two later outcomes. This second alternative suggests that prevention or treatment of depression could lower risk for later onset of conditions. So far, two separate intervention trials have attempted to lower the risk of later heart attack among those with a first attack by treating the patients' comorbid depression (Berkman et al. 2003; Glassman et al. 2002; Sheps et al. 2003). The trials have shown that it is safe and effective to treat the depression, but so far, there has been little demonstrable effect on lowering the risk for later heart attack.

FOLLOW-UP AFTER 23 YEARS

In spring 2004 the Baltimore ECA follow-up surveyed the sample one more time—a 23-year follow-up. The emphasis had shifted increasingly toward health and mental health conditions important in middle-aged and elderly people, because the youngest person in the sample cohort (i.e., a subject who was 18 in 1981) was now older than 40 years. The mental health foci were depression and cognitive health. The foci for medical conditions included those shown in Table 2–2. The project included enhanced measures of physical functioning, including some performance-based measures as well as self-report measures. The project took advantage of the advances of the Human Genome Project by asking respondents to donate blood for genetic studies on candidate genes that have not been identified yet. We also assayed for potential mediators of the risk processes shown in Figure 2–3, for example, cholesterol, C-reactive protein, and other measures, to eventually determine whether depression is associated with higher values and whether that then contributes to raised risk for heart attack. We intended also to obtain measures related to allostatic load. The project goal is to follow the sample completely, through the life span of each and every member of the cohort. As of this writing (spring 2005), we have located and interviewed 1,055 subjects, a number we project to be about 75% of survivors from the 1993–1994 follow-up.

REFERENCES

Addington A, Gallo J, Ford D, et al: Epidemiology of unexplained fatigue and major depression in the community: the Baltimore ECA follow-up, 1981–1994. Psychol Med 31:1037–1044, 2001

American Psychiatric Association: Diagnostic and Statistical Manual of Mental Disorders, 3rd Edition. Washington, DC, American Psychiatric Association, 1980

Anda R, Williamson D, Jones D, et al: Depressed affect, hopelessness, and the risk of ischemic heart disease in a cohort of U.S. adults. Epidemiology 4:285–294, 1993

Armenian HK, Lilienfeld AK: Incubation period of disease. Epidemiol Rev 5:1–15, 1983

Armenian HK, Pratt LA, Gallo JJ, et al: Psychopathology and symptomatic arthritis: the 13-year follow-up of the Baltimore Epidemiologic Catchment Area sample. Unpublished study, 1996

Badawi MA, Eaton WW, Myllyluoma J, et al: Psychopathology and attrition in the Baltimore ECA follow-up 1981–1996. Soc Psychiatry Psychiatr Epidemiol 34:91–98, 1999

Barefoot JC, Helms MJ, Mark DB, et al: Depression and long-term mortality risk in patients with coronary artery disease. Am J Cardiol 78:613–617, 1996

Barker DJP: Fetal origins of coronary heart disease. BMJ 311:171–174, 1995

Berkman LF, Blumenthal J, Burg M, et al: Effects of treating depression and low perceived social support on clinical events after myocardial infarction: the Enhancing Recovery in Coronary Heart Disease Patients (ENRICHD) randomized trial. JAMA 289:3106–3116, 2003

Berkson J: Limitations of the application of fourfold table analysis to hospital data. Biometrics 2:47–53, 1946

Bogner HR, Gallo JJ, Sammel MD, et al: Urinary incontinence and psychological distress among community dwelling older adults. J Am Geriatr Soc 50:489–495, 2002

Bovasso GB: Cannabis abuse as a risk factor for depressive symptoms. Am J Psychiatry 158:2033–2037, 2001

Boyd JH, Burke JD, Gruenberg EM, et al: The exclusion criteria of DSM-III: a study of the co-occurrence of hierarchy-free syndromes. Arch Gen Psychiatry 41:983–989, 1984

Bruce ML, Leaf PJ, Rozal GPFL, et al: Psychiatric status and 9-year mortality data in the New Haven Epidemiologic Catchment Area Study. Am J Psychiatry 151:716–721, 1994

Bucholz KK, Shayka JJ, Marion SL, et al: Is a history of alcohol problems or of psychiatric disorder associated with attrition at 11-year follow up? Ann Epidemiol 6:228–234, 1996

Carnethon MR, Kinder LS, Fair JM, et al: Symptoms of depression as a risk factor for incident diabetes: findings from the National Health and Nutrition Examination Epidemiologic Follow-Up Study, 1971–1992. Am J Epidemiol 158:416–423, 2003

Christie KA, Burke JD, Regier DA, et al: Epidemiologic evidence for early onset of mental disorders and higher risk of drug abuse in young adults. Am J Psychiatry 145:971–975, 1988

Cohen P, Cohen J: The clinician's illusion. Arch Gen Psychiatry 41:1178–1182, 1984

Cooper-Patrick L, Gallo J, Powe N, et al: Mental health service utilization by African Americans and whites: the Baltimore Epidemiologic Catchment Area Follow-up. Med Care 37:1034–1045, 1999

Cottler LB, Zipp JF, Robins LN, et al: Difficult-to-recruit respondents and their effect on prevalence estimates in an epidemiologic survey. Am J Epidemiol 125:329–339, 1987

Crum RM, Brown C, Liang KY, et al: The association of depression and problem drinking: analyses from the Baltimore ECA follow-up study. Addict Behav 26:765–773, 2001

Dohrenwend BP, Dohrenwend BS: Perspectives on the past and future of psychiatric epidemiology: the 1981 Rema Lapouse lecture. Am J Public Health 72:1271–1279, 1982

Eaton WW: The NIMH Epidemiologic Catchment Area Program: implementation and major findings. Int J Methods Psychiatr Res 4:103–112, 1994a

Eaton WW: A ten-year retrospective on the NIMH Epidemiologic Catchment Area (ECA) Program (editorial). Int J Methods Psychiatr Res 4:88–91, 1994b

Eaton WW: General population follow-up studies, in Epidemiology and Health Services. Edited by Armenian HK, Shapiro S. New York, Oxford University Press, 1998, pp 83–105

Eaton WW, Kessler LG (eds): Epidemiologic Field Methods in Psychiatry: The NIMH Epidemiologic Catchment Area Program. Orlando, FL, Academic Press, 1985

Eaton WW, Regier DA, Locke BZ, et al: The Epidemiologic Catchment Area Program of the National Institute of Mental Health. Public Health Rep 96:319–325, 1981

Eaton WW, Kramer M, Anthony JC, et al: The incidence of specific DIS/DSM-III mental disorders: data from the NIMH Epidemiologic Catchment Area Program. Acta Psychiatr Scand 79:163–178, 1989

Eaton WW, Anthony JC, Tepper S, et al: Psychopathology and attrition in the Epidemiologic Catchment Area surveys. Am J Epidemiol 135:1051–1059, 1992

Eaton WW, Badawi M, Melton B: Prodromes and precursors: epidemiologic data for primary prevention of disorders with slow onset. Am J Psychiatry 152:967–972, 1995

Eaton WW, Armenian HK, Gallo JJ, et al: Depression and risk for onset of type II diabetes: a prospective, population-based study. Diabetes Care 19:1097–1102, 1996

Eaton WW, Anthony JC, Gallo J, et al: Natural history of DIS/DSM major depression: the Baltimore ECA follow-up. Arch Gen Psychiatry 54:993–999, 1997

Eaton WW, Muntaner C, Bovasso G, et al: Socioeconomic status and depressive syndrome: the role of inter- and intragenerational mobility, government assistance, and work environment. J Health Soc Behav 42:277–294, 2001

Ferketich AK, Schwartzbaum JA, Frid DJ, et al: Depression as an antecedent to heart disease among women and men in the NHANES I study. National Health and Nutrition Examination Survey. Arch Intern Med 160:1261–1268, 2000

Ford DE, Mead LA, Chang PP, et al: Depression is a risk factor for coronary artery disease in men: the precursors study. Arch Intern Med 158:1422–1426, 1998

Gallo JJ, Armenian HK, Ford DE, et al: Major depression and cancer: the 13-year follow-up of the Baltimore Epidemiologic Catchment Area Sample. Cancer Causes Control 11:751–758, 2000

Gavard JA, Lustman PJ, Clouse RE: Prevalence of depression in adults with diabetes. Diabetes Care 16:1167–1178, 1993

Glassman AH, O'Connor CM, Califf RM, et al: Sertraline treatment of major depression in patients with acute MI or unstable angina. JAMA 288:701–709, 2002

Golden SH, Williams JE, Ford DE, et al: Depressive symptoms and the risk of type 2 diabetes: the Atherosclerosis Risk in Communities study. Diabetes Care 27:429–435, 2004

Kawakami N, Shimizu H, Takatsuka N, et al: Depressive symptoms and occurrence of type 2 diabetes among Japanese men. Diabetes Care 22:1071–1076, 1999

Kessler RC: Building on the ECA: The National Comorbidity Survey and the Children's ECA. Int J Methods Psychiatr Res 4:81–94, 1994

Kouzis AC, Eaton WW: Emotional disability days: prevalence and predictors. Am J Public Health 84:1304–1307, 1995

Kouzis AC, Eaton WW: Psychopathology and the development of disability. Soc Psychiatry Psychiatr Epidemiol 32:379–386, 1997

Kouzis AC, Eaton WW: Psychopathology and the initiation of disability payments. Psychiatr Serv 51:908–913, 2000

Kouzis AC, Eaton WW, Leaf P: Psychopathology and mortality in the general population. Soc Psychiatry Psychiatr Epidemiol 30:165–170, 1995

Krieger N: Epidemiology and the web of causation: has anyone seen the spider? Soc Sci Med 39:887–903, 1994

Kuh D, Ben-Shlomo Y (eds): A Life Course Approach to Chronic Disease Epidemiology. Oxford, England, Oxford University Press, 1997

Larson SL, Owens PL, Ford DE, et al: Depressive disorders, dysthymia risk of stroke: a thirteen year follow-up from the Baltimore ECA. Stroke 32:1979–1983, 2001

Leaf PJ, German PS, Spitznagel EL, et al: Sampling: the institutional survey, in Epidemiologic Field Methods in Psychiatry: The NIMH Epidemiologic Catchment Area Program. Edited by Eaton WW, Kessler LG. Orlando, FL, Academic Press, 1985, pp 49–66

Lilienfeld DE, Stolley PD: Foundations of Epidemiology. New York, Oxford University Press, 1994

Lustman PJ, Griffith LS, Glouse RE: Depression in adults with diabetes: results of 5-year follow-up study. Diabetes Care 11:605–612, 1988

Mendes de Leon CF, Krumholz HM, Seeman TS, et al: Depression and risk of coronary heart disease in elderly men and women: New Haven EPESE, 1982–1991. Established Populations for the Epidemiologic Studies of the Elderly. Arch Intern Med 158:2341–2348, 1998

Pratt LA, Ford DE, Crum RM, et al: Depression, psychotropic medication and risk of heart attack: prospective data from the Baltimore ECA follow-up. Circulation 94:3123–3129, 1996

Regier DA: ECA Contributions to national policy and further research. Int J Methods Psychiatr Res 4:73–80, 1994

Regier DA, Myers JK, Kramer M, et al: The NIMH Epidemiologic Catchment Area (ECA) Program: historical context, major objectives, and study population characteristics. Arch Gen Psychiatry 41:934–941, 1984

Regier DA, Hirschfeld RMA, Goodwin FK, et al: The NIMH Depression Awareness, Recognition, and Treatment Program: structure, aims, and scientific basis. Am J Psychiatry 145:1351–1357, 1988

Robins LN, Regier DA: Psychiatric Disorders in America: The Epidemiologic Catchment Area Study. New York, The Free Press, 1991

Robinson RG: Neuropsychiatric consequences of stroke. Annu Rev Med 48:217–229, 1997

Robinson RG, Starr LB, Kubos KL, et al: A two-year longitudinal study of post-stroke mood disorders: findings during the initial evaluation. Stroke 14:736–741, 1983

Robinson RG, Starr LB, Lipsey JR, et al: A two-year longitudinal study of post-stroke mood disorders: dynamic changes in associated variables over the first six months of follow-up. Stroke 15:510–517, 1984

Rosenblatt A, Mehta KM, Romanoski A, et al: Major depression and cognitive decline after 11.5 years: findings from the ECA study. J Nerv Ment Dis 191:827–830, 2003

Rothman KJ: Induction and latent periods. Am J Epidemiol 114:253–259, 1981

Rothman KJ: Modern Epidemiology. Boston, MA, Little, Brown, 1986

Rugulies R: Depression as a predictor for coronary heart disease: a review and meta-analysis. Am J Prev Med 23:51–61, 2002

Saydah SH, Brancati FL, Golden SH, et al: Depressive symptoms and the risk of type 2 diabetes mellitus in a U.S. sample. Diabetes Metab Res Rev 19:202–208, 2003

Sesso HD, Kawachi I, Vokonas PS, et al: Depression and the risk of coronary heart disease in the Normative Aging Study. Am J Cardiol 82:851–856, 1998

Shapiro S, Skinner EA, Kessler LG, et al: Utilization of health and mental health services, three Epidemiologic Catchment Area sites. Arch Gen Psychiatry 41:971–978, 1984

Sheps DS, Freedland KE, Golden RN, et al: ENRICHD and SADHART: implications for future biobehavioral intervention efforts. Psychosom Med 65:1–2, 2003

Shrout PE: The NIMH Epidemiologic Catchment Area Program: broken promises and dashed hopes? Int J Methods Psychiatr Res 4:113–122, 1994

Swartz KL, Pratt LA, Armenian HK, et al: Mental disorder and the incidence of migraine headaches in a community sample: results from the Baltimore Epidemiologic Catchment Area follow-up study. Arch Gen Psychiatry 57:945–950, 2000

Torrey EF, Peterson MR: Slow and latent viruses in schizophrenia. Lancet 2(7819):22–24, 1973

Von Korff M, Cottler L, George LK, et al: Nonresponse and nonresponse bias in the ECA surveys, in Epidemiologic Field Methods in Psychiatry: The NIMH Epidemiologic Catchment Area Program. Edited by Eaton WW, Kessler LG. Orlando, FL, Academic Press, 1985, pp 85–98

Wassertheil-Smoller S, Applegate WB, Berge K, et al: Change in depression as a precursor of cardiovascular events. SHEP Cooperative Research Group (Systolic Hypertension in the Elderly). Arch Intern Med 156:553–561, 1996

Whalley LJ, Starr JM, Athawes R, et al: Childhood mental ability and dementia. Neurology 55:1455–1459, 2000

Whooley MA, Browner WS: Association between depressive symptoms and mortality in older women. Study of Osteoporotic Fractures Research Group. Arch Intern Med 158:2129–2135, 1998

Risk Factors

Linking Fetal Experience to Adult Disease

Examples From Schizophrenia

Mark G. A. Opler, Ph.D., M.P.H.

Michaeline A. Bresnahan, Ph.D., M.P.H.

George Davey Smith, D.Sc.

Ezra S. Susser, M.D., Dr.P.H.

THIS CHAPTER DISCUSSES the application of life course epidemiology to study fetal influences on adult diseases. We identify the most effective designs currently in use and propose that these be complemented by other approaches in a process we term *translation and reverse translation*. Our examples come mainly from research on the fetal origins of schizophrenia, but the discussion is meant to have a broader import. Therefore, we focus on designs and dilemmas that are relevant to studying fetal influences on any adult disease.

In a current definition, *life course epidemiology* is "the study of long-term biological, behavioural, and psychosocial processes that link adult health and disease risk to physical or social exposures acting during gestation, childhood, adolescence, earlier in adult life, or across generations" (Kuh and Ben-Shlomo 2004, p. 778).

This requires positing and testing causal explanations for the connections between experience at an earlier stage and disease at a later stage of the life course. For example, one may posit a causal chain in which one event leads to another, creating a sequence that ultimately influences disease risk; or an exposure at a critical early point in development that is manifest as disease in later life; or dynamic reciprocal relationships between specific social and biological experiences over the life course.

Many life course epidemiologists have placed special emphasis on fetal development as a critical period, premised on the idea that adult health may be affected by exposures during embryogenesis. A wide range of conditions has been implicated as having fetal origins, including cardiovascular, metabolic, and brain disorders. In the United States, epidemiological studies of schizophrenia have pioneered this effort (Wyatt and Susser 2000), while in the United Kingdom and elsewhere, studies of cardiovascular disease have led its development (Barker 1998).

The observational approaches to study risk factors for disease developed after World War II have proven to be remarkably adaptable for the broader questions posed by life course research. The cohort study in particular has been stretched to accommodate studies linking fetal exposures to adult diseases. Nonetheless, when used for this purpose, the cohort design presents formidable barriers that have to be circumvented and reduce the strength of causal inference. Foremost among these barriers is that our ability to observe prenatal experience is limited, requiring investigators to search for "windows" onto prenatal life outside the usual scope of observation or recollection. Another is that fetal exposures and adult outcomes may be separated by several decades. In part for this reason, we propose the use of complementary strategies alongside the cohort design.

We begin by discussing the particular types of cohort designs that have proved effective for studying fetal origins of schizophrenia and present selected results from such studies. We next discuss how this research may be further advanced using genetic research to help validate (or refute) these results, animal research to elucidate biological pathways, and historical studies of time trends to further test the coherence of findings. The chapter concludes by arguing for an iterative process of translation and reverse translation.

COHORT DESIGNS TO STUDY FETAL ORIGINS OF ADULT DISEASE

The cohort design is a versatile strategy, and many variants can be differentiated (Susser et al. 2005). We describe two particular types of cohort study that have been most useful in studies of fetal origins. One is the *natural experiment*, in which the key advantage is in the isolation of the effect of interest from other effects or in epidemiological parlance in control of confounding. Another is the *prenatal cohort with archived biological specimens*, which derives its strength from the precision of the prenatal exposure data. Cohorts with special exposures, including environmental and genetic exposures, are also useful but are not discussed here (Brown et al. 2000; Susser 1999; Susser and Bresnahan 2002).

Natural Experiments

In a natural experiment, people are selected into the exposed or unexposed group by some event that is largely or entirely outside their own control. Like an ordinary experiment, the event is imposed upon some subjects but not others. Unlike an ordinary experiment, the event is a natural one, in the sense that it is not created by the investigator. Natural experiments have been devised to study both environmental and genetic causes.

A natural experiment of an environmental exposure is typically based upon an unanticipated disaster such as a famine, an earthquake, or a hurricane (Susser 1991). It can also be based around a beneficial event (Costello et al. 1996). The design is most applicable when an event subjects a population to a well-characterized, circumscribed, time-limited exposure.

One example of a natural experiment, the Dutch Famine Study, illustrates the advantages and disadvantages of this approach. This study had its roots in the Nazi occupation of Holland during World War II. In the later stages of the war, a strike by railroad workers brought transportation to a halt. The Nazis retaliated by blockading all shipments, including food supplies, into the western part of the country, which at the time was one of the most densely populated parts of the world. With resources already strained, the blockade precipitated a severe famine. The natural experiment that this tragic confluence of events afforded is virtually unique; a famine that was well defined in time and space in a large, urban society that was otherwise well fed, had widespread access to health care, and conducted extensive record keeping.

The studies that were conducted on the effects of prenatal exposure to the famine, crossing from conception to birth and into adulthood, used observational data across the life span and required the efforts of multiple generations of researchers. Several studies are ongoing (Stein et al. 2004). The original studies by Stein et al. (1975) assessed the effects of prenatal famine on neurodevelopment, particularly mental retardation and reduced IQ. Several studies had demonstrated an association of low birth weight with impaired mental development and low IQ (Barker 1966; Drillien 1970), and there also was some evidence that prenatal nutritional deficiency could lead to low birth weight. Of course these associations could be noncausal, reflecting, for example, a common antecedent such as adverse social circumstances. In the natural experimental setting of the Dutch famine, prenatal famine (in the third trimester) did lead to lower birth weight, but no effect of prenatal famine (in any trimester) was seen on either IQ or other measures of mental performance. The lack of coherence between the findings from prior observational studies and this natural experiment reflects a key issue in life course epidemiology—that with a large number of interrelated putative causal factors acting across the life course, it is difficult to differentiate causal factors from confounded markers of disease risk (Kramer, in Kuh and Ben-Shlomo 2004; see also Ben-Shlomo and Davey Smith 1991).

The Dutch Famine Study did, however, support earlier reports suggesting that inadequate maternal nutrition contributed to risk of central nervous system anomalies such as spina bifida and anencephaly, which were related to conception during the most severe stages of the famine (Stein and Susser 1975). Subsequent epidemiological studies and, ultimately, randomized control trials demonstrated that this finding was a clue to a true causal connection. Periconceptual folate supplements reduced the risk of neural tube defects (Medical Research Council, Vitamin Study Research Group 1991; Smithells et al. 1983).

This study set the stage for a generational succession wherein the son of the two primary investigators of the original study (E. Susser) followed cohorts into adulthood in order to study early prenatal exposure to the famine as a risk factor for schizophrenia. Using national psychiatric registries, rates of schizophrenia were found to be approximately doubled for individuals conceived at the height of the famine. Early gestational exposure to famine conferred risk for schizophrenia, whereas late gestational exposure did not. Other studies extending these findings to schizophrenia spectrum personality disorders also showed a twofold increase in risk for early gestational exposure to famine (Susser et al. 1998).

The Dutch Famine Studies are notable for the use of a natural experiment and improved timing and classification of exposure as compared with previous work. They illustrate how a prenatal exposure may be related to different neurodevelopmental outcomes over the life course—in this instance, a congenital neurodevelopmental outcome (neural tube defects), a late adolescent psychiatric outcome (schizophrenia spectrum personality disorder), and an adult psychiatric outcome (schizophrenia per se). However, the degree to which specific underlying mechanisms can be further investigated in this population is limited. For example, although specific micronutrient deficiencies are hypothesized to be of potential importance, it is difficult to study them separately from the broader effects of nutritional deprivation. In order to obtain greater resolution with respect to exposure status, other designs are required.

Prenatal Cohorts With Archived Specimens

This specialized type of cohort study has three essential features. The first is the recruitment of women into a cohort early in pregnancy. To this we must enjoin a second feature, the collection of prenatal biological specimens that have been archived for future analysis of prenatal exposures. The third feature is that the follow-up of the offspring must extend well into adulthood with thorough diagnosis of the disease outcome (e.g., schizophrenia).

Two large prenatal cohorts that proved amenable to this type of study were founded in the United States during the 1950s: the Childhood Health and Development Study and the National Collaborative Perinatal Project. These studies recruited large numbers of pregnant women and collected biological specimens at prenatal visits. Studies of the fetal origins of schizophrenia were built upon both of these cohorts. (The cohorts are now also being used to investigate fetal origins of a wide spectrum of other diseases [Susser and Terry 2003]). One example is the Prenatal Determinants of Schizophrenia (PDS) study built upon the Child Health and Development Study. The original cohort included a total of 19,044 live births in a prepaid health plan in Alameda County between the years of 1959 and 1967 (van den Berg et al. 1988). In the PDS, starting in 1981, individuals treated for psychiatric disorders were identified from a health plan database of inpatient, outpatient, and pharmacy records, allowing potential cases to be sought for a thorough diagnostic interview. Using either diagnostic interview data or chart review, 71 cases of schizophrenia and related spectrum disorders were identified between 1981 and 1997 (Susser et al. 2000).

A wide range of prenatal information is available for study in the PDS. Data taken during maternal interviews at prenatal visits include information on obstetric health, general medical health, and demographic information. Most relevant to the present discussion, maternal serum samples were collected and stored in the form of aliquots at $-20°C$ in anticipation of future studies. These archived prenatal specimens were used in the PDS in a nested case control design in which control subjects were selected from the cohort and matched to cases on the basis of several factors (for details, see Susser et al. 2000).

Several findings have now been reported from the PDS based on serological data. For example, these data were used to test the hypothesis that prenatal influenza is a risk factor for schizophrenia (Brown et al. 2004). Previously, numerous ecological studies and record-based reports had suggested an association, but the results were overall inconclusive. A serological analysis from the PDS found that exposure to influenza during the first half of pregnancy was associated with a threefold increase in risk of schizophrenia spectrum disorders, whereas no increase was seen following exposure during the second half of pregnancy. Although the number of cases of schizophrenia and related spectrum disorders with the required prenatal sera was limited (64 cases and 128 matched control subjects), and this result is certainly not definitive, it provides the best evidence thus far in favor of a causal connection.

As a second example, serological data were used to test the hypothesis that prenatal exposure to lead is a risk factor for schizophrenia. Lead has been known as a neurotoxic agent for centuries. It has long been associated with psychosis following acute exposures in adults, and more recently with deficits in intelligence, impaired attention, and juvenile delinquency following chronic prenatal and perinatal exposure (Dietrich et al. 2001; Needleman et al. 1979). Although some studies have followed samples with prenatal exposures into adolescence (Ris et al. 2004), there is a dearth of literature on long-term effects, particularly on the subsequent risk of mental disorders during adulthood. This was the first study to examine prenatal lead—or any other chemical—exposure as a risk factor for schizophrenia.

The principal technique for assessing lead exposure in studies of prenatal exposure is through direct measurements on maternal blood. The PDS had stored sera, not whole blood containing the lead-sequestering erythrocytes required for direct measurements in small volumes. Techniques for direct measurement of lead could not be employed. However, a biological marker of lead exposure, δ-aminolevulinic acid (δ-ALA), may be detected in urine, plasma, and serum using high-pressure liquid chromatography with fluorescence detection.

Feasibility studies were conducted to assess the utility of this technique in small volumes of stored maternal serum. It was determined that second trimester serum was likely to be the best indicator of prenatal exposure because both lead and corresponding δ-ALA levels were believed to be relatively stable at midpregnancy. Second trimester samples were available for 44 cases and 75 matched control subjects. A single aliquot of second trimester serum was made available for each subject. A cutoff value was used to divide the sample into exposed and unexposed subjects. Samples were coded and blinded with respect to case status. Using this approach, lead exposure as measured by elevated δ-ALA was associated with about a twofold increase in risk of schizophrenia spectrum disorders in this sample (OR=2.3; 95% CI=1.0, 4.3; P=0.05). The small numbers of subjects contributed to the wide confidence limits, and like the influenza result, this finding is considered suggestive, far from conclusive.

In addition, because this study used a biological marker of exposure, serum δ-ALA, rather than direct measurement of lead, an increase in risk of schizophrenia cannot necessarily be ascribed to lead exposure. An intriguing alternative hypothesis is that serum δ-ALA itself may be the exposure of interest. In experimental models, δ-ALA has been shown to be neurotoxic, interfering with γ-aminobutyric acid neurotransmission (Cory-Slechta 1995).

Both the influenza and lead findings from the PDS illustrate how prenatal cohorts with archived biological specimens can take a leap forward in terms of defining and ascertaining exposure status and timing. At the very least, they allow researchers to say with more certainty than before that certain classes of exposure (e.g., infectious agents and environmental toxins) are risk factors that merit more detailed investigation. Yet as we have emphasized, although both these findings are intriguing and biologically plausible, neither is definitive. Several challenges remain, including the need for larger sample sizes with greater statistical power and the need to verify that results are indeed due to the exposure of interest during the developmental period of interest (i.e., not due to confounding).

The lack of statistical power could be addressed by establishing larger cohorts of this type as well as using more advanced technology for collection, storage, and more precise analysis of prenatal specimens. A number of authors have suggested that in order to realize the full potential of life course research, a series of large-scale, longitudinal, "conception-to-death" cohorts are required (e.g., Eaton 2002; Susser and Terry 2003). Beginning in the prenatal period and continuing periodic follow-up across the life course will create an observational laboratory for examining developmental trajectories. Cohort studies that at least approximate this design have already been initiated, although none have yet been followed into adulthood (Golding 1990; Trasande and Landrigan 2004; see also www.ncs.gov, www.fhi.no/tema/morogbarn/kortproteng.html, and www.ssi.dk/sw9314.asp).

A more intractable problem is to rule out confounding and establish that an association signifies a true causal connection. We suggest that for studies linking fetal exposures to adult disease, achieving this goal will ultimately require turning to other approaches that can help to confirm (or refute) a causal connection. In the following sections we discuss three complementary methods that can be helpful in this regard. Then we discuss some further approaches to strengthening causal inference.

COMPLEMENTARY METHODS

- -

Given the problem of confounding, which tends to be exacerbated in studies that cannot directly observe the exposure of interest, it is important to employ other strategies that are not subject to the same confounding bias. These strategies do not have to be—in fact, cannot be—free of any bias, but they can be free of the bias most likely to create artifact in the cohort studies. In this section we discuss approaches based on genetic associations, historical time trends, and animal studies, all of which can help to confirm (or refute) a causal connection suggested by a cohort study.

Mendelian Randomization

The current epidemiological literature is intensely exploring ways in which genetic findings can be used to corroborate findings on environmental risk factors. One such approach has been referred to as *Mendelian randomization* (Katan 2004). The name refers to the random assortment of genes from parents to offspring that occurs during gamete formation and conception, which is the basis of what has come to be called Mendel's second law—the law of independent assortment. The association between risk of a disease and a genetic variant that mimics the biological link between a proposed exposure and disease is not generally susceptible to the reverse causation or confounding that may distort interpretations of conventional observational studies.

Several cases in which the phenotypic effects of polymorphisms are well documented provide encouraging evidence of the explanatory power of Mendelian randomization (Davey Smith and Ebrahim 2003, 2004). We discussed earlier the finding from the Dutch Famine Study that periconceptual maternal famine exposure was associated with increased risk of offspring neural tube defects (Stein et al. 2004). Based on the findings of randomized, controlled trials that periconceptual folate supplementation reduces risk of such defects, we would interpret this as indicating that maternal folate depletion, consequent of the famine, increased the risk of offspring neural tube defects. Mendelian randomization approaches would come to the same conclusion. Briefly, a variant of a gene involved in folate metabolism (the thermolabile variant of the enzyme methylene tetrahydrofolate reductase [MTHFR]) is associated with lower enzymatic activity. Mothers who are homozygous for this variant have double the risk of having offspring with a neural tube defect of mothers not carrying this variant (Botto and Yang 2000). Fathers who are homozygous for this variant have no elevation in risk of having offspring with a neural tube defect, indicating that, as with folate intake, this is a maternal effect. These data point to maternal folate deficit as a potential important cause of neural tube defects, and this is what randomized, controlled trials have shown. Perhaps if the Mendelian randomization method had been available in the past, this understanding of a potential way to prevent neural tube defects could have been reached earlier than was the case.

The MTHFR polymorphism is already being used in an analogous fashion to examine whether prenatal folate was the operative factor in the findings on schizophrenia from the Dutch famine studies (Lewis et al. 2005). However, we now turn to another example to illustrate the potential as well as some of the limitations of this approach for schizophrenia research.

Consider the hypothesis we alluded to earlier, that the effects of δ-ALA itself could explain the association reported from the PDS on prenatal lead exposure (which was measured indirectly via serum δ-ALA) and schizophrenia. Several genetic polymorphisms have been identified in *ALA-D*, the enzyme responsible for metabolizing δ-ALA. This enzyme is also the biochemical target for lead-induced elevations of serum δ-ALA. The two major isoforms, *ALA-D1* and *ALA-D2*, have several functional differences, including different affinities for lead; the *ALA-D2* form has a higher affinity than *ALA-D1*.

We have suggested that high levels of maternal δ-ALA might elevate the risk of schizophrenia in offspring. If one of the polymorphisms in *ALA-D* were shown to be associated with this intermediate phenotype (elevated δ-ALA) and also with the disease (schizophrenia), then the finding would support the hypothesis that elevated δ-ALA is a risk factor for schizophrenia.

However, many complexities may be associated with the use of Mendelian randomization, and several of them pertain to this example. First, in a seeming contradiction, although the *ALA-D2* form is associated with higher affinities for lead and elevated levels of blood lead, two studies report that *ALA-D2* carriers have lower levels of δ-ALA and better performance on neuropsychological tests as compared with *ALA-D1* homozygotes (Bellinger et al. 1994; Kim et al. 2004). This suggests that maternal *ALA-D2* carriers are likely to experience fewer elevations in δ-ALA during development, thereby reducing risk of exposure in their offspring, but the available data on the relationship are limited thus far.

A second complexity is that of genetic pleiotropy—that is, *ALA-D* genotype may alter the risk of schizophrenia via other pathways, regardless of its effects on δ-ALA levels. A third complexity is canalization, whereby adaptive responses may reduce the effect of the genotype on the intermediate phenotype.

The underlying premise of this approach is very similar to that of the natural experiment. As noted earlier, natural experiments have been devised to study genetic causes, including twin studies, adoption studies, and many other kinds. Certain types of genetic association studies may also be considered a kind of natural experiment (Susser et al. 2005). All these studies, in any event, include a central feature of a natural experiment—that is, individuals cannot choose their genes. The clustering of environmental exposures that we typically find in ordinary populations is not found for genetic alleles. Although these designs carry other problems for causal inference, they are *different* problems. The results are complementary in the sense that they cannot be produced by the *same* bias. By contrast, a long string of cohort studies could produce the same artifactual finding due to the same bias.

Historical Time Trends

The examination of time trends in disease occurrence may also contribute to the search for and confirmation of environmental risk factors acting during gestation. When trying to spot the footprints of prenatal environmental factors in secular trends, we necessarily focus on the experiences of generations. An early life exposure that is shared by some generations and not others will manifest in changes in the rates of disease across birth years and is best appreciated in analyses comparing age-specific disease rates over successive generations. For example, people born in 1901–1910, 1911–1920, and 1921–1930 might be compared with respect to their disease rate at ages 20–24. By comparing an array of successive generations we are able to detect the deferred effects of a change in exposure that occurred at some point in the life cycle antecedent to the age-specific disease rates being examined.

One approach is to examine time trends for clues to the presence of early life exposures that influence the risk of an adult disease. A generation analysis alone, however, is insufficient to establish that generation (or "cohort") effects are responsible for a disease trend. It is also necessary to rule out the possibility of confounding by factors acting around the time of disease occurrence—or "period" effects—including changes affecting case definition and detection. A method referred to as *age-period-cohort analysis* is used for this purpose (for a full discussion, see Susser et al. 2005). This is often difficult, and an age-period-cohort analysis may yield indeterminate results. Yet in several important instances, the generation effects have been clear enough to provide clues to early life (although not prenatal) effects on major diseases; two classic examples are tuberculosis and peptic ulcer (Frost 1939; Susser 1982; Susser and Stein 2002).

Another approach is to use time trends to confirm (or refute) a specific finding. Coherence of trends over time in both rates of disease and a candidate prenatal environmental exposure may provide supporting, although not definitive, evidence for causality. The use of time trends to explore a causal hypothesis might be suggested in circumstances in which the exposure prevalence is changing over time. A confirmatory test of a causal hypothesis may be best achieved in circumstances in which there are readily evident changes in both exposure prevalence and disease rates over time. Inferences based on such analyses alone must be guarded, but again, they can provide important evidence from another line of investigation that has *different* sources of bias from the cohort study.

One example of this strategy is a study that examined various hypotheses relating cannabis use and schizophrenia, modeling the effects of cannabis use on the incidence and prevalence of schizophrenia over the life span in eight birth cohorts (Degenhardt et al. 2003). This example also illustrates that a disease trend across generations may be explained not only by exposures during gestation but also by cumulative exposures prior to the onset of disease common to the generation (e.g., cannabis, urban living). The authors used empirical evidence as the basis for assumptions regarding the natural history of schizophrenia (e.g., age of onset, chronicity) and cannabis use (e.g., the age-specific prevalence of use in successive cohorts), and the projected trends were compared with current information on schizophrenia time trends. In this instance, the evidence was not compatible with the causal hypothesis and suggested using caution in the interpretation of cohort-study data indicating that cannabis use is a risk factor for schizophrenia. A similar conclusion was recently drawn from a systematic review of observational studies that paid particular attention to the potential role of confounding factors (Macleod et al. 2004).

Comparison of time-trend and individual data might also turn out to be feasible with respect to the hypothesis that prenatal lead exposure is related to risk of schizophrenia. Unlike the cannabis hypothesis, the time trends for the candidate risk factor may at least be in broad synchrony with trends in the rates of schizophrenia. In high-income societies, the rates of schizophrenia appear in some studies to be declining for persons born following the time of regulations that reduced lead levels in gasoline and paint. A rigorous study relating these two time trends would, however, be quite challenging. It would require the use of locally detailed information on environmental lead exposure and reliable schizophrenia rates for these localities. It would also have to consider confounding by postnatal exposure and correlates of lead exposure such as urbanicity.

Animal Models of Prenatal Exposures

Just as prenatal events are difficult, although clearly not impossible, to explore through observational methods, the biological pathways connecting exposure to disease processes are similarly complicated. When considering molecular- or cellular-level events during earliest periods of brain growth and development in the context of the life course, experimental approaches using animal models may be preferable in certain instances. Animal models permit focus on specific molecular events and may be useful when attempting to tease out the effects of an exposure from its possible biochemical intermediates. Returning to the example of lead exposure and elevated δ-ALA, it is difficult to separate these factors and study them independently using population-based methods and unfeasible in the cohorts that are currently available. Experimental models could be designed to provide a clearer understanding of the effects of δ-ALA at key points during the course of fetal development, independently of the effects of lead (e.g., studying the effects of doses of δ-ALA in pregnant dams and their offspring). In cases such as this, experiments may produce supportive evidence that can help investigators design future epidemiological studies, allowing relevant aspects of the exposure–disease relationship to be isolated.

Lipska and Weinberger (2000) discussed models of schizophrenia, stating that they may be used to investigate an exposure, model the symptoms of the disorder, or explore potential treatments. The information they yielded, particularly about changes in nervous system growth consequent to exposure, may greatly benefit observational studies, particularly because they suggest pathways and help clarify issues of exposure definition (e.g., timing and nature of relevant exposure).

This can be illustrated by work on lead and neurodevelopment. Developmental toxicologists have long used rodents to investigate both the acute and chronic effects of lead exposure, using adult, juvenile, and neonatal animals. Although early studies were inconclusive, later studies began to test physiological and behavioral outcomes and utilize more rigorous study designs focusing on specific neurotransmitter systems (Booze and Mactutus 1985; Golter and Michaelson 1975). There are currently a number of transmitter systems that are altered in adult animals following pre- and perinatal lead exposure, including two that may be dysregulated in schizophrenia: glutamate and dopamine.

Guilarte et al. (1994) demonstrated that neonatal lead exposure results in impaired spatial learning, as well as decreases in expression and function of NMDA (N-methyl-D-aspartic acid)-glutamate receptor subunits. They suggested that reduced synaptic plasticity in the hippocampus is the principal mechanism by which lead exposure causes changes in cognitive function. Because the behavioral and molecular effects of lead exposure they documented appear to be reversible via postnatal somatosensory stimulation, this is a highly plausible general mechanism for several intermediate and long-term behavioral outcomes described in human studies of exposure to lead.

Dopamine metabolism may also be affected by lead exposure. Cory-Slechta et al. (1992) reported that early postnatal exposure to lead in rats increased dopamine receptor sensitivity throughout life. Although levels of dopamine and DOPAC (3,4-dihydroxyphenylacetic acid, a major metabolite) in the nucleus accumbens are not significantly different in lead-exposed groups, receptor number and sensitivity are elevated during maturation. Several authors have suggested that dopamine synthesis may become impaired consequent to early lead exposure, followed by systemic alteration in presynaptic dopamine synthesis, in time followed by compensatory effects involving postsynaptic sites and presynaptic autoreceptors (Lasley and Lane 1988).

Altered dopamine and NMDA-glutamate receptor function have been implicated in the pathogenesis of schizophrenia based on pharmacological, imaging, and postmortem findings (Laruelle et al. 2003). Both may merit additional study in the context of exposure to lead as a potential risk factor for schizophrenia. New experimental models of lead exposure may utilize behavioral assessments relevant to paradigms for schizophrenia, such as prepulse inhibition or reversal learning, believed to mimic the functional impairments of schizophrenia and other psychotic disorders. By doing so in tandem with neurochemical and neurophysiological assessments throughout development, a more complete functional picture may help guide future observational studies, particularly in identifying likely intermediate outcomes and indicating which specific systems are vulnerable.

As noted earlier, in addition to the direct effects of lead on receptor expression and function, general mechanisms that account for potentially neurotoxic secondary effects (e.g., δ-ALA exposure) must also be considered. These studies may be particularly relevant to epidemiological designs. If we were to learn that δ-ALA, rather than lead, produced the effects thought to be relevant to schizophrenia pathogenesis, this would direct us to a more proximal measure of the exposure—that is, to measure maternal δ-ALA itself rather than lead exposure.

OTHER APPROACHES TO STRENGTHENING INFERENCE FROM OBSERVATIONAL STUDIES

Improved Measurement of Confounding Factors

In many observational studies only limited effort is taken to classify confounding factors accurately, particularly when the potential for confound-

TABLE 3–1. Association between plasma vitamin C levels and coronary heart disease incidence: Women's Heart and Health Study

Age	EPIC confounders	Life course socioeconomic position	Fully adjusted
0.70 (0.60, 0.82)	0.73 (0.62, 0.87)	0.87 (0.73, 1.05)	0.91 (0.75, 1.10)

Note. The relative risk in the European Prospective Investigation into Cancer and Nutrition (EPIC) study was 0.7 (0.51, 0.95) in men and 0.63 (0.45, 0.90) in women for the same difference in plasma vitamin C level as in the above study. Thus, the age-adjusted effect estimate is very similar to that from the EPIC study. In the EPIC study, adjustment for confounders had little influence on the association. However, when further adjustment was made for life course confounders, the association was virtually abolished, and a small degree of residual confounding due to measurement error in the included confounders would account for the small effect on the fully adjusted model.
Source. Lawlor et al. 2005.

ing across the life course is taken into account. For example, many observational studies have suggested that vitamin C protects against coronary heart disease because vitamin C intake or vitamin C levels are inversely associated with future risk of the disease (e.g., Khaw et al. 2001). These studies have adjusted for a small number of potential confounding factors and have not taken into account the fact that adverse social circumstances and behavioral risk profiles across the life course are related to adulthood vitamin C intake and levels (Lawlor et al. 2004). In one study that explicitly considered the importance of life course confounding it was demonstrated that findings of similar magnitude to those in earlier studies could be obtained, such that higher vitamin C levels were related to lower coronary heart disease risk (Table 3–1). Adjusting for precisely the same—but limited—set of confounders that had been adjusted for in the best known of the previous studies (Khaw et al. 2001) yielded the same magnitude result seen in that study. However, additional adjustment for confounders acting across the life course essentially abolished the association (Lawlor et al. 2005). The null effect seen in the observational study adjusted for life course confounders is similar to the null effects seen in randomized, controlled trials of vitamin C supplementation (Heart Protection Study Collaborative Group 2002).

In the psychiatric epidemiology literature, there are examples of similar differences between studies that are and are not adequately adjusted for life course confounders. For example, many studies have shown a strong dose–

TABLE 3–2. Relative risk of suicide for different levels of smoking: univariate and multivariate analysis (logistic regression analysis) with 95% confidence intervals

	Univariate		Multivariate*	
Nonsmokers	1.00	—	1.00	—
Smokers (1–10 cigarettes/day)	1.39	0.97, 1.97	1.08	0.75, 1.55
Smokers (11–20 cigarettes/day)	1.59	1.10, 2.29	0.87	0.58, 1.30
Smokers (>20 cigarettes/day)	3.03	1.72, 5.34	0.98	0.53, 1.82
P for trend	0.02		0.76	

Note. *Adjustment for risky use of alcohol, drug use, contact with child welfare, parental divorce, low emotional control, psychiatric diagnosis at conscription, medication for nervous problems, and education.

response association between smoking and suicide that is robust to adjustment for a small number of potential confounding factors acting during adult life (Davey Smith et al. 1992; Miller et al. 2000). However, the one study with detailed information on early life factors that may precede both smoking and suicide risk found a dramatic attenuation of the association on adjustment (Table 3–2; Hemmingsson and Kriebel 2003). This example demonstrates the power of taking a life course approach when considering the potential effect of confounding.

Sensitivity Analyses to Assess Residual Confounding

Sensitivity analyses can be undertaken to give an indication of the probable effect of measurement error for included confounders and of unmeasured confounders; methods have been described in detail elsewhere (Greenland 1996). For unmeasured confounders, various plausible values for the strength of associations between the unmeasured confounder and outcome and of unmeasured confounders with exposure can be used, and a series of fully adjusted exposure-outcome associations can be estimated. If these estimated associations are little attenuated, unmeasured confounders are unlikely to be a major problem. An alternative way to present these sensitivity analyses is to report the strength of an association between all potential unmeasured confounders with exposure and outcome that would be needed to attenuate an association to the null value.

Specificity of an Association

Specificity refers to the idea that an association is more likely to be causal if an exposure is related to one outcome, and this was one of Bradford Hill's indicators of causality. It has lost favor over recent decades: for example, a standard textbook of epidemiology states that "Specificity does not confer greater validity to any causal influence regarding the exposure effect…. The criterion is useless and misleading" (Rothman and Greenland 1998, p. 25). In support of this, it is pointed out that smoking is related to many causes of death, but this fact does not exonerate it as a cause of lung cancer (Rothman and Greenland 1998). Smoking, however, is not a single exposure—tobacco smoke contains a wide variety of factors, each of which might be specifically associated with different outcomes. Smoking is unusual in this regard. The view that specificity is an unimportant criterion of causation has been challenged because in many cases an exposure is a plausible cause of just one or a few outcomes; observing associations with both the hypothesized outcomes and with other outcomes decreases the likelihood of the former being causal (Weiss 2002). For example, in 1986 Pettiti and colleagues showed that hormone replacement therapy was apparently "protective" against deaths from accidents and violence (as well as cardiovascular disease) in observational studies, a finding resistant to statistical adjustments. This suggested that both hormone replacement therapy–outcome associations were residually confounded. This report has been rarely cited and failed to quell the interest in promoting hormone replacement therapy as a preventive intervention for cardiovascular disease risk. However, the reports of randomized, controlled trials that fail to show any cardioprotective effect of hormone replacement therapy suggest that the implications of this lack of specificity—that the hormone replacement therapy–outcome association was generated by a variety of social and behavioral factors that were also associated with other causes of death, such as accidents and violence, rather than a biological protector effect—should have been considered. In reports of many epidemiological studies, only the association between exposure and the single outcome of interest is given, which does not allow specificity to be examined. This practice should be depreciated.

CONCLUSION: TRANSLATION AND REVERSE TRANSLATION

The remarkable versatility of the cohort design is once again evident in its adaptation for studying fetal influences on adult disease. Two types of cohort study, natural experiments and prenatal cohorts with archived specimens, have already yielded important results that may ultimately lead to the discovery of causes and means of prevention. Every area of inquiry described in this chapter will benefit from further refinements in the techniques and designs of such cohort studies. In the case of infectious agents, the strains that cause the greatest increases in risk, the molecular components of infection that affect the developing brain, and the timing of exposure may be further specified. The biochemical events consequent to lead exposure must be examined, along with a wider variety of chemical exposures, and the proximal effects of exposure eventually teased apart and differentiated from more distal physiological responses. Yet even with these improvements incorporated into cohort studies, the results are unlikely to be sufficient to prove the case.

We believe that these further investigations using the cohort design are clearly warranted, but they must also be combined with complementary approaches. Replication or extension of findings under the same design always carries the hazard of replicating an artifact. When we cannot directly measure the fetal exposure of interest, even in maternal serum, this presents a profound challenge. We therefore propose a strategy of translation and reverse translation, using alternating cycles of experimental and observational methods to test, refine, and validate hypotheses.

The most common use of the term *translational research* refers to the application of results from basic research to the development of new treatments, typically in the form of clinical drug trials. Some authors have suggested that application of results from clinical observation to the design of basic experiments is equally important (Insel and Fernald 2004; Marincola 2003), whereas in the social sciences, translation implies the application of basic theory to studies of behavioral interventions and policy making (Corrigan et al. 2003). In keeping with the general intention of the term, we suggest that translational research be broadly defined as the strategy of testing findings obtained from one type of study conducted at a specific level of organization (e.g., population-based studies, basic experiments, or clinical observations) in another investigation conducted at a different level of organization, perhaps using another disciplinary approach. In the case of fetal influences on schizophrenia and other adult diseases, there are now several cases in which epidemiological findings could be refined, possibly by using animal models to better characterize potentially relevant exposures at the molecular level during fetal development (e.g., maternal δ-ALA as a potential risk factor for schizophrenia).

Following this initial translation, investigators must then determine if the newly specified finding is valid when tested via other approaches. We are terming this second part of this process *reverse translation*, premised on the idea that a finding thus refined should be carefully reinterpreted and applied at the original level of organization. In the case of epidemiological findings given added resolution by experimental models, the significance of a new theory should ultimately be tested at the population level to determine its value. Interdisciplinary collaborations will play an important role in the future of this endeavor, as will the training and development of a new cohort of interdisciplinary researchers. In the next decade, these investigators will embark on studies that translate findings between the observational and experimental approaches, incorporating genotype to environment to effective prevention of mental illness throughout the life course.

REFERENCES

Barker DJP: Low intelligence: its relation to length of gestation and rate of foetal growth. Br J Prev Soc Med 20:58–66, 1966

Barker DJP: Mothers, Babies and Health in Later Life. Edinburgh, Churchill Livingstone, 1998

Bellinger D, Hu H, Titlebaum L, et al: Attentional correlates of dentin and bone lead levels in adolescents. Arch Environ Health 49:98–105, 1994

Ben-Shlomo Y, Davey Smith G: Deprivation in infancy or adult life: which is more important for mortality risk? Lancet 337:530–534, 1991

Booze RM, Mactutus CF: Experimental design considerations: a determinant of acute neonatal toxicity. Teratology 31:187–191, 1985

Botto LD, Yang Q: 5,10-Methylenetetrahydrofolate reductase gene variants and congenital anomalies: a HuGE Review. Am J Epidemiol 151:862–877, 2000

Brown AS, Schaefer CA, Wyatt RJ, et al: Maternal exposure to respiratory infections and adult schizophrenia spectrum disorders: a prospective birth cohort study. Schizophr Bull 26:287–295, 2000

Brown AS, Begg MD, Gravenstein S, et al: Serologic evidence for prenatal influenza in the etiology of schizophrenia. Arch Gen Psychiatry 61:774–780, 2004

Corrigan PW, Bodenhausen G, Markowitz F, et al: Demonstrating translational research for mental health services: an example from stigma research. Ment Health Serv Res 5:79–88, 2003

Cory-Slechta DA: Relationships between lead-induced learning impairments and changes in dopaminergic, cholinergic, and glutamatergic neurotransmitter system functions. Annu Rev Pharmacol Toxicol 35:391–415, 1995

Cory-Slechta DA, Pokora MJ, Widzowski DV: Postnatal lead exposure induces supersensitivity to the stimulus properties of a D_2–D_3 agonist. Brain Res 598:162–172, 1992

Costello EJ, Angold A, Burns BJ, et al: The Great Smoky Mountains Study of Youth: goals, design, methods, and the prevalence of DSM-III-R disorders. Arch Gen Psychiatry 53:1129–1136, 1996

Davey Smith G, Ebrahim S: "Mendelian randomization": can genetic epidemiology contribute to understanding environmental determinants of disease? Int J Epidemiol 32:1–22, 2003

Davey Smith G, Ebrahim S: Mendelian randomization: prospects, potentials, and limitations. Int J Epidemiol 33:30–42, 2004

Davey Smith G, Phillips AN, Neaton JD: Smoking as "independent" risk factor for suicide: illustration of an artefact from observational epidemiology? Lancet 340:709–712, 1992

Degenhardt L, Hall W, Lynskey M: Testing hypotheses about the relationship between cannabis use and psychosis. Drug Alcohol Depend 71:37–48, 2003

Dietrich KN, Ris MD, Succop PA, et al: Early exposure to lead and juvenile delinquency. Neurotoxicol Teratol 23:511–518, 2001

Drillien CM: The small-for-date infant: etiology and prognosis. Pediatr Clin North Am 17:9–24, 1970

Eaton W: The logic for a conception-to-death cohort study. Ann Epidemiol 12:445–451, 2002

Frost WH: The age selection of mortality from tuberculosis in successive decades. Am J Hygiene 30:91–96, 1939

Golding J: Children of the nineties: a longitudinal study of pregnancy and childhood based on the population of Avon (ALSPAC). West Engl Med J 105:80–82, 1990

Golter M, Michaelson IA: Growth, behavior, and brain catecholamines in lead-exposed neonatal rats: a reappraisal. Science 187:359–361, 1975

Greenland S: Basic methods for sensitivity analysis of biases. Int J Epidemiol 25:1107–1116, 1996

Guilarte TR, Miceli RC, Jett DA: Neurochemical aspects of hippocampal and cortical Pb^{2+} neurotoxicity. Neurotoxicology 15:459–466, 1994

Heart Protection Study Collaborative Group: MRC/BHF Heart Protection Study of antioxidant vitamin supplementation in 20536 high-risk individuals: a randomised placebo-controlled trial. Lancet 360:23–33, 2002

Hemmingsson T, Kriebel D: Smoking at age 18–20 and suicide during 26 years of follow-up: how can the association be explained? Int J Epidemiol 32:1000–1005, 2003

Insel TR, Fernald RD: How the brain processes social information: searching for the social brain. Annu Rev Neurosci 27:697–722, 2004

Katan MB: Commentary: Mendelian randomization, 18 years on. Int J Epidemiol 33:10–11, 2004

Khaw KT, Bingham S, Welch A, et al: Relation between plasma ascorbic acid and mortality in men and women in EPIC-Norfolk prospective study: a prospective population study. European Prospective Investigation Into Cancer and Nutrition. Lancet 357:657–663, 2001

Kim HS, Lee SS, Lee GS, et al: The protective effect of delta-aminolevulinic acid dehydratase 1–2 and 2–2 isozymes against blood lead with higher hematologic parameters. Environ Health Perspect 112:538–541, 2004

Kuh D, Ben-Shlomo Y (eds): Introduction, in A Life Course Approach to Chronic Disease Epidemiology, 2nd Edition. Oxford, England, Oxford University Press, 2004

Laruelle M, Kegeles LS, Abi-Dargham A: Glutamate, dopamine, and schizophrenia: from pathophysiology to treatment. Ann N Y Acad Sci 1003:138–158, 2003

Lasley SM, Lane JD: Diminished regulation of mesolimbic dopaminergic activity in rat after chronic inorganic lead exposure. Toxicol Appl Pharmacol 95:474–483, 1988

Lawlor DA, Davey Smith G, Bruckdorfer KR, et al: Those confounded vitamins: what can we learn from the differences between observational versus randomised trial evidence? Lancet 363:1724–1727, 2004

Lawlor DA, Smith GD, Rumley A, et al: Associations of fibrinogen and C-reactive protein with prevalent and incident coronary heart disease are attenuated by adjustment for confounding factors. British Women's Heart and Health Study. Thromb Haemost 93:955–963, 2005

Lewis SJ, Zammit S, Gunnell D, et al: A meta-analysis of the MTHFR C677T polymorphism and schizophrenia risk. Am J Med Genet 135B:2–4, 2005

Lipska BK, Weinberger DR: To model a psychiatric disorder in animals: schizophrenia as a reality test. Neuropsychopharmacology 23:223–239, 2000

Macleod J, Oakes R, Copello A, et al: Psychological and social sequelae of cannabis and other illicit drug use by young people: a systematic review of longitudinal, general population studies. Lancet 363:1579–1588, 2004

Marincola FM: Translational medicine: a two-way road. J Transl Med 1:1, 2003

Medical Research Council, Vitamin Study Research Group: Prevention of neural tube defects: results of the Medical Research Council Vitamin Study. Lancet 338:131–137, 1991

Miller M, Hemenway D, Bell NS, et al: Cigarette smoking and suicide: a prospective study of 300,000 male active-duty Army soldiers. Am J Epidemiol 151:1060–1063, 2000

Needleman HL, Gunnoe C, Leviton A, et al: Deficits in psychological and classroom performance of children with elevated dentine lead levels. N Engl J Med 300:689–695, 1979

Petitti DB, Perlman JA, Sidney S: Postmenopausal estrogen use and heart disease. N Engl J Med 315:131–132, 1986

Ris MD, Dietrich KN, Succop PA, et al: Early exposure to lead and neuropsychological outcome in adolescence. J Int Neuropsychol Soc 10:261–270, 2004

Rothman KJ, Greenland S: Modern Epidemiology, 2nd Edition. Philadelphia, PA, Lippincott Williams & Wilkins, 1998

Smithells RW, Nevin NC, Seller MJ, et al: Further experience of vitamin supplementation for prevention of neural tube defect recurrences. Lancet 1:1027–1031, 1983

Stein AD, Zybert PA, van de Bor M, et al: Intrauterine famine exposure and body proportions at birth: the Dutch Hunger Winter. Int J Epidemiol 33:831–836, 2004

Stein Z, Susser M: The Dutch famine 1944–1945, and the reproductive process, I: effects or six indices at birth. Pediatr Res 9:70–76, 1975

Stein ZA, Susser M, Saenger G, et al: Famine and Human Development: The Dutch Hunger Winter of 1944–1945. New York, Oxford University Press, 1975

Susser E: Life course cohort studies of schizophrenia. Psychiatr Ann 29:161–165, 1999

Susser E, Bresnahan M: Epidemiologic approaches to neurodevelopmental disorders. Mol Psychiatry 7 (suppl):S2–S3, 2002

Susser M, Stein Z: Civilization and peptic ulcer. Int J Epidemiol 31:13–17, 2002

Susser E, Terry MB: A conception-to-death cohort. Lancet 361:797–798, 2003

Susser ES, Hoek HW, Brown AS: Neurodevelopmental disorders after prenatal famine: the story of the Dutch Famine Study. Am J Epidemiol 147:213–216, 1998

Susser ES, Schaefer CA, Brown AS, et al: The design of the prenatal determinants of schizophrenia study. Schizophr Bull 26:257–273, 2000

Susser E, Schwartz S, Morabia A, et al: Psychiatric Epidemiology: Searching for the Causes of Mental Disorders. New York, Oxford University Press, 2005

Susser M: Period effects, generation effects and age effects in peptic ulcer mortality. J Chronic Dis 35:29–40, 1982

Susser M: What is a cause and how do we know one? A grammar for pragmatic epidemiology. Am J Epidemiol 133:635–648, 1991

Trasande L, Landrigan PJ: The National Children's Study: a critical national investment. Environ Health Perspect 112:A789–A790, 2004

van den Berg BJ, Christianson RE, Oechsli FW: The California Child Health and Development Studies of the School of Public Health, University of California at Berkeley. Paediatr Perinat Epidemiol 2(3):265–282, 1988

Weiss NS: Can the "specificity" of an association be rehabilitated as a basis for supporting a causal hypothesis? Epidemiology 13:6–8, 2002

Wyatt RJ, Susser ES: U.S. birth cohort studies of schizophrenia: a sea change. Schizophr Bull 26:255–256, 2000

Epidemiological Phenotype Hunting

Panic Disorder and Interstitial Cystitis

Myrna M. Weissman, Ph.D.

The work presented in this chapter was funded by a National Alliance for Schizophrenia and Depression Senior Investigator Award (M.M. Weissman); grants MH2874 (M.M. Weissman) and MH35792 (D.F. Klein, A.J. Fyer); and training grant 5T32-MH13043 (R. Gross) from the National Institute of Mental Health. Genotyping services were provided by the Center for Inherited Disease Research, which is fully funded through federal contract N01-HG-65403 from the National Institutes of Health to The Johns Hopkins University.

The data are derived, in part, from work presented in the following manuscripts:

- Fyer AJ, Weissman MM: Genetic linkage study of panic: clinical methodology and description of pedigrees. Am J Med Genet 88:173–181, 1999
- Hamilton SP, Fyer AJ, Durner M, et al: Further genetic evidence for a panic disorder syndrome mapping to chromosome 13q. Proc Natl Acad Sci 100:2550–2555, 2003
- Weissman MM, Fyer AJ, Haghighi F, et al: Potential panic disorder syndrome: clinical and genetic linkage evidence. Am J Med Genet 96:24–35, 2000
- Weissman MM, Gross R, Fyer A, et al: Interstitial cystitis and panic disorder. Arch Gen Psychiatry 61:273–279, 2004

THIS CHAPTER DESCRIBES how we used epidemiological and clinical observations and large multigenerational pedigrees with careful diagnostic assessments, collected blind to their genotyping, to develop hypotheses about a possible new phenotype of panic disorder. The possible syndromes or phenotypes included kidney/bladder problems, serious headache/migraine, thyroid problems, and/or mitral valve prolapse (MVP). We tested these hypothesis in data collected from a genome scan (linkage study) and followed the findings in a case–control study to understand the kidney/bladder problems, which may represent a possible new phenotype.

It is generally agreed that psychiatric disorders are heterogeneous and that different clinical expressions of the disorder are likely to be genetically heterogeneous. Each phenotype or subtype of the disorder may have a different familial aggregation, clinical course, and/or etiology. There have been many efforts to try to define genetically homogeneous subtypes in psychiatry. These studies usually have used different expressions of the disorder such as symptom patterns, severity, age of onset, or comorbidity with other psychiatric disorder to define the phenotype (Maser and Cloninger 1990). Genetic/family studies of psychiatric disorders with few exceptions (Hudson et al. 2003) have usually ignored medical conditions in individuals and/or families, which may aggregate with the disorder of interest. Epidemiological evidence for an increased comorbidity of a psychiatric disorder with some medical condition has been considered misclassification due to an overlap of symptoms or the medical consequence or the cause of the psychiatric disorder.

This chapter describes our search for a possible new phenotype of panic disorder and its comorbidity with other medical conditions within families. We describe the epidemiology of panic disorder and its comorbidity with medical conditions. We then describe the genetic linkage findings, which suggested a potential new genetic syndrome involving panic disorder and several medical conditions. Finally, we describe a case–control study to refine the medical phenotype that seemed to be part of a possible new panic syndrome.

PANIC DISORDER

Panic disorder is a familial, possibly genetic disorder with a lifetime prevalence of about 1%–3% cross-nationally, age of onset in the early 20s, increased risk in women, discrete clinical manifestation occurring across diverse cultures, and responsiveness to several biological challenges (Coryell 1997; Fyer and Weissman 1999; Gorman et al. 1997, 2000; Knowles and

Weissman 1995; Perna et al. 1995, 1996; Vieland et al. 1993, 1996; Weissman et al. 1997). Numerous family studies using direct interviews of relatives show that panic disorder is highly familial. The absolute rates in relatives vary by methods of assessment. However, the familial nature of panic is consistent in all family studies, conducted in different countries with about a seven- to eightfold relative risk of panic disorder in the first-degree relatives of probands with the disorder as compared with the relatives of control subjects (Weissman 1993). Heritability, based on four twin studies, is estimated to be about 49% (Hettema et al. 2001). Panic disorder is considered a complex genetic disorder.

The symptoms of panic disorder include recurrent episodes of sudden, unpredictable apprehension and associated autonomic symptoms involving several systems: cardiorespiratory (shortness of breath, chest pain, palpitations, faintness, choking, smothering, hyperventilation); neurological (dizziness, unsteadiness, derealization, paresthesia, tremulousness); gastrointestinal (nausea, abdominal distress); and autonomic (hot and cold flashes, sweating) as well as cognitive (fear of dying). Because these symptoms mimic several medical conditions, patients with panic disorder are high users of medical services and often receive diagnoses other than panic. Other medical conditions are usually ruled out before a diagnosis of panic disorder is made.

A large-scale, community-based epidemiological study in the United States found an increased association of panic disorder with reports of cardiovascular/cerebrovascular problems (Miniati et al. 1998; Weissman et al. 1990), a history of seizures (Neugebauer et al. 1993), irritable bowel syndrome (Lydiard et al. 1994), and migraine (Stewart et al. 1994). The association of panic disorder has always been reported with one medical problem and not clusters of problems within individuals or families. Moreover, family history or medical records were not available in the epidemiological surveys, so that information of the extent and details of the medical problem was limited. Tentative findings on medical comorbidity in large epidemiological samples are supported by clinical studies that show an increased rate of MVP (Crowe et al. 1980, 1982; Gorman et al. 1988) and possible accompanying arrhythmia and an increased risk of cardiovascular disorder and of mortality due to cardio- or cerebrovascular disease in patients with panic disorder (Gräsbeck et al. 1996; Heninger 1998; Sullivan et al. 2004; Weissman et al. 1990; Wilkinson et al. 1998). Also reported is an increased risk of panic disorder in patients with irritable bowel syndrome (Lydiard et al. 1994) and a possible clinical overlap between specific anxiety attacks and complex partial seizures (Devinsky et al. 1989; Edlund et al. 1987; Weilburg et al. 1987). In the absence of pathophysiological hypotheses, and given the limitations of all the clinical and epidemiological studies, these associations are usually dismissed as an artifact of symptom overlap and/or misdiagnosis. None of the family studies have determined whether these or other medical disorders co-aggregate with panic disorder or have an increased familial risk independent of panic in individual family members of probands with panic disorder.

GENETIC LINKAGE STUDY

Our initial findings of the comorbidity between panic disorder and several medical conditions come from our collaborative genetic linkage study of panic disorder. The criteria for inclusion, including methodology, sampling, and diagnostic criteria, and the rationale for our procedures are detailed in Fyer and Weissman (1999) and are briefly summarized here. Families, whether from clinical or nonclinical settings, were accepted into the genetic linkage study if on initial screening they appeared to have at least three relatives affected with panic disorder in several generations and relatives who were available and willing to participate. All clinical data and final best-estimate diagnoses were obtained blind to family structure or diagnosis and to individual genotype. All willing subjects had blood drawn.

Clinical Assessment

The essential features of the clinical assessment were 1) clinically experienced interviewers; 2) a diagnostic interview based on the Schedule for Affective Disorders and Schizophrenia–Lifetime Version modified for the study of anxiety disorders (Mannuzza et al. 1986) that included major Axis I disorders and detailed information on panic and anxiety disorders; 3) a comparable family history assessment based on the Family Informant Schedule and Criteria (Fyer and Weissman 1999); 4) a detailed narrative case history written by the interviewer that served as a check on the plausibility of the diagnosis, its severity, and comorbidity; and 5) a medical checklist and request for pertinent medical records.

All data collected from interview, family history, narrative summaries, and medical records were considered as provisional, to be used by senior clinicians to arrive at a final best estimate of the diagnosis. Diagnosis information was compiled and blinded for name and family by research assistants, and at least two clinical investigators independently diagnosed each individual based on all available data. Any cases that had a discrepant diagnosis were reviewed at a meeting; additional information was collected if necessary and a consensus diagnosis was made. Subjects were classified into having definite, probable, possible, or any panic disorder unaffected or unknown (Fyer and Weissman 1999).

Flagged Cases

To enable us to identify cases that may have occurred in conjunction with potentially confounding conditions and/or may suggest interesting phenotypes, medical conditions were routinely flagged during the best estimate procedure. Our hypothesis in analyzing the flagged cases was that such cases were clustered in a family, they may constitute a genetically different subtype, and thus we would analyze families with these conditions separately. Flagged cases also could be false-positives or phenocopies, in which case we would classify them as "unknown" in our analysis. Any evidence of MVP, neurological diseases, head injuries, headaches or serious migraines, thyroid conditions, substance use, or any other condition that seemed unusual or possibly relevant was flagged. During the course of completing best estimate diagnoses, we noted numerous cases that involved unusual bladder/kidney problems. We began systematically flagging these cases and reviewed all the previous cases to see whether any cases with bladder or kidney problems had been overlooked.

As we collected these cases based on the literature and our observation, we hypothesized that the unusual bladder/kidney problems, thyroid problems, serious headaches/migraines, and MVP that we were seeing may be part of the same syndrome running in families rather than individuals and that these conditions could be pleiotropic effects—that is, genes producing many different phenotypes (see Hodgkin 1998). We conducted the first analysis of the genetic linkage study in the first 34 multiplex families, comprising 476 relatives in which 19 families had this potential syndrome—that is, at least one family member had a bladder/kidney problem. Any relative with any of these medical conditions was diagnosed as affected (Weissman et al. 2000).

We hypothesized that there may exist a subgroup of panic families with these medical conditions, which, for simplicity, we called the "syndrome." Subsequently we reclassified the families as with or without the "syndrome" and extended the phenotype for analysis to include the medical conditions listed previously. All these classifications were done before the genetic analysis and were made blind to marker data. We then examined our linkage results, looking for significant differences between families with and without the "syndrome" (using several definitions of the "syndrome"—i.e., testing for genetic heterogeneity). When the families with and without bladder/

kidney problems were separated from each other, one marker—D13S779 (ATA26D07)—yielded a lod score of over 3 in the families with bladder/ kidney problems. This score went up to 4.2 in these families when we diagnosed any individual with any one of the "syndrome" conditions as affected. These results were statistically significant even after applying an extremely conservative Bonferroni correction for multiple tests.

The second genome scan we conducted included 587 individuals in 60 multiplex pedigrees (including the original 19 "syndrome" families), segregating panic disorder and bladder/kidney conditions (Hamilton et al. 2003). The chromosome 13 findings were corroborated by multipoint findings and extended our previous results from 19 to 60 families. Several other regions showed elevated scores when one analytic method was used but not the other. These results suggested that there are genes on chromosome 13q that influence susceptibility to a pleiotropic syndrome that includes panic disorder, bladder problems, severe headaches, MVP, and thyroid conditions.

REFINING THE PHENOTYPE

Because kidney/bladder problems provided the highest lod scores, we enlisted a board certified urologist to try to understand what the problems were and to review our case material (see Weissman et al. 2000 for case note description of the bladder problem). This review led to the hypothesis that interstitial cystitis might best describe the kidney/bladder problems (see Weissman et al. 2004 for full description).

Interstitial Cystitis

Interstitial cystitis is a chronic, debilitating bladder syndrome of unknown etiology and no generally accepted treatment (Warren and Keay 2002). There have been several attempts to estimate the prevalence of interstitial cystitis in the United States (Held et al. 1990). The largest, most systematic set of data based on self-report from the National Household Interview study provided a lifetime prevalence of 0.5% after weighting to the U.S. population by age, race, and gender (Jones and Nyberg 1997). Like panic disorder, interstitial cystitis is more commonly found in females but has an older age of onset, with a median age of onset at 40 years (Curham et al. 1999; Simon et al. 1997). The role of genetic susceptibility has not been thoroughly investigated. One small twin study found considerably higher concordance in monozygotic versus dizygotic twins. Five of the eight monozygotic and none of the 26 dizygotic pair twins had confirmed interstitial cystitis (Warren et al. 2001). Findings from a small family study suggest higher rates of interstitial cystitis in the first-degree relative of patients with the syndrome compared with population control subjects (Hanno 1994).

Interstitial cystitis symptom presentation varies but most commonly includes urinary frequency and urgency, nocturia, severe pain on bladder filling (typically relieved with voiding), and sterile urine (Hanno 1994; Hanno et al. 1999). Interstitial cystitis encompasses a major portion of the chronic pelvic pain syndrome (Agarwal et al. 2001; Kusek and Nyberg 2001), which includes a large group of urological patients with bladder and/or pelvic pain, irritative voiding symptoms, and negative urine cultures and cytology tests (Propert et al. 2000). In males it is characterized by impairing clinical symptoms typical of chronic prostatitis (pain on voiding and erectile dysfunction) without evidence of bacteria cultured in the prostatic secretions (Krieger et al. 1999; Ku et al. 2001). A syndrome remarkably analogous to interstitial cystitis called feline interstitial cystitis occurs in domestic cats. Studies of cats and humans suggest central nervous system involvement including subtle abnormalities of the hypothalamic-pituitary-adrenal axis and significant increase in tyrosine hydroxylase immunoreactivity in the locus coeruleus (Buffington et al. 1999; Lutgendorf et al. 2002; Peeker et al. 2000; Westropp et al. 2003).

Currently available treatments for interstitial cystitis are based primarily on observational data and a few clinical trials. Included are cystoscopic hydrodistention of the bladder, amitriptyline, antihistamine (oral hydroxyzine), pentosan polysulfate sodium, and intravesical dimethyl sulfoxide therapy (Parkin et al. 1997; Theoharides and Sant 1997). These treatments may improve symptoms, but there is insufficient information to know whether treatment modifies the long-term course (Rovner et al. 2000). Interstitial cystitis is considered to be a local manifestation of a systemic disease, possibly an autoimmune disorder, but this is controversial. Systematic studies of large samples of patients with interstitial cystitis have found increased rates of autoimmune diseases as well as migraine headaches and hypothyroid disease (Alagiri et al. 1997; Koziol 1994). Recently, the National Institute of Diabetes and Digestive and Kidney Diseases requested research applications in basic cellular, molecular, and genetic studies of interstitial cystitis.

Case–Control Study

We developed a case–control study involving interstitial cystitis patients in collaboration with the Department of Urology at Columbia University

(Weissman et al. 2004). Whereas panic disorder had been well characterized in the genetic linkage study by direct interviews with subjects, the urological problem had been found only by medical history checklists and/or records. We wanted to determine whether interstitial cystitis diagnosed by state-of-the-art urological examinations would yield similar results to the linkage study regarding individual and familial aggregation of the "syndrome" condition. The hypothesis was that patients with interstitial cystitis diagnosed by urodynamic and/or cystoscopy and their first-degree relatives would have increased rates of the "syndrome" condition. These findings would both validate that the bladder problems observed in the linkage study could be interstitial cystitis and would provide further support for the panic syndrome. One hundred forty-six probands (67 with interstitial cystitis and 79 with other urological problems) and 815 first-degree relatives were studied. The information from probands was obtained by direct interview, and the information on first-degree relatives was obtained by family history. We consecutively entered probands from chart lists to avoid selection bias. The interview, family history, and best estimate diagnoses were obtained blind to urological and psychiatric diagnosis in probands. The best estimate diagnoses were made by the same diagnostician in the linkage study, using the same criteria.

We found that the lifetime prevalence of panic disorder was significantly higher (more than fourfold) among patients with interstitial cystitis compared with control subjects. Patients with interstitial cystitis had higher lifetime prevalence of the syndrome, defined as having at least one of the disorders (more than twofold; Table 4–1).

First-degree relatives of probands with interstitial cystitis compared with control subjects were significantly more likely to have panic disorder, thyroid disorder, urological problems, and the "syndrome" (Table 4–2). These results in first-degree relatives did not change substantially when probands with panic disorder were removed from the analysis and when the gender of proband was controlled for in the analysis.

We concluded that the increased frequency of seemingly disparate disorders in patients with interstitial cystitis and their first-degree relatives was consistent with the genetic linkage findings in families with panic disorder. The findings suggested that the bladder problems observed in the linkage study may be interstitial cystitis. The hypothesis that there is a familial, possibly pleiotropic syndrome that includes interstitial cystitis, panic disorder, thyroid disorders, and possibly MVP and chronic headaches/migraine deserves further investigation.

TABLE 4–1. Panic disorder and other "syndrome" conditions in probands with and without interstitial cystitis (IC)

Disorder	Proband is IC-positive (n=67) % (No.)	Proband is IC-negative (n=79) % (No.)	OR	95% CI	P level
Panic disorder	26.9 (18)	7.6 (6)	4.05	1.22, 13.40	0.02
Mitral valve prolapse	33.8 (22)	22.7 (17)	1.88	0.74, 4.80	0.19
Thyroid disorder	17.9 (12)	7.8 (6)	6.13	1.50, 25.10	0.01
Chronic headaches/migraines	28.8 (19)	25.3 (20)	0.63	0.25, 1.62	0.34
"Syndrome disorder"[a]	72.3 (47)	48.7 (37)	2.22	0.89, 5.54	0.09

Note. Odds ratios (ORs) and 95% confidence intervals (CIs) signify the increased likelihood that probands with IC (vs. those without IC) have the disorder listed in the first column, controlling for age and gender. *N* for each disorder outcome was 140–146 due to missing data.

[a]*Syndrome disorder* was defined as the lifetime presence of at least one of the following: panic disorder, mitral valve prolapse, thyroid disorder, or chronic headaches/migraines.

Source. Weissman et al. 2004.

TABLE 4–2. Lifetime disorders in first-degree relatives of probands with and without interstitial cystitis (IC), excluding probands with panic disorder

Disorder in first-degree relatives	Proband is IC-positive (probands, $n=49$; relatives, $n=235$) Rate/100	Proband is IC-negative (probands, $n=73$; relatives, $n=466$) Rate/100	OR	95% CI	P level
Panic disorder[a]	4.0	1.5	3.32	1.19, 9.22	0.02
Mitral valve prolapse	8.3	6.2	1.22	0.55, 2.68	0.62
Thyroid disorder	9.0	3.5	2.89	1.33, 6.28	0.007
Chronic headaches/migraines	8.6	6.7	1.33	0.57, 3.08	0.51
Urological problems[b]	15.2	7.4	2.01	1.04, 3.89	0.04
"Syndrome disorder" (including panic disorder)[c]	38.4	24.1	1.95	1.13, 3.38	0.02

Note. Odds ratios (ORs) and 95% confidence intervals (CIs) signify the increased likelihood of having the disorder for first-degree relatives of probands with (vs. without) IC. Correlation among family members was accounted for by using generalized estimating equations (GEE) with an exchangeable correlation matrix. Age and gender of relatives and gender of proband were controlled in the GEE analyses. For each disorder, 29 (4.1%) of the 701 relatives were excluded from the analysis because of unknown age and/or gender, and an additional number (range, 3–89 [0.4%–12.7%]) were excluded because their disorder status could not be ascertained.

[a]Panic disorder in first-degree relatives was broadly defined and included panic attack.
[b]Bladder or kidney problem (excluding bladder cancer).
[c]*Syndrome disorder* was defined as the lifetime presence of at least one of the following: panic disorder, mitral valve prolapse, thyroid disorder, or chronic headaches/migraines.

Source. Weissman et al. 2004.

CONCLUSION

We have attempted to present an approach to using epidemiological and clinical observation, including medical and psychiatric conditions, for finding possible new phenotypes. Findings on the increased risk of the "syndrome" in patients with interstitial cystitis and their relatives is consistent with the findings of the genetic linkage study but are still quite tentative. A family history study alone cannot validate a genetic syndrome or confirm pleiotropy. However, several novel avenues are suggested for further understanding the relationship between panic disorder and interstitial cystitis and for examining the other disorders that are part of the "syndrome."

Potential clinical implications of this finding include identification of new pharmacological interventions for interstitial cystitis targeting specific neurotransmitter receptors (Steers 2001a, 2001b). Serotonin reuptake blockers, which are effective in panic disorder, might inhibit serotonergic activation of mast cells and modulate exaggerated bladder activity through downregulation of central postsynaptic serotonin receptors (Holsboer 1999; Theoharides 2001).

Similar studies attempting to characterize the other hypothesized medical conditions we noted, such as MVP, thyroid, and migraines, and their relationship to panic disorder could be undertaken in cardiac, endocrinological, and neurological clinics using a similar case–control design. Other disorders such as irritable bowel syndrome, chronic fatigue syndrome, celiac disease, and fibromyalgia may be part of the syndrome (Carta et al. 2002; Clauw et al. 1997; Epstein et al. 1999; Russo 2003).

A family interview and medical examination study, as contrasted with the less expensive but much less definitive family history study we undertook, would also be useful. Moreover, we only assessed first-degree relatives in the case–control study, whereas the genetic linkage study included multiplex families spanning several generations with the syndrome. Thus, disorders in the extended family likely have been missed by our including only first-degree relatives. Pleiotropy would not require that all elements of the expression of the phenotype be present in an individual.

The final message we obtained from this phenotype hunt is that "genes do not divide at the neck." Genes are indifferent to professional specialties. Genetic studies of psychiatric disorders should routinely include assessments of medical disorders, and this is beginning to occur (Hudson et al. 2003). Genetic studies of medical conditions are not immune to this problem. Genetic studies of interstitial cystitis, MVP, thyroid, and migraine also might well include assessment of panic disorder and other psychiatric conditions.

REFERENCES

Agarwal M, O'Reilly PH, Dixon RA: Interstitial cystitis: a time for revision of name and diagnostic criteria in the new millennium? BJU Int 88:348–350, 2001

Alagiri M, Chottiner S, Ratner V, et al: Interstitial cystitis: unexplained associations with other chronic disease and pain syndromes. Urology 49 (suppl):52–57, 1997

Buffington CA, Chew DJ, Woodworth BE: Feline interstitial cystitis. J Am Vet Med Assoc 215:682–687, 1999

Carta MG, Hardoy MC, Boi MF, et al: Association between panic disorder, major depressive disorder and celiac disease: a possible role of thyroid autoimmunity. J Psychosom Res 53:789–793, 2002

Clauw DJ, Schmidt M, Radulovic D, et al: The relationship between fibromyalgia and interstitial cystitis. J Psychiatr Res 31:125–131, 1997

Coryell W: Hypersensitivity to carbon dioxide as disease-specific trait marker. Biol Psychiatry 41:259–263, 1997

Crowe RR, Pauls DL, Slymen DJ, et al: A family study of anxiety neurosis. Morbidity risk in families of patients with and without mitral valve prolapse. Arch Gen Psychiatry 37:77–79, 1980

Crowe RR, Gaffney G, Kerber R: Panic attacks in families with mitral valve prolapse. J Affect Disord 4:121–125, 1982

Curham GC, Speizer FE, Hunter DJ, et al: Epidemiology of interstitial cystitis: a population based study. J Urol 161:549–552, 1999

Devinsky O, Sato S, Theodore WH, et al: Fear episodes due to limbic seizures with normal ictal scalp EEG: a subdural electrographic study. J Clin Psychiatry 50:28–30, 1989

Edlund MJ, Swann AC, Clothier J: Patients with panic attacks and abnormal EEG results. Am J Psychiatry 144:508–509, 1987

Epstein SA, Kay G, Clauw D, et al: Psychiatric disorders in patients with fibromyalgia: a multicenter investigation. Psychosomatics 40:57–63, 1999

Fyer AJ, Weissman MM: Genetic linkage study of panic: clinical methodology and description of pedigrees. Am J Med Genet 88:173–181, 1999

Gorman JM, Goetz RR, Fyer M, et al: The mitral valve prolapse–panic disorder connection. Psychosom Med 50:114–122, 1988

Gorman JM, Browne ST, Papp LA, et al: Effects of antipanic treatment on response to carbon dioxide. Biol Psychiatry 42:982–991, 1997

Gorman JM, Kent JM, Sullivan GM, et al: Neuroanatomical hypothesis of panic disorder, revised. Am J Psychiatry 157:493–505, 2000

Gräsbeck A, Rorsman B, Hagnell O, et al: Mortality of anxiety syndrome in a normal population: the epidemiology of anxiety and depressive syndromes (V). Neuropsychobiology 33:118–126, 1996

Hamilton SP, Fyer AJ, Durner M, et al: Further genetic evidence for a panic disorder syndrome mapping to chromosome 13q. Proc Natl Acad Sci 100:2550–2555, 2003

Hanno PM: Diagnosis of interstitial cystitis. Urol Clin North Am 21:63–66, 1994

Hanno PM, Landis JR, Matthews-Cook Y, et al: The diagnosis of interstitial cystitis revisited: lessons learned from the National Institutes of Health Interstitial Cystitis Database study. J Urol 161:553–557, 1999

Held PJ, Hanno PM, Wein AJ, et al: Epidemiology of interstitial cystitis, in Interstitial Cystitis. Edited by Hanno PM, Staskin DR, Krane RJ, et al. London, Springer-Verlag, 1990, pp 29–48

Heninger GR: Catecholamines and pathogenesis in panic disorder (commentary). Arch Gen Psychiatry 55:522–523, 1998

Hettema JM, Neale MC, Kendler KS: A review and meta-analysis of the genetic epidemiology of anxiety disorders. Am J Psychiatry 158:1568–78, 2001

Hodgkin J: Seven types of pleiotropy. Int J Dev Biol 42:501–505, 1998

Holsboer F: The rationale for corticotropin-releasing hormone receptor (CRH-R) antagonists to treat depression and anxiety. J Psychiatr Res 33:181–214, 1999

Hudson JI, Mangweth B, Pope HG, et al: Family study of affective spectrum disorder. Arch Gen Psychiatry 60:170–177, 2003

Jones CA, Nyberg L: Epidemiology of interstitial cystitis. Urology 9 (suppl):2–9, 1997

Knowles AJ, Weissman MM: Panic disorder and agoraphobia: psychiatric genetics, in Review of Psychiatry, Vol. 14. Edited by Oldham JM, Riba M. Washington, DC, American Psychiatric Press, 1995, pp 383–404

Koziol JA: Epidemiology of interstitial cystitis. Urol Clin North Am 21:7–20, 1994

Krieger JN, Nyberg L Jr, Nickel JC: NIH consensus definition and classification of prostatitis. JAMA 282:236–237, 1999

Ku JH, Kim ME, Lee NK, et al: The prevalence of chronic prostatitis-like symptoms in young men: a community-based survey. Urol Res 29:108–112, 2001

Kusek JW, Nyberg LM: The epidemiology of interstitial cystitis: is it time to expand our definition? Urology 57 (suppl):95–99, 2001

Lutgendorf SK, Kreder KJ, Rothrock NE, et al: Diurnal cortisol variations and symptoms in patients with interstitial cystitis. J Urol 167:1338–1343, 2002

Lydiard R, Greenwald S, Weissman MM, et al: Panic disorder and gastrointestinal symptoms: findings from the NIMH Epidemiologic Catchment Area Project. Am J Psychiatry 151:64–70, 1994

Mannuzza S, Fyer AJ, Klein DF, et al: Schedule for Affective Disorders and Schizophrenia—Lifetime Version modified for the study of anxiety disorders (SADS-LA): rationale and conceptual development. J Psychiatr Res 20:317–325, 1986

Maser JD, Cloninger RC (eds): Comorbidity of Mood, Anxiety Disorders. Washington, DC, American Psychiatric Press, 1990

Miniati M, Mauri M, Dell'Osso L, et al: Panic-agoraphobic spectrum and cardiovascular disease. CNS Spectrums 3:58–62, 1998

Neugebauer R, Weissman MM, Ouellette R, et al: Comorbidity of panic disorder and seizures: affinity or artifact? J Anxiety Disord 7:21–35, 1993

Parkin J, Shea C, Sant GR: Intravesical dimethyl sulfoxide (DMSO) for interstitial cystitis: a practical approach. Urology 49(suppl):105–107, 1997

Peeker R, Aldenborg F, Dahlstrom A, et al: Increased tyrosine hydroxylase immunoreactivity in bladder tissue from patients with classic and nonulcer interstitial cystitis. J Urol 163:1112–1115, 2000

Perna G, Cocchi S, Bertani A, et al: Sensitivity to 35% CO_2 in healthy first-degree relatives of patients with panic disorder. Am J Psychiatry 152:623–625, 1995

Perna G, Bertani A, Caldirola D, et al: Family history of panic disorder and hypersensitivity to CO_2 in patients with panic disorder. Am J Psychiatry 153:1060–1064, 1996

Propert KJ, Schaeffer AJ, Brensinger CM, et al: A prospective study of interstitial cystitis: results of longitudinal follow-up of the Interstitial Cystitis Data Base cohort. J Urol 163:1434–1439, 2000

Rovner E, Propert KJ, Brensinger C, et al: Treatments used in women with interstitial cystitis: the Interstitial Cystitis Data Base (ICDB) Study experience. Urology 56:940–945, 2000

Russo E: A new approach to autoimmune diseases. The Scientist 5:30–32, 2003

Simon LJ, Landis JR, Erickson DR, et al: The interstitial cystitis data base study: concepts and preliminary baseline descriptive statistics. Urology 49 (suppl):64–75, 1997

Steers WD: Interstitial cystitis: past and future. Urology 57 (suppl):101–102, 2001a

Steers W: Potential targets in the treatment of urinary incontinence. Rev Urol 3 (suppl):S19–S26, 2001b

Stewart W, Breslau N, Keck PE: Comorbidity of migraine and panic disorder. Neurology 44(suppl):S23–S27, 1994

Sullivan GM, Kent JM, Kleber M, et al: Effects of hyperventilation on heart rate and QT variability in panic disorder pre- and post-treatment. Psychiatr Res 125:29–39, 2004

Theoharides TC, Sant GR: Hydroxyzine therapy for interstitial cystitis. Urology 49 (suppl):108–110, 1997

Theoharides TC, Sant GR: New agents for the medical treatment of interstitial cystitis. Exp Opin Investig Drugs 10:521–526, 2001

Vieland VJ, Hodge SE, Lish JD, et al: Segregation analysis of panic disorder. Psychiatr Genet 3:63–71, 1993

Vieland VJ, Goodman DW, Chapman T, et al: A new segregation analysis of panic disorder. Am J Med Genet 67:147–153, 1996

Warren JW, Keay SK: Interstitial cystitis. Curr Opin Urol 12:69–74, 2002

Warren JW, Keay SK, Meyers D, et al: Concordance of interstitial cystitis in monozygotic and dizygotic twin pairs. Urology 57 (suppl):22–25, 2001

Weilburg JB, Bear DM, Sachs G: Three patients with concomitant panic attacks and seizure disorder: possible clues to the neurology of anxiety. Am J Psychiatry 144:1053–1056, 1987

Weissman MM: Family genetic studies of panic disorder. J Psychiatr Res 27:69–78, 1993

Weissman MM, Markowitz J, Ouellette R, et al: Panic disorder and cardiovascular/cerebrovascular problems: results from a community survey. Am J Psychiatry 147:1504–1508, 1990

Weissman MM, Bland RC, Canino GJ, et al: The cross national epidemiology of panic disorder. Arch Gen Psychiatry 54:305–309, 1997

Weissman MM, Fyer AJ, Haghighi F, et al: Potential panic disorder syndrome: clinical and genetic linkage evidence. Am J Med Genet 96:24–35, 2000

Weissman MM, Gross R, Fyer AJ, et al: Interstitial cystitis and panic disorder: a potential genetic syndrome. Arch Gen Psychiatry 61:273–279, 2004

Westropp JL, Welk KA, Buffington CAT: Small adrenal glands in cats with feline interstitial cystitis. J Urol 170:2494–2497, 2003

Wilkinson DJC, Thompson JM, Lambert GW, et al: Sympathetic activity in patients with panic disorder at rest under laboratory mental stress and during panic attacks. Arch Gen Psychiatry 55:511–520, 1998

Fundamental Social Causes

The Ascendancy of Social Factors as Determinants of Distributions of Mental Illnesses in Populations

Bruce G. Link, Ph.D.

Jo C. Phelan, Ph.D.

IN THE PUBLICATION of his 1988 award-winning address to the American Psychopathological Association, Leonard Heston (1988) provided an assessment of the current status of environmentally oriented research and a prescription to address the ills he found in that research. His assessment went like this: "The facts make it clear that searches for specific environmental factors external to the body juices are likely to prove dead ends. Such research has been done too long and too intensely with no result" (p. 212). His prescription for extricating the field from this very undesirable situation was simple—a redistribution of resources to "hardball biology" (p. 212).

Of course, Heston was absolutely correct in his observation that there had been a long-standing fascination with the role of the environment in shaping rates of psychopathology. The classic texts that began the field of psychiatric epidemiology focused on social and economic adversity. Hollingshead and Redlich's (1958) *Social Class and Mental Illness* not only drew attention to the strong connection between socioeconomic status (SES) and treated rates of mental illness but also documented dramatic differences in the quality of treatment that people of different socioeconomic circumstances encountered. In the concluding chapter ("Sociologists' Sightlines") of the classic Midtown Manhattan Study, Srole et al. (1962) sought to explain distributions of psychopathology by social factors through three interrelated processes: 1) the poverty complex, 2) the role-discontinuity predicament, and 3) the stigmatize-rejection mechanism. Of course, Alexander Leighton (1959) focused our attention on social disorganization and the stresses and strains it imposed on individual goal-striving in the classic Stirling County Study. In the current era, the basic findings that motivated this earlier generation are still with us. For example, Kessler et al. (1994) found monotonic associations between educational attainment and several psychiatric disorders. Odds ratios for people with fewer than 12 years of education as compared with people with 16 or more are 1.79 for any affective disorder, 2.10 for any substance abuse, and 3.79 for having three or more disorders of any kind. Findings like these (Kohn et al. 1998) have continued to motivate some of us who have sought progress in addressing such classic questions as the social causation–social selection issue (Dohrenwend et al. 1992) and the connection between stressful circumstances and psychopathology (Dohrenwend 1998). In his book *Adversity, Stress and Psychopathology*, which was based on papers presented at the American Psychopathological Association, Dohrenwend concatenated evidence concerning environmental adversity in such a way as to challenge designations such as "dead end" and "with no result."

For the time being, however, we intend to leave this important debate to construct a different theory about the prominence of social factors in health and mental health. To do so we shift our focus from the mental disorders to other disorders and broaden our scope of vision to include epidemiological trends across decades. We do so to gain perspective; then we bring that perspective back to the mental disorders and to the importance of social factors in the onset and course of mental illnesses. We begin with this prediction: no matter what factors happen to be most important in generating associations between SES and mental illnesses at present, social causation factors will predominate in the time ahead. This depends on two conditions: 1) that we develop the capacity to reduce the prevalence of mental disorders through prevention or treatment and 2) that we distribute the benefits of that newfound capacity unequally such that people with more knowledge, money, power, prestige, and beneficial social connections benefit more than people who have fewer of these resources. Our proposition contains an intended irony. It says that even if Heston's prescription for a dramatic redistribution of resources to hard ball biology is fully implemented, and even if that redistribution brings the great advances it claims to herald, the importance of social factors will be ascendant in the long run. To the extent that new biological knowledge allows control over the incidence and course of mental illnesses, people with more resources will be better able to benefit from this newfound capacity, and thus social factors will dominate as causes. A successful biology will construct the fundamental importance of social factors. The evidence supporting this line of reasoning begins with the strong and relatively consistent association between SES and the onset and outcome of physical illness.

HEALTH DISPARITIES IN PHYSICAL ILLNESS BY SOCIOECONOMIC STATUS AND RACE

There exists a well-established and extremely robust association linking both morbidity and mortality to educational attainment, occupational standing, and income (Antonovsky 1967; Kunst et al. 1998; Sorlie et al. 1995). This association was present in the early nineteenth century in Mulhouse, France; in Rhode Island in 1865; in Chicago in the 1930s (see Antonovsky 1967); and in Europe and the United States today (Kunst et al. 1998; Lantz et al. 1998; Sorlie et al. 1995). Figure 5–1 provides adjusted death rates per 100,000 people age 25–64 in the United States in 2001 by educational status. For both men and women, adjusted death rates are vastly higher in people with fewer than 12 years of education compared with people with 13 years or more. Life expectancy for African Americans has been dramatically lower than for whites ever since such data became available in the United States. As Figure 5–2 shows, these disparities are with us today with all-cause age-adjusted death rates being dramatically higher for blacks than for whites. What explains the persistence of these disparities? Why should SES and race/ethnicity have such enduring and widespread associations with mortality?

Broadly speaking, two sorts of explanations have been offered and debated. Social causation explanations blame the adversity or stress associated with lower SES. Social selection explanations see genetic vulnerability as leading to illness and disability that impairs individuals' ability to attain socioeconomic resources. A slightly different selection explanation sees genes as strong influences on factors such as intelligence or on personality dimensions such as conscientiousness that in turn determine both health and SES.

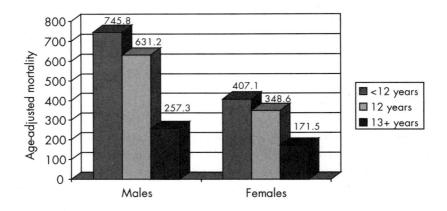

FIGURE 5–1. All-cause age-adjusted death rates per 100,000 people ages 25–64 years, by education: 2001.

Source. Health United States 2003, U.S. Department of Health and Human Services, National Center for Health Statistics.

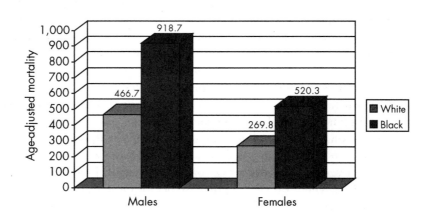

FIGURE 5–2. All-cause age-adjusted death rates per 100,000 people ages 25–64 years, by race: 1998.

Source. Health United States 2003, U.S. Department of Health and Human Services, National Center for Health Statistics.

This is a long-standing debate that we believe has been dramatically altered with regard to physical illness by changing circumstances. In order to construct an explanation that fits these circumstances we turn attention to evidence of trends in the improvement in health over the past half-century.

THE RELEVANCE OF IMPROVING HEALTH

Figure 5–3 shows a dramatic rise in life expectancy at birth from only 47 years in 1900 to 77 years in 2000. For some of us, this dramatic change occurred roughly within the relatively short time span from when our parents were born to when our children were born. Although some large part of this improvement is due to dramatic declines in infant mortality, it is also true that life expectancy has increased for people who are much older. For example, the average man turning 65 in 2000 can expect to live almost a year longer than the average man turning 65 in 1990. This is a remarkable change in a very short period of time. These improvements apply to many, many causes of death, including some of the major killers of our time. Age-adjusted death rates per 100,000 people due to heart disease have plummeted from 587 in 1950 to 258 in 2000. For stroke the figures are equally dramatic, with rates falling from 181 per 100,000 in 1950 to 61 in 2000. For all cancers combined, age-adjusted rates rose through 1990 but since then have begun to drop significantly. For infectious diseases such as influenza or pneumonia, age-adjusted death rates have dropped from 48 per 100,000 in 1950 to 24 in 2000.

What is driving these dramatic improvements in health? Clearly some very powerful processes are at work and having a remarkably strong impact on population health. Whatever these powerful processes are, is it not possible that they have some relevance for explaining health disparities by SES and race? If we seriously consider such a possibility, we can return to the factors that were the centerpieces of previous explanations for health disparities and ask whether they are the same as those driving improvements in population health. Let us begin with genetic factors that lie behind some forms of selection explanations for health disparities. Genes cannot have changed so rapidly and in such a uniformly positive direction as to have created the enormous improvements in population health that we just documented. Moreover, if one considers the relevance of traits that might be influenced by genes, such as intelligence or conscientiousness, one would have to posit enormous and implausible gains in these traits over the past 50–100 years. When we turn to the mainstay of social causation explanations for disparities, we encounter similar problems. One would have to

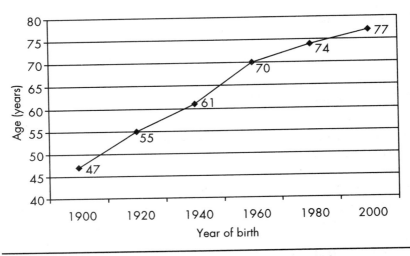

FIGURE 5–3.   U.S. life expectancy at birth: 1900–2000.
Source.   Health United States 2003, U.S. Department of Health and Human Services, National Center for Health Statistics.

posit that the prevalence of stress or adversity has declined dramatically over the past several decades and that this decline had a powerful impact on illnesses as diverse as heart disease, flu, and—since 1990—all cancers combined. It seems clear that whatever is driving improvements in population health, it is not coterminous with the factors that have explained health disparities by SES and race.

So what is driving the dramatic improvements in population health? Of course it is not just one, but *many* things. For example, recent declines in age-adjusted rates of lung cancer are probably influenced by the lagged effects of declines in smoking rates in earlier decades. The rapid decline in mortality due to HIV and AIDS in the United States is probably related to the new antiretroviral drugs that were developed and disseminated in the late 1990s. The precipitous decline in mortality due to Hodgkin's disease since the 1960s is probably due to the development of chemotherapy regimens that are able to cure the disease. In addition, there are screenings for various diseases; public health efforts to increase consumption of fruits and vegetables, promote exercise, and eradicate smoking; and other measures such as pollution control, flu shots, seat belts, cholesterol drugs, angioplasty, and so on. Thus the improvement in population health is likely due to different factors for different diseases, yet the confluence of all these things has had an enormously positive impact on population health. Over the past century human beings have dramatically increased their capacity to control disease and death.

THE CORE PROPOSITION: CONTROLLING DISEASE AND CREATING DISPARITIES

Our core proposition is thus: that it is our enormously expanded capacity to control disease and death, in combination with existing social and economic inequality, that creates health disparities according to race and SES. This occurs because the benefits of our newfound capacity to control disease and death are distributed according to resources of knowledge, money, power, prestige, and beneficial social connections. People who are advantaged with respect to such resources thus benefit more and experience lower death rates than do those who are not so advantaged. Disparities are the result.

This explanation is a central part of the theory of fundamental social causes. Because our proposition derives from that theory we briefly develop a broader rationale for the theory and then turn to evidence that bears on our core proposition.

FUNDAMENTAL SOCIAL CAUSES OF HEALTH DISPARITIES

The fundamental social causes explanation begins with the graded relationship between indicators of SES and health (Link and Phelan 1995, 1996, 2000). Clearly, biological mechanisms must be involved in the SES–disease association. Just as clearly, other mechanisms involving behaviors and environmental exposures must also be present—disease does not flow directly from income, educational, or occupational status into the body. Nevertheless, the effect of SES on mortality cannot be understood by focusing solely on the mechanisms that happen to link the two at any particular time.

Imagine a causal model with SES as the distal factor linked to death by more proximal risk factors. If the proximal risk factors are eliminated, we would expect the SES–mortality association to disappear. On the contrary, however, there have been several important instances in which major proximal risk factors were eliminated while SES disparities in mortality persisted. Consider the situation in Europe and the United States in the nineteenth century, when major causes of death included diseases such as cholera, diphtheria, measles, smallpox, and tuberculosis and the principal risk factors were poor sanitation, contaminated water, and substandard and crowded living conditions. People of lower SES were more exposed to these conditions and experienced much higher death rates as a consequence (Chapin 1924; Villerme 1840). Sanitation was vastly improved, water systems were made safe, housing conditions dramatically improved, and effective vaccines were developed, and people now rarely die of cholera, diphtheria, measles, small pox, or tuberculosis in the United States and western Europe. One might have thought that the association between SES and disease would have disappeared because the mechanisms that linked the two were eliminated or blocked. Yet new risk factors (such as chemical pollutants) arose, new knowledge about risk factors (such as smoking) emerged, and new treatment technologies (such as medicines that reduce cholesterol) were developed, and those who commanded the most resources were best able to avoid the risks and take advantage of the protective factors, resulting in the emergence of an SES gradient in these factors. The list of circumstances shaped by SES-related resources is enormously long and not confined to the standard behavioral risk factors typically measured in risk-factor epidemiology (e.g., smoking, exercise, diet). For example, Luftey and Freese (in press) used an ethnographic approach to study the management of diabetes once it has developed and showed how the organization of clinics (one provider versus rotating providers), the physician expectations of patient capacity to use the newest diabetes control techniques, the patients' access to insurance, and many other circumstances resulted, on average, in an advantaged circumstance for patients with better resources. As the authors pointed out, it is when circumstances like these are reproduced over many other situations (e.g., ones related to health behaviors, preventive health care, and the full range of existing diseases) that the robust association between SES-related resources and health emerges. As new discoveries expand our ability to control disease processes, additional items will be added to the list of health-enhancing circumstances, and according to our theory, people who command more resources will, on average, be advantaged in gaining access to and benefiting from these discoveries. Thus, the association between SES and disease is reproduced dynamically through an evolving and complex set of intervening mechanisms that change with time and differ from place to place.

According to the fundamental-cause idea, this dynamic reproduction of the association between SES and disease occurs because flexible resources of knowledge, money, power, prestige, and beneficial social connections allow the association to be reproduced in widely varying circumstances and at very different times. Flexible resources are important in at least two ways. First, resources directly shape individual health behaviors by influencing whether people know about, have access to, can afford, and are supported in their efforts to engage in health-enhancing behaviors. Second, resources shape access to broad contexts such as neighborhoods, occupations, and social networks that vary dramatically in associated profiles of risk and protective factors. Housing that poor people can afford is more likely to be located near noise, pollution, and noxious social conditions; blue-collar occupations tend to be more dangerous than white-collar occupations; and high-status jobs are more likely to include health care as a benefit. Thus, the processes implied by the fundamental-cause perspective operate at both individual and contextual levels.

EVIDENCE FOR THE FUNDAMENTAL SOCIAL CAUSES HYPOTHESIS

Test #1: Socioeconomic Associations With More- and Less-Preventable Causes of Death

We say that SES disparities arise because people of higher SES use flexible resources to avoid risks and adopt protective strategies. It follows that the SES gradient should be more pronounced for diseases we can do something about—those for which there are known and modifiable risk and protective factors. Phelan et al. (2004) constructed a test of the theory of fundamental causes by identifying situations in which it is difficult to use resources to prolong life—when even the richest or most powerful person on earth cannot use resources to escape death. Such situations exist when one considers death from diseases that we do not yet know how to prevent or treat. If the use of resources is critical in prolonging life, then when resources associated with higher status are useless, high SES should confer little advantage, and the usually robust SES–mortality association should be reduced.

Phelan et al. (2004) tested this prediction using the National Longitudinal Mortality Study and ratings they developed to measure the preventability of death from specific causes. The National Longitudinal Mortality Study (Sorlie et al. 1995) is a large, prospective study that uses combined samples of selected current population surveys that are then linked to the National Death Index to determine occurrences and causes of death in a follow-up period of approximately 9 years. Reliable ratings (intraclass correlation 0.85) of the preventability of death were made by two physician-epidemiologists. Causes were categorized into high-preventability and low-preventability groups, with common high-preventability causes being cerebrovascular diseases; chronic obstructive pulmonary disease; ischemic heart disease; malignant neoplasm of the trachea, bronchus, and lung; and pneumonia and influenza and common low-preventability causes being arrhythmias and malignant neoplasms of the pancreas, female breast, and prostate. Gradients according to SES indicators of education and income were then examined separately for high- and low-preventability causes. Consistent with predictions derived from the fundamental-cause theory, Phelan et al. (2004) found that the SES–mortality association is significantly stronger for highly preventable causes of death than for less preventable causes of death. For example, for individuals between 45 and 64 years of age, the relative risk of death associated with a difference between an eighth-grade education and more than a college education is 2.00 for high-preventability causes as opposed to 1.21 for low-preventability causes. Similarly, the relative risk of death associated with having an income less than $5,000 compared with having one of more than $50,000 in the same age group is 2.81 for high-preventability causes and 1.86 for low-preventability causes.

Test #2: Time Trends in Socioeconomic Status and Race Disparities in Mortality

If our core proposition is true, we should find that disparities according to SES and race emerge when new health-enhancing information or technology is obtained. Examples of diseases for which death has become dramatically more preventable include heart disease, Hodgkin's disease, lung cancer, and colon cancer. On the other hand, if death from a disease remains difficult or impossible to prevent, as it is for brain and ovarian cancer, disparities will not change dramatically with time.

Consider first the mortality trends for low-preventability diseases. Figure 5–4 presents age-adjusted death rates for brain cancer per 100,000 men in the United States between 1950 and 1999. Consistent with the idea that we have not yet learned how to prevent death from this disease, the death rates remain steady or even climb slightly with time. Death rates for blacks are lower than those for whites, and the difference remains relatively constant through time. Age-adjusted death rates for females are lower than those for males, but the picture through time and the difference between blacks and whites are very similar. Figure 5–5 shows age-adjusted death rates for ovarian cancer. Again, consistent with the idea that we have not yet learned how to prevent death from this disease, age-adjusted death rates remain relatively constant through time, as do the modestly lower rates experienced by blacks as compared to whites.

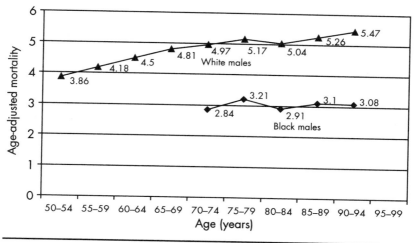

FIGURE 5–4. Brain cancer age-adjusted death rates per 100,000 males: 1950–1999.

Source. U.S. Department of Health and Human Services, Centers for Disease Control and Prevention, National Center for Health Statistics Office of Analysis, Epidemiology, and Health Promotion Compressed Mortality File (CMF) compiled from CMF 1968–88, Series 20, No. 2A 2000, CMF 1989–98, Series 20, No. 2F 2003.

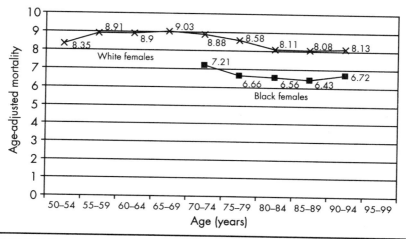

FIGURE 5–5. Ovarian cancer age-adjusted death rates per 100,000 females: 1950–1999.

Source. U.S. Department of Health and Human Services, Centers for Disease Control and Prevention, National Center for Health Statistics Office of Analysis, Epidemiology, and Health Promotion Compressed Mortality File (CMF) compiled from CMF 1968–88, Series 20, No. 2A 2000, CMF 1989–98, Series 20, No. 2F 2003.

Consider next some examples of diseases for which great strides have been made in prevention and treatment. In order to capture the enormous changes that have taken place since the 1950s in a disease such as heart disease, it is instructive to imagine oneself reflecting on the evidence available at that time. This can be achieved by returning to the work of one of the most prominent cardiovascular disease epidemiologists of the latter half of the twentieth century, who was just beginning his career in the early 1960s. Writing in 1964, Leonard Syme characterized the descriptive epidemiology of heart disease by indicating that the disease occurs "far more frequently among whites than Negroes" and that "there seems to be little evidence of a systematic relationship between social class and coronary disease except perhaps in England where the rate appears to increase with socioeconomic status" (Syme 1964, p. 81). Consistent with the rates in England, Syme's nicely executed case control study of heart disease in North Dakota revealed a higher risk in white-collar as opposed to blue-collar or farm workers. Figure 5–6 tells part of the story of what has happened since Syme wrote in the early 1960s. First, consistent with our learning to prevent death from this disease, age-adjusted rates clearly declined rapidly between 1950 and 2000. Second, whereas rates of death for blacks and whites were shown to be quite similar in 1950, disparities favoring whites over blacks emerged over time. At present, death rates due to heart disease are much higher in individuals with lower levels of education. Together the evidence is consistent with the idea that when we develop the wherewithal to address a disease, groups that are relatively more resource rich (whites, people with higher levels of education) and less likely to experience discrimination benefit more fully from that knowledge.

Monitoring mortality rates by SES is problematic because no indicators of status were identified on death certificates until recently. To allow some assessment of trends by SES over time, Singh and colleagues (2002a) employed principal components analysis to develop socioeconomic scores from 1990 census data for every county in the United States. The scores were based on 11 variables measuring county-level SES. Although all 11 variables loaded on one component, the three most important variables in defining that component were median family income, family poverty rate, and the percentage of the population with more than 12 years of education. Singh et al. (2002b) examined the stability of the county socioeconomic measure using data from the 1970 and 1980 census and found them to be quite stable.

Using quintiles derived from the socioeconomic scores, Singh's group found dramatic evidence of changing associations between SES and two major cancer killers, lung cancer and colon cancer. Figure 5–6 shows age-

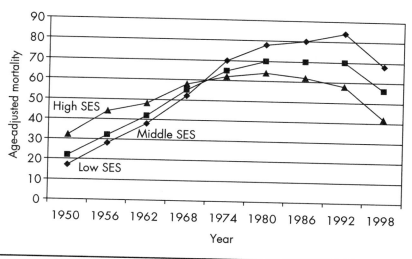

FIGURE 5–6. Age-adjusted lung cancer mortality in men ages 25–64 years between 1950 and 1998, by socioeconomic status (SES) of county of residence.

Source. Adapted from Singh et al. 2002b.

adjusted lung cancer rates for three quintiles (highest, middle, and lowest) for men ages 25–64 years. As the figure shows, rates were substantially higher in the highest-SES counties in 1950. Once evidence about the harmful effects of smoking emerged in the late 1950s and early 1960s, mortality in the highest-SES counties began to flatten out, whereas rates in the poorest counties continued to rise. By 1998 the association between county SES and lung cancer reversed completely, such that the highest rates were now in the lowest-SES counties. The situation for women is not as dramatic as for men, but a more modest version of the same reversal seems to be under way—women from high-SES counties had the highest rates of lung cancer mortality until the late 1980s but by 1998 had the lowest rates.

Figure 5–7 shows age-adjusted mortality rates due to colon cancer in women (ages 25–64 years) in three quintiles (highest, middle, and lowest). As the figure shows, women living in low-SES counties enjoyed dramatically lower rates of colon cancer mortality in 1950. As our capacity to prevent death from this disease increased in the ensuing decades, women in high-SES counties experienced a dramatic decline in death rates, whereas women in low-SES counties did not. A similar circumstance occurred among men, such that at the current time overall rates are modestly higher in low-SES counties than in high-SES counties.

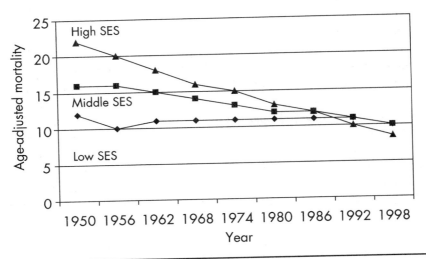

FIGURE 5–7. Age-adjusted colon cancer mortality in women ages 25–64 years between 1950 and 1998, by socioeconomic status (SES) of county of residence.

Source. Adapted from Singh et al. 2002b.

CONCLUSIONS CONCERNING THE TESTS

When considered together, these trends offer substantial support for our second test of the fundamental-cause theory. For two diseases for which there is no effective prevention or cure—brain cancer and ovarian cancer—we find no indication that disparities by race or SES have emerged over time. In sharp contrast, evidence concerning several other major killers indicates that disparities arose when new knowledge and technology gave us the capacity to prevent death from these diseases. People from groups that are relatively resource rich (whites and people from high-SES counties) were more likely to benefit from this newfound capacity, thereby creating disparities in the current era. To the extent that disparities are created in this manner, explanations must take account of our enormously expanded capacity to control disease and death *and* they must focus on who benefits from that capacity.

Clearly, this fundamental-cause explanation and the data that support it have implications for other theories that seek to explain disparities. Critically, any explanation that posits a factor that is constant over time runs into difficulties in accounting for disparities that change with time. Some examples of such explanations are genetic factors, relative deprivation, or the stress associated with low-SES position. If, for example, one were to posit a genetic basis for current racial disparities in coronary artery disease, one would have to explain why the same gene or set of genetic factors failed to produce disparities in earlier eras. Similarly, if relative deprivation and the anger, resentment, and envy associated with being lower in the social hierarchy explains the currently higher rates of heart disease in lower-SES persons, why did the same processes not operate in the past? One would have imagined that people lower in the hierarchy in 1950 would have experienced the same anger, resentment, and envy with the same pathological consequences. If it is the stress associated with a relatively low position that produces race and SES disparities in heart disease or colon cancer now, why did those same stress processes not produce the same disparities in earlier era? None of these explanations accounts for changes in disparities over time.

In order to account for disparities by race and SES we need to recognize the tremendous improvement in population health that has occurred over the past several decades, and we need to ask who benefits from that improvement. Thus the critical question for understanding disparities is: "Who gets what in terms of risk and protective factors, and why do they get it?" The fundamental-cause explanation focuses attention on flexible resources of knowledge, money, power, prestige, and beneficial social connections that can be used to harness advantages and avoid disadvantages in changing circumstances.

IMPLICATIONS FOR DISPARITIES IN THE DISTRIBUTION OF PSYCHIATRIC DISORDERS

As with the physical illnesses, there are strong inverse gradients between SES and many mental illnesses. However, from the perspective put forward here, this is where the similarity ends. Although age-adjusted mortality rates have declined dramatically, and people are now experiencing many more years of life free from physical disability, the same sort of sea change has not occurred for the mental illnesses. We have made tremendous strides in the treatment of mental illnesses, but our current ability to prevent or cure at least the most common ones has not led to large declines in prevalence that we can detect with the best designs and methods available to us. Indeed, the best evidence from true prevalence studies finds current rates to be very high. Moreover, evidence about secular changes, although subject to substantial debate, finds rates of depression to be either higher in more recent cohorts or at least no different than in the older cohorts that preceded them (Klerman 1989; Murphy et al. 2000). It follows that whatever is causing any SES or race disparities that exist at the current time is something other than our capacity to decrease the prevalence of these illnesses and the maldistribution of that capacity in the population.

It is just a matter of time until this situation changes. Unless the massive national investment in neurobiology and genetics fails, we *will* gain the capacity to influence the onset and course of common but serious mental illnesses, and given that large disparities in access to mental health treatment according to SES and race/ethnicity exist at the current time (Alegria et al. 2002; Hollingshead and Redlich 1958; Lorant et al. 2003), we can almost certainly expect that any new knowledge about how to prevent or cure mental illnesses will be maldistributed by these same factors in the time ahead. In this way, social inequalities will become major determinants of disease distribution in an era of successful prevention and treatment. They will add to or combine with the factors that currently produce associations between SES and the mental illnesses. Some readers may doubt the ultimate success of neurobiological and genetic approaches in reducing the prevalence of mental illnesses—it is *possible* that our enormous investment in these approaches will fail. If so, social factors will not be ascendant for the reasons we have speculated about here. Instead, the situation shall remain much as it is: robust associations between SES and many mental disorders will be explained through processes of social stress or social selection across the life course. The importance of social status has been with us since the inception of our field, it is with us today, and if the reasoning represented herein is apt, it will be become an even more prominent cause in the time ahead.

REFERENCES

Alegria M, Canino G, Rios R, et al: Mental health care for Latinos: inequalities in use of specialty mental health services among Latinos, African Americans, and non-Latino whites. Psychiatr Serv 53:1547–1555, 2002

Antonovsky A: Social class, life expectancy and overall mortality. Milbank Mem Fund Q 45:31–73, 1967

Chapin CV: Deaths among taxpayers and non-taxpayers income tax, Providence, 1865. Am J Public Health 4:647–651, 1924

Dohrenwend B: Overview of evidence for the importance of adverse environmental conditions in causing psychiatric disorders, in Adversity, Stress and Psychopathology. Edited by Dohrenwend B. New York, Oxford University Press, 1998, pp 523–538

Dohrenwend BP, Levav I, Shrout P, et al: Socioeconomic status and psychiatric disorder: the causation-selection issue. Science 255:946–952, 1992

Heston L: What about the environment? in Relatives At Risk for Mental Disorder. Edited by Dunner D, Gershon E, Barrett J. New York, Raven, 1988, pp 205–213

Hollingshead A, Redlich F: Social Class and Mental Illness. New York, John Wiley and Sons, 1958

Kessler R, McGonagle K, Zhao S, et al: Lifetime and 12-month prevalence of DSM-III-R psychiatric disorders in the United States: results from the National Comorbidity Study. Arch Gen Psychiatry 51:8–19, 1994

Klerman GL: The current age of youthful melancholia: evidence for increase in depression among adolescents and young adults, in Annual Progress in Child Psychiatry and Child Development. Edited by Chess S, Hertzig M. Philadelphia, PA, Brunner/Mazel, 1989, pp 333–335

Kohn R, Dohrenwend B, Mirotznik J: Epidemiological findings on selected psychiatric disorders in the general population, in Adversity, Stress, and Psychopathology. Edited by Dohrenwend BP. New York, Oxford University Press, 1998, pp 235–284

Kunst AE, Feikje G, Mackenbach JP, et al: Occupational class and cause specific mortality in middle aged men in 11 European countries: comparison of population based studies. BMJ 316:1636–1642, 1998

Lantz PM, House JS, Lepkowski JM, et al: Results from a nationally representative prospective study of U.S. adults. JAMA 279:1703–1708, 1998

Leighton A: My Name is Legion: The Stirling County Study of Psychiatric Disorder and Social Environment, Vol 1. New York, Basic Books, 1959

Link BG, Phelan JC: Social conditions as fundamental causes of disease. J Health Soc Behav (Special Issue):80–94, 1995

Link BG, Phelan JC: Understanding sociodemographic differences in health: the role of fundamental social causes. Am J Public Health 86:471–473, 1996

Link BG, Phelan JC: Evaluating the fundamental cause explanation for social disparities in health, in The Handbook of Medical Sociology, 5th Edition. Edited by Bird CE, Conrad P, Freemont AM. Upper Saddle River, NJ, Prentice Hall, 2000, pp 33–46

Lorant V, Kampfl D, Seghers A, et al: Socio-economic differences in psychiatric inpatient care. Acta Psychiatr Scand 107:170–177, 2003

Luftey K, Freese J: Toward some fundamentals of fundamental causality: socioeconomic status and health in the routine clinic visit for diabetes. Am J Sociol (in press)

Murphy J, Laird N, Monson R, et al: A 40-year perspective on the prevalence of depression: the Stirling County Study. Arch Gen Psychiatry 57:209–215, 2000

Phelan JC, Link BG, Diez-Roux A, et al: "Fundamental causes" of social inequalities in mortality: a test of the theory. J Health Soc Behav 45:265–287, 2004

Singh G, Miller B, Hankey B, et al: Changing area socioeconomic patterns in U.S. cancer mortality, 1950–1998, part I: all cancers among men. J Natl Cancer Inst 94:904–915, 2002a

Singh G, Miller B, Hankey B: Changing area socioeconomic patterns in U.S. cancer mortality, 1950–1998, part II: lung and colorectal cancers. J Natl Cancer Inst 94:916–925, 2002b

Sorlie PD, Backlund E, Keller J: U.S. mortality by economic, demographic, and social characteristics: the National Longitudinal Mortality Study. Am J Public Health 85:949–956, 1995

Srole L, Langner T, Michael S, et al: Mental Health in the Metropolis: The Midtown Manhattan Study. New York, McGraw-Hill, 1962

Syme SL, Hyman M, Enterline P: Sociocultural factors and coronary heart disease. Sociol Inq 35:81–91, 1964

Villerme L: Tableau d'Etat Physique et Moral des Ouvriers, Vol 2. Paris, France, Jules Renouard et Cie, 1840

Mood Disorders

Mood Disorders and the Heart

Joseph R. Carbone, M.D.

Jack M. Gorman, M.D.

Jeanne Goodman

Megan B. Willems, M.D.

THROUGHOUT HISTORY, poets and others have long associated sadness and other negative emotions with the heart. Expressions such as a "broken heart" have long been in use and can be seen throughout many cultures. A 1937 paper by Malzberg noted an increase in cardiovascular deaths in patients with the form of major depression formerly referred to as *involutional melancholia* (Malzberg 1937), but unfortunately, no real interest was aroused in the rest of the medical scientific community at the time. Only recently has the medical scientific community begun to appreciate a link between emotions and heart disease. In the 1960s clinicians and scientists began talking about a so-called type A personality, which they believed was associated with a higher risk of developing heart disease. This gave rise to a real interest on the part of the medical scientific community in the exploration of the possible relationship between negative affective states and heart disease, and various lines of research have been unfolding.

Initially, research focused almost exclusively on the role of depression in the development of heart disease. Depression has been identified as an independent risk factor in the development of ischemic heart disease. Other research has looked more closely at the relationship between hostility and heart disease. Still other work has focused on the role of anxiety as a possible risk factor. The results have been exciting and mixed. Although depression appears to be a major risk factor in the development of heart disease, some have questioned the strength of this association. Research is now raising the question of whether comorbid anxiety is really responsible for the apparent association between depression and heart disease. Research into the possible mechanisms of the association between negative affective states and heart disease has also been very exciting. Possible links being explored include altered platelet function, autonomic nervous system dysregulation, and increased serum cortisol levels.

The importance of gaining a greater understanding into the relationship between mood disorders and the heart cannot be overstated. Each year morbidity and mortality related to cardiac disease account for enormous pain and suffering worldwide as well as staggering economic costs. Many of the victims are people at the peak of their productivity. Certainly the more that can be understood about the etiology of these disorders, the greater the potential gains for society. In addition, a greater understanding of the relationship between mood disorders and the heart will give us a better understanding of the complex interrelationships between psychological and physiological processes, referred to frequently as "mind–body connection," and help us more effectively prevent needless suffering.

DEPRESSION

Much of the initial work in the area of mood disorders and the heart has focused on the role of depression. As stated earlier, depression has been identified as an independent risk factor for the development of heart disease. In addition, depression has been found to be associated with a greatly increased risk for the development of additional morbidity and mortality in those with preexisting cardiac disease. Studies indicate relative risks of 1.5–4.0 of incident coronary disease in community samples and relative risks of 2–6 for adverse events, including myocardial infarction (MI) and death, in patients with preexisting coronary disease or acute coronary syndromes. At least 15 major studies have examined the association between cardiac disease and depression. The studies looking at the association between depression and heart disease can be grouped into four categories:

1. Studies that explore depression as an independent risk factor for the development of heart disease;
2. Studies that look at the increase in morbidity and mortality in patients with preexisting heart disease who are also depressed;
3. Studies that explore the treatment of depression in patients with comorbid heart disease; and
4. Studies that explore the possible pathophysiological mechanisms linking depression and heart disease.

Depression as an Independent Risk Factor for Development of Heart Disease

The Western Collaborative Group Study (Rosenman et al. 1975), although it examined type A personality and not depression, was truly the pioneering study in the area of mood disorders and the heart. The type A personality comprises a variety of traits including free-floating anxiety and hostility. In their study, Rosenman and his colleagues looked prospectively at subjects who met the criterion for type A personality and studied the incidence of ischemic heart disease. They found that in subjects 39–49 years of age with type A personality traits, the odds ratio for developing coronary heart disease (CHD) was 1.87, and in those ages 50–59 years with type A personality traits, the odds ratio was 1.98.

The Baltimore cohort of the Epidemiologic Catchment Area (ECA) program (Pratt et al. 1996) revealed an odds ratio of 4.54 for MI in subjects having a history of major depression compared with those with no history of depression. The Precursors Study (Ford et al. 1998) looked at 1,190 male medical students over the course of four decades and found the relative risk of developing coronary artery disease (CAD) and MI in subjects with clinical depression was 2.12.

The National Health Examination Study (Anda et al. 1993) looked at 2,832 subjects for a mean follow-up of 12.4 years. Subjects with depressed affect and hopelessness were found to have a relative risk of 1.5 of developing fatalities secondary to CAD. Subjects with moderate levels of hopelessness were found to have a relative risk of 1.6, and those subjects having high levels of hopelessness were found to have a relative risk of 2.1. An increased risk for the development of CAD without death was also found.

The Cardiovascular Health Study (Schulz et al. 2000) looked at 5,201 subjects whom the investigators followed for 6 years. The authors concluded that depressive symptoms were an independent risk factor for mortality. In their study of a community sample consisting of 730 subjects whom they followed for 27 years, Barefoot and Schroll (1996) found a relative risk of 1.71 for the development of MI in subjects with depression. They also found a relative risk of 1.59 for deaths from all causes in subjects with depression.

The Stirling County Study (Murphy et al. 1985, 1987) looked at 1,003 community-dwelling subjects followed for 16 years. The study looked at standardized found mortality ratios, which the authors defined as the ratio of observed deaths to expected deaths. They found the standardized mortality ratio due to cardiovascular deaths to be 2.1 in men with depression and 1.2 in women with depression.

The National Health and Nutrition Examination Study I (NHANES I; Ferketich et al. 2000) looked at depressed men and women over a 10-year period. The investigators determined multivariable-adjusted relative risk of subjects' developing a nonfatal event. The relative risk approached 2 in both the male and female subjects.

Depression as a Risk Factor for Increased Morbidity and Mortality in Patients With Preexisting Heart Disease

The work of Hance et al. (1996) and Frasure-Smith et al. (1993) has been crucial in examining the presence of depression in patients with comorbid heart disease. Their studies have shown a greater than 15% prevalence of depression in patients diagnosed with CAD and post-MI (Frasure-Smith et al. 1993) and a close to 35% prevalence of depression in patients after coronary artery bypass graft (CABG; Hance et al. 1996).

The Penninx Study (Penninx et al. 2001), one of the most frequently referred-to studies in the area, was performed in the Netherlands. In this study the authors examined a population of 450 patients with comorbid depression and heart disease. They followed this population for a period of 4 years. They found a relative risk of 1.6 of subsequent mortality in patients diagnosed with minor depression and a relative risk of 3.0 of subsequent mortality in patients diagnosed with major depression. The Glostrup Study (Hagerup 1974) similarly looked at 730 patients with comorbid depression and heart disease. These patients were followed during a 27-year period. The investigators found significant increases in the relative risk of greater than 1.5 both for the development of an acute MI and for total mortality in patients with comorbid depression.

The Post-Infarction Late Potential Study (Ladwig et al. 1991) looked at a population of 60 male patients with comorbid affective disorders and their survival after acute MI. They found the prevalence of patients diagnosed with major depression after acute MI to be three times greater than that of the general population and the presence of major depression to be a significant predictor of cardiac death. The Goteburg Study (Welin et al. 1995) found an overall risk of nonfatal events related to CHD of close to 2 in depressed women and greater than 1.5 in depressed men.

A very important study performed by Strik et al. (2003) examined the role of anxiety as well as depression in patients with comorbid cardiac disease. They concluded that anxiety may be a more important variable in the development of additional cardiac morbidity and mortality and use of clinical resources than depression. They went on to suggest that where depression appears to be a crucial variable influencing the development of additional morbidity, mortality, and use of clinical resources, it may actually be anxiety comorbid with the depression that is the cause of complications. This is a very important study because it actually compared the effects of depression and anxiety on comorbid cardiac disease. It is interesting to note, however, that neither the Stirling County Study nor the Baltimore ECA follow-up found an increase in cardiovascular mortality among patients with anxiety disorders.

Frasure-Smith et al. (1993) studied the effect of depression on prognosis in the first 6 months after MI. They found "a significantly elevated risk of mortality" in patients with depression. One of their findings is that depression is as great a risk factor for additional adverse cardiac events as left ventricular dysfunction and history of previous MI. In another study, Frasure-Smith et al. (1995) used the National Institute of Mental Health Diagnostic Interview Schedule to diagnose depression and the Beck Depression Inventory to determine the severity of symptoms of depression. They assessed depression approximately 7 days after an MI and conducted a follow-up assessment 18 months later. They found that the majority of deaths due to cardiac causes occurred in patients they had diagnosed as being depressed. In addition, they found that the majority of deaths occurred in patients who had experienced 10 or more premature ventricular contractions (PVCs) per hour. The results of their studies led them to conclude that depression is a significant risk factor for mortality in patients diagnosed with depression in the hospital following an MI and that there appears to be an "arrhythmic mechanism" linking depression and death in patients who are depressed following an MI.

In another study, Lesperance et al. (2000) looked at a group of 430 patients following an episode of angina in order to assess the relationship between depression and recurrent cardiac events. They found a much higher rate of cardiac death or nonfatal MI in the patients determined to have depression than in the nondepressed patients. Barefoot et al. (1996) looked at the relationship between long-term mortality risk and baseline Zung depression scores in patients with CAD. They found that the patients could be divided into three major categories: moderately to severely depressed, mildly depressed, and nondepressed. Patients with moderate to severe depression were much more likely to die of cardiac death than either patients with mild depression or patients who were not depressed. The patients with mild depression were intermediate in the risk of cardiac death between those with moderate to severe depression and those who were not depressed. The authors also found this relationship to hold for more than 10 years following the acute MI.

In looking at survival free of recurrent cardiac events after CABG, Connerney et al. (2001) found that the presence of major depressive disorder ranked with low ejection fraction and female gender as a major predictor of cardiac morbidity and mortality following CABG. The risk ratio for both depression and low ejection fraction was 2.3 and the risk ratio for female gender was 2.4.

Treatment of Depression in Patients With Comorbid Heart Disease

The Enhancing Recovery in Coronary Heart Disease Study (ENRICHD; Carney et al. 2004), a large, multicenter, randomized, controlled trial, explored the use of psychosocial interventions and cognitive behavioral therapy in treating patients with comorbid major or minor depression who had recently had an acute MI. Approximately 3,000 individuals were studied, and sertraline was used as needed. Overall, treatment was found to have no benefit in reducing post-MI mortality. The study actually demonstrated poorer results among women who had had a recent MI and received psychosocial support. In a recent review of the data the ENRICHD investigators found that "patients whose depression is refractory to cognitive behavior therapy and sertraline, two standard treatments for depression, are at high risk for late mortality after myocardial infarction" (Carney et al. 2004, p. 466).

The Montreal Heart Attack Readjustment Trial (M-HART; Frasure-Smith 1995; Frasure-Smith et al. 1997) looked at patients who had sustained an MI and had either poor social supports or depression. The patients were randomized to intervention and control groups. They were monitored by telephone, and psychosocial support was provided if patients were distressed. Psychosocial support was given in the form of home visits and problem solving. Nurses were trained to provide interventions. Cardiovascular mortality was examined at 12 months. It was found that women who had received intervention had a higher cardiovascular mortality rate than women who did not receive any intervention (9% vs. 5%). The mortality rate for men studied was about the same, at slightly greater than 2% whether or not intervention was provided.

The Sertraline Antidepressant Heart Attack Randomized Trial (SADHART; Glassman et al. 2002) represented a particularly bold initiative to study the effect of sertraline, a selective serotonin reuptake inhibitor (SSRI), on the treatment of depression in patients with acute coronary syndromes including recent MI and unstable angina. In fact, although the study did not show a worsening of cardiac status with sertraline, the results were inconclusive regarding benefits. No adverse effect of any kind was shown to result from the administration of sertraline. Surprisingly, however, sertraline did not separate from placebo on the main outcome measure—reduction in Hamilton Depression Scale score—except in a post hoc analysis in which a group of patients with recurrent and severe depression was separated from the rest of the group. There were trends for sertraline to be superior to placebo in preventing cardiac and all-cause mortality, but most of these comparisons failed to reach statistical significance. Still, compared with the psychosocial treatments in the ENRICHD and M-HART studies that may have actually worsened the outcome for some patients, the SADHART study suggests that antidepressant therapy may have benefits and should be studied further. We return to the SADHART study later in our consideration of mechanisms of action. Another treatment study, on a smaller scale than the others but no less interesting, involved the work of Musselman et al. (2000) at Emory University, who showed that treatment of depression decreases platelet reactivity. With the latter being an essential element in the pathophysiology of heart disease as well as stroke, this work is extremely important.

Pathophysiology Underlying the Link Between Depression and Heart Disease

Possible mechanisms linking depression with cardiac disease include altered platelet and endothelial cell function. Studies performed by Musselman et al. (1996) have demonstrated that patients with depression have increased baseline platelet reactivity. Musselman has also demonstrated a decrease in platelet reactivity following the treatment of the depression. Shimbo et al. (2002) demonstrated exaggerated serotonin-mediated platelet reactivity in depressed patients. Laghrissi-Thode et al. (1997) have demonstrated elevations of platelet factor 4 (PF4) and beta-thromboglobulin (β-TG) in patients with depression and ischemic heart disease. They were able to show a decrease in the secretion of PF4 and β-TG by platelets after treatment of patients with paroxetine (Pollock et al. 2000). This was the same SSRI used by Musselman in her studies. Laghrissi-Thode's group was not able to demonstrate a reduction in the secretion of PF4 and β-TG in response to the administration of nortriptyline. This is a very important finding because it suggests that it is not the treatment of the depression alone that results in a normalization of platelet function, but that such normalization is dependent on the type of antidepressant used. This would specifically suggest that serotonin-mediated platelet function is the aspect of increased platelet reactivity that needs to be targeted in order to reduce a depressed patient's risk of developing cardiac disease.

The increase in platelet reactivity in patients with depression is felt by some to be related to an increase in intraplatelet calcium mobilization (Konopka et al. 1996; Kusumi et al. 1991, 1994) The increase in calcium mobilization is crucial to platelet reactivity. Essentially, the binding of agonists such as serotonin at the platelet membrane results in a series of postreceptor events leading to the mobilization of calcium. The latter is essential for the subsequent change in platelet shape and release of substances from platelet granules resulting in platelet adhesion and aggregation (Eckart et al. 1993; Nemeroff and Musselman 2000).

Platelets, which are reservoirs in the circulation for serotonin, have many of the same serotonin receptors as are found in the central nervous system. Therefore, it is not surprising that abnormalities in serotonin function that have been linked to depression also occur in platelets and that serotonin reuptake inhibitor antidepressants have similar effects on serotonin receptors in the brain and on platelets. It has been postulated that in patients with depression there is a hyperactivity of the signaling system activated by the binding of serotonin to the 5-HT_{2A} receptor on the platelet surface (Delisi et al. 1998; Nemeroff and Musselman 2000; Schins et al. 2003). The resulting hyperactivity of this postreceptor signaling system would explain the increase in intraplatelet calcium found in these patients and would explain mechanistically the resulting increase in platelet reactivity. The hyperactivity of this system is therefore postulated to occur along with the upregulation of 5-HT_{2A} receptors found on the platelets of depressed patients. This would be consistent with our current understanding of the neurobiology of depression in which it has been found that there is an upregulation of central 5-HT_{2A} receptors. In addition, there is a decrease, or downregulation, in the concentration of central 5-HT serotonin transporter receptors (Owens and Nemeroff 1994), and this is found in the platelets of depressed patients as well (Kusumi et al. 1991). The hypothesis that there is a hyperactivity of the post 5-HT_{2A} receptor signaling system in the platelets of depressed patients would be consistent with the work of Shimbo et al. (2002), which demonstrates increased serotonin-mediated platelet reactivity but not increased platelet reactivity in response to adenosine diphosphate binding.

For completeness, it should be added that in his review of the literature Mendelson (2000) concluded that the increase in $5\text{-}HT_2$ receptor density in the platelets of depressed patients is more of a consistent finding in those who are suicidal rather than in depressed patients in general. He also concluded that in some depressed patients the aggregation of platelets in response to 5-HT binding is actually inhibited. It is unclear how to reconcile Mendelson's conclusions with the findings previously discussed.

A study indicating abnormal endothelial cell function in patients with depression was carried out by Rajagapalan et al. (2001). They looked at the vasodilation of the brachial artery in young subjects with and without depression. They found that normal vasodilation mediated by blood flow through the artery was impaired in the subjects with depression. They concluded that this was evidence of endothelial dysfunction in the patients with depression. Increased platelet and endothelial cell reactivity are important factors in the etiology of acute coronary syndromes and can therefore serve as a pathophysiological link between depression and the development of heart disease.

A platelet substudy was conducted as part of the SADHART study, in which the effect of the SSRI sertraline on the release of markers of platelet and endothelial activity was studied. It was found that fewer markers were released with sertraline treatment than with placebo. Markers studied included prostaglandin 4, β-TG, platelet/endothelial cell adhesion molecule–1, P-selectin, thromboxane B2, 6-ketoprostaglandin F_{1a}, vascular cell adhesion molecule–1, and E-selectin.

Another possible link between depression and heart disease involves a decrease in heart rate variability (HRV), also known as heart period variability, beat-to-beat variability, and normal sinus arrhythmia. HRV is an aspect of autonomic nervous system functioning. Gorman and Sloan (2000) reported that there is a decrease in HRV in patients with a variety of negative affective states. Treatment implications, as alluded to earlier, are exciting in that medications, including the serotonin reuptake inhibitors, have been shown to increase HRV in the setting of negative affective states (Agelink et al. 2002; Balogh et al. 1993; McFarlane et al. 2001; Tucker et al. 1997). For example, Tucker et al. (1997) reported paroxetine's ability to increase HRV. This particular study was performed in the setting of panic disorder but has immediate implications for the possible treatment of patients with comorbid depression and heart disease. The SSRI sertraline has been found to increase HRV as well (McFarlane et al. 2001).

We know that depression involves alterations in the brain, such as changes in neurotransmitter levels. If depression can result in cardiac disease and affect morbidity and mortality in patients with preexisting heart disease, then it might be concluded that depression's impact on the heart might be mediated through the brain. For this to occur there would have to be evidence that the brain actually has the ability to control the heart. It is well known that the brain does this through vasomotor centers located in the medulla oblongata. In addition, the autonomic nervous system, originating in the brain, is known to be crucial for the functioning of the heart. Indeed, HRV has been defined as "the standard deviation of successive R to R intervals in sinus rhythm and is thought to reflect the balance between sympathetic and parasympathetic input to the heart" (Nemeroff et al. 1998), and as previously noted, Gorman and Sloan (2000) and others have pointed out that HRV is decreased in depression, hostility, anxiety, and panic.

Other work by Gorman, Sloan, Bigger, Bagiella, and colleagues (Shapiro et al. 1993, 1994, 1996; Sloan et al. 1994) has focused on the reaction of the transplanted heart to stress. The implications and ramifications of this particular work are important because the transplanted heart gives us a unique window through which to view the interaction between brain and heart. Specifically, the transplanted heart, unlike the native heart, is a heart devoid of direct innervation by the brain. This gives us a very rich opportunity to see how the heart functions without direct brain connections. The transplanted heart is still subject to indirect brain influences via circulating catecholamines, for example, but the direct innervation is absent. When Gorman and others investigated the reactions of subjects to stress using mathematical problem-solving paradigms, the subjects with transplanted hearts did not have the same changes in heart function as the subjects with native hearts. For example, heart rate reactivity was decreased. The normal, adaptive increases in heart rate reactivity, with an increase in heart rate, seen in response to stress was slower in patients with transplanted hearts. The patient with a transplanted heart gives us an even richer opportunity to more fully understand the interactions between brain and heart because although the new heart is not connected by nerves to the subject's brain, the native sinoatrial node is routinely left in place. Therefore, its reactions to the stress-provoking mathematical exercises can also be monitored, and these reactions can show us how the brain-innervated heart would react. In subjects with transplanted hearts given the mathematical exercises, the native sinoatrial node responded with the adaptive increases in heart rate, whereas the transplanted heart's sinoatrial node was slower to react. Therefore, the presence of circulating catecholamines and other neurotransmitters was not sufficient to produce the same increase in heart rate as was found in the native sinoatrial node. The presence of such a response could only occur with direct innervation by the brain as shown by the reactions of the native sinoatrial node. It would be reasonable to infer from this line of work that negative affective states such as depression, hostility, anxiety, and panic, which have been shown to result in alterations of brain function, could, through such alterations, adversely affect the normal functioning of the heart, particularly in response to stress.

Nashoni et al. (2004) studied a cohort of physically healthy depressed patients and compared them with heart transplant patients who were not depressed. Both groups were compared with a control group of physically healthy subjects without depression. It was hypothesized that based on the HRV literature, the physically healthy depressed patients would have HRV values somewhere in between those of the nondepressed heart transplant patients and those of the nondepressed, physically healthy control subjects. This is essentially what they found. It appears, therefore, that depression somehow results in a kind of functional denervation of the heart. This is thought to be due to an autonomic imbalance with a decrease in vagal tone.

As previously mentioned, treatments of depression can increase HRV. This, again, is not true of every treatment. A notable exception is the use of some tricyclic antidepressants, particularly nortriptyline (Pollock et al. 2000), which can actually decrease HRV, possibly due to their anticholinergic effects. This would be consistent with the theory that vagal tone is decreased in patients with depression and other negative affective states. Indeed, chemically there would already be a decrease in cholinergic transmission that would theoretically be exacerbated by the use of a strongly anticholinergic medication such as amitriptyline.

Other work by Nashoni et al. (2001) demonstrated an increase in HRV following the treatment of depression with electroconvulsive therapy. Thus, one might hypothesize that it is the actual treatment of depression that somehow improves cardiac autonomic balance and normalization of HRV unless a strongly anticholinergic antidepressant is used. One might speculate that even in patients treated with a strongly anticholinergic agent, there might still be some increase in HRV above pretreatment levels but that a full normalization is prevented by the anticholinergic properties of the medication. Alternatively, there might be a common mechanistic pathway by which different antidepressant treatments might improve HRV independent of whether depression is fully treated. Clearly, further studies are needed to sort this out.

Zellweger et al. (2004) pointed out in their review of CAD and depression that the finding most frequently replicated in patients with comorbid CAD and depression is a higher mortality rate after an acute MI. One of the reasons for this higher mortality rate could be an autonomic dysregulation, and one of the manifestations of this dysregulation is decreased HRV. Another manifestation of autonomic dysregulation might be the propensity of depressed patients to develop ventricular arrhythmias. Carney et al. (1993) studied ventricular tachycardia in patients with comorbid depression and heart disease and found that patients with depression and comorbid heart disease have a higher prevalence of ventricular tachycardia than patients with CAD who are not depressed. Welin (2000) found depression to be more common in patients with ventricular arrhythmia. Theoretically, this propensity to develop ventricular tachycardia could explain the higher mortality rate found in these patients following an acute MI. This is consistent with the work of Frasure-Smith et al. (1995) mentioned previously, in which their finding of increased cardiac mortality among post-MI patients found to have 10 or more PVCs per hour led them to propose that "an arrhythmic mechanism" may be the physiologic link between depression and cardiac mortality.

Another mechanism by which depression and other negative affective states may lead to increased cardiovascular morbidity and mortality is suggested by the work of Carels et al. (1999), who focused on the relationship between so-called emotional reactivity and myocardial ischemia. They found that patients with CAD who characterized themselves as having strong emotional responses to even minor daily stressors actually had demonstrable myocardial ischemia associated with their negative emotional responses. The authors monitored patients with ambulatory electrocardiograms and subjected them to mental stress tests. Subjects who had been found to have high emotional reactivity in response to the stress demonstrated ST segment depression, whereas subjects characterized as having low emotional reactivity did not demonstrate myocardial ischemia in response to the same challenges. Moreover, the subjects who were characterized as having high emotional reactivity and associated myocardial ischemia in response to the mental stress tests were more likely to report anxiety and/or depression. The investigators concluded that the high emotional reactivity might, therefore, be the psychological link between anxiety and depression and cardiac events and that this can be targeted with interventions aimed at reducing the risk of additional cardiac events in patients with CAD.

Another possible mechanism linking depression and heart disease has to do with an entity studied extensively by Greenwald, Alexopoulos, Krishnan, Rapp, and others referred to as *vascular depression*. This entity is thought to represent a unique type of depression that generally begins late in life. Unlike depression beginning before geriatric years, there is usually no personal or family history of depression in patients with vascular depression. The incidence is equal among males and females. Clinically, apathy is present to a greater extent than dysphoria. The patients also have vascular risk factors. Several abnormalities are seen on magnetic resonance imaging (MRI) scans in patients with vascular depression, including white matter lesions and hyperintensities in gray matter. Such abnormalities can be indicative of small vessel disease (Alexopoulos et al. 1997; Greenwald et al. 1996; Rapp et al. 2005). Patients with this type of brain abnormality would most likely also have CAD and heart disease. The idea that a person can present with depression as a result of vascular disease suggests the possibility that, instead of being two separate entities, the depression and heart disease may actually represent different manifestations of the same common pathological processes. If this were the case, then it would not make sense to refer to depression as a risk factor for heart disease; rather, vascular disease would be seen as a risk factor for both depression and heart disease.

A problem with this proposed mechanism is that it does not appear to apply to the usual primary depression. If depression and heart disease were results of the same common pathological processes, then one might argue that all patients with depression might be expected to have comorbid heart disease, and such is not the case. Therefore it could be stated that this mechanism might explain the relationship between only one specific subtype of depression, vascular depression, and heart disease. Nevertheless, it could be postulated that patients with primary depression who subsequently develop heart disease may have pathology in the cerebral vasculature that is not gross enough to be picked up on routine MRI scans and that such patients also have depression on a vascular basis. Indeed, there might be vascular pathology affecting the brain vessels and resulting in alterations of brain functioning sufficient to cause depression before enough vessel disease is present to adversely affect cardiac functioning. It might just be that the brain mechanisms essential to the regulation of mood are more sensitive to early vascular disease than the heart is, and therefore the heart disease might take longer to manifest. This would result in the false impression that the depression is a risk factor for the later onset of heart disease. Instead, the depression would be the first manifestation of the same vascular pathology that only later on results in obvious heart disease. Clearly, further research into a possible vascular basis of primary depression would be useful in helping to clarify our understanding of what is truly occurring and might result in newer insights into the etiology and treatment of depression.

Recent work has focused on the possibility that increased cortisol levels may be a link between depression and cardiac disease. The reasoning behind this is that depression has long been found to be associated with increased cortisol levels. It is also known that a variety of conditions common in patients with CHD as well as some of the medications prescribed for these patients can be associated with elevated cortisol secretion. A recent study looking at 24-hour urinary cortisol levels in medical outpatients with CHD found that those patients having the highest cortisol levels were twice as likely to be depressed when CHD patients having lower cortisol levels (Otte et al. 2004).

From ancient times, a relationship between sadness and heart disease has been hinted at but often dismissed as poetic and not scientific. It is now clear, however, that depression plays a clear role in increased risk for cardiovascular morbidity and mortality. Moreover, the physiological relationships for these "heart–brain" relationships are increasingly being elucidated. Although treatment studies have yielded conflicting and sometimes counterintuitive findings—such as the finding that psychosocial interventions may worsen cardiac outcomes in women—it is now reasonable to anticipate that some modulation of dysphoric state might reduce the burden of cardiovascular disease. Indeed, depression appears to be as potent a risk factor for poor cardiovascular outcomes as some of the more "traditional" cardiac risk factors such as hyperlipidemia, obesity, and hypertension. Hence, much larger studies examining depression as a cardiovascular risk factor are clearly warranted.

HOSTILITY AND HEART DISEASE

The link between hostility and CHD has been studied for decades. Although it remains unclear whether hostility predicts coronary events, several studies have shown that high levels of anger are associated with an increased risk of subsequent CHD events (Chang et al. 2002; Knox et al. 1998; Williams et al. 2000). This review discusses the general themes that prevail in the body of literature regarding hostility and cardiovascular disease.

Hostility as a Risk Factor for Incidence or Prognosis of Coronary Heart Disease

Recent prospective cohort studies examine how anger influences the development of cardiovascular disease. The nature of these prospective studies can provide information about the effect of hostility on *incidence* of CHD events. The connection between feelings of anger and subsequent MI is compelling, because it has been reported that 36,000 (2.4% of 1.5 million) heart attacks are precipitated annually in the United States by anger (Verrier and Mittleman 1996). The general prospective cohort study design involves obtaining a measurement of hostility from the target population using either structured interview or self-report techniques followed by observation of subsequent CHD events over time. Analysis is then performed for correlation between levels of hostility and CHD events.

A recent study involving 12,986 participants enrolled in the Atherosclerosis Risk in Communities study examined prospectively the association between trait anger and the risk of CHD incidence (Barefoot et al. 1995). The participants were white and black men and women between the ages of 45 and 64 years. Incident CHD events occurred in the follow-up period of 53 months (median). The results showed that individuals with high trait anger were at a two-times-greater risk of CHD events (multivariate-adjusted hazard ratio 1.54 with 95% confidence interval). These results point to a strong association between levels of trait anger and incidence of CHD. Although the study provided the opportunity to recruit and examine a large number of subjects, it is important to mention the possibility of selection bias. These participants may have agreed to participate in the study for fear of future CAD based on their own health risk factors or familial history of heart disease. Therefore, these individuals may already have been at higher risk for cardiovascular disease, and these results may not be generalized to the broader population. Other studies have also reported the link between hostility and incidence of disease. Barefoot et al. (1995) performed a 25-year follow-up study of 409 men and 321 women and found that hostility scale scores were associated with increased risk of incident acute MI when controlling for traditional risk factors (i.e., alcohol consumption, cigarette smoking, body mass index).

Anger may have different effects on the onset versus progression of disease. Several studies show the pronounced effect of hostility among persons with preexisting CHD. For example, one study involving 23,522 male health professionals who responded to a mailed questionnaire showed that increased frequency of feeling angry was significantly associated with elevated risk of recurrent coronary disease (Eng et al. 2003). Chaput et al. (2002) showed hostility to be an independent risk factor for recurrent CHD events. Irritability, easy arousal of anger, and type A behavior may be associated with elevated rates of CHD-related hospitalization and mortality among men with preexisting disease (Koskenkuo et al. 1988). Goodman et al. (1997) approached this issue from a physiologic perspective. In their study, 41 patients with single-vessel or multivessel CAD underwent percutaneous transluminal coronary angioplasty (PTCA). These same patients were assessed by means of the structured interview for the hostility component of type A behavior pattern. Results showed that patients with high total hostility ratings were almost 2.5 times more likely to have restenosis than those with low hostility scores. This led the investigators to initiate a coronary-prone behavior modification program for patients with persistent, same-site restenosis after PTCA. Similar programs have been reported to be efficacious. For example, the Recurrent Coronary Prevention Project (Thoresen et al. 1982) compared treatment groups and showed that patients receiving behavioral modification attempting to alter type A behavior pattern experienced a reduced rate of recurrence.

It should be noted that the definition of CHD events may vary across studies. An incident CHD event has been defined as any of the following: acute MI, fatal CHD, silent MI, cardiac revascularization procedure, unstable angina, CABG surgery, PTCA, and others. Additionally, different studies employed various measurements of hostility. The most commonly used assessment scales for anger are the Minnesota Multiphasic Personality Inventory, which includes the Cook-Medley Hostility Scale, and the Spielberger Trait Anger Scale. Therefore, there may be significant variations among studies that would need further clarification and standardization before clear conclusions can be drawn and generalizability confirmed.

In prospective cohort studies, which are clearly of great use when examining incidence of disease, it is important to decide upon a follow-up period that is long enough to yield significant results. Although it can be difficult to achieve, the best studies will obtain data regarding the individual's experience of anger and proceed to observe his or her health over at least 5 years. It would be useful for future studies to obtain these data earlier in the subject's life (before age 50 years) so that the effects of long-term hostility (or type A personality, which includes hostile affect) on cardiovascular health can be specifically examined.

Coping With Anger: Significance of Coping Style

Some studies have focused less on the individual's level of hostility and more on how he or she handles feelings of anger. Anger-In and Anger-Out measures, assessed in the Spielberger Scale, have been used to determine whether there is a difference in effects on coronary disease based on how anger is expressed. When expressing anger, it may be focused outward on other people or objects (anger-out) or directed inward (anger-in).

Conflicting data exist regarding the issue of coping style. Among provoked persons, extreme anger expression (anger-out) has been related to greater blood pressure and heart rate activity (Siegman et al. 1992; Suarez and Williams 1990) as well as risk of hypertension, yet another study showed low levels of expression are linked to increased cardiovascular reactivity as well (Everson et al. 1998; Harburg et al. 1991). Kawachi et al. (1994a) conducted the most recent comprehensive study addressing this issue, recruiting 51,529 male subjects from the Health Professional Follow-Up Study, a prospective study of chronic disease. Based on results from the Spielberger Anger-Out Scale, anger expression seemed to be somewhat protective against nonfatal MI; compared with men with low scores on the Anger-Out Scale, men with moderate levels of anger-out expression had nearly half the risk of nonfatal MI.

Future studies addressing the hostility–cardiovascular disease link should investigate the role of coping style. It is possible that both extremes in coping style may be detrimental. Kawachi et al. (1994b) have shown that higher Anger-Out scores seem to provide protection against incident CHD. How does anger-in affect incidence? Further understanding of the relationship between modes of anger expression and risk for CHD would be beneficial so that appropriate behavioral treatments may be employed.

Potential Mechanisms Behind the Hostility–Coronary Heart Disease Link

There is a significant amount of literature demonstrating the association between hostility and coronary disease. Therefore it is likely that some underlying mechanism, or combination of mechanisms, is responsible for this connection. There are five main proposals of potential mechanisms that exist in the literature: the health behaviors model, arousal of sympathetic activity, platelet activation, trigger hypothesis, and immune response. Each is discussed here.

Health Behaviors Model

The health behaviors model suggests that hostility serves as a marker for behaviors that increase risk for disease; anger itself does not directly influence coronary health but rather is associated with other behaviors that put the individual at risk. Leiker et al. (1988) used the Cook and Medley Hostility scale in conjunction with the TestWell self-report and found that high hostility scorers reported poorer health habits, specifically regarding physical fitness, self-care, drug use, and driving. Although this theory has validity, it is important to consider that most studies addressing the hostility–CHD link control for health risk factors such as smoking and alcohol consumption, thus eliminating these as potential confounding variables. This strategy must be maintained in future studies.

Arousal of Sympathetic Activity

A second explanation for the correlation between high levels of anger and coronary disease proposes that chronic anger arouses sympathetic activity. For example, in groups of men and women given emotionally demanding tasks that induce hostility and anger expression, these feelings are indicative of enhanced reactivity (higher blood pressures and heart rate; Vitaliano et al. 1993). Activation of the hypothalamic-pituitary-adrenal axis results in elevated levels of serum catecholamines that can adversely affect blood pressure, heart rate, and free fatty acids. The hypothesis suggests that heightened catecholamine secretion induced by anger may damage the endothelium and heart muscle (Haft 1974) and also play a role in the development of atherosclerotic lesions. Studies have also confirmed that the presence of catecholamines is associated with increased platelet adhesion and aggregation (Haft 1981). As discussed later, platelets may also be involved in the hostility–CHD link.

Platelet Activation

Increased platelet activation has been associated with adverse secondary events after MI or coronary angioplasty. It is thus important to examine a possible association between hostility and platelet activation. In one study, 32 patients with CHD were tested for platelet activation by whole blood flow cytometry, and platelet activation was measured in blood exiting a bleeding time wound as well as in venous blood stimulated in vitro with collagen (Markovitz 1998). In addition, the Type A Structured Interview was used to assess potential for hostility in these same patients. Results showed that platelet activation was related to hostility, consistent with other studies indicating a relationship between platelet activation and psychological factors. Other studies have examined emotional effects on plasma coagulation and fibrinolysis. One study obtained blood samples before, during, and after mental stress-inducing exercises and showed increased von Willebrand factor antigen, increased factor VIII coagulant activity, and increased fibrinogen concentration during stress (Jern et al. 1989). These results suggest that mental stress has significant effects on plasma coagulation and could thus be a risk factor for cardiovascular disease. Whether such results can be generalized to include hostility is unclear.

Trigger Hypothesis

The trigger hypothesis has most likely been proposed in response to the evidence that in 4%–18% of cases of MI, emotional stress has been reported to occur immediately before the onset of symptoms. Mittleman et al. (1995) stated the trigger theory as follows: "A proposed mechanism for triggering of myocardial infarction by anger is that onset occurs when a vulnerable but not necessarily stenotic atherosclerotic plaque disrupts in response to hemodynamic stresses; thereafter, hemostatic and vasoconstrictive forces determine whether the resultant thrombus becomes occlusive" (p. 1724). Indeed, atherosclerosis has been shown to have an effect on the vasomotor response of coronary arteries to mental stress. The normal vasomotor response to mental stress involves no change or dilation of the large coronary arteries. However, in 26 patients who performed mental arithmetic under stressful conditions during catheterization, it was shown that patients with atherosclerosis demonstrated paradoxical constriction during mental stress, particularly at points of stenosis (Yeung et al. 1991). Perhaps it is these vasoconstrictive forces that may result in an occlusive thrombus, as proposed by Mittleman's group. Further support of the trigger hypothesis is suggested in the Mittleman et al. results by the fact that aspirin, and perhaps β-adrenergic blockers, reduced the relative risk of MI onset after anger. It could be that these agents may decrease the likelihood of plaque disruption and acute occlusive thrombus formation in response to an outburst of anger. Therefore, the risk factors that would be present during an episode of anger in an unmedicated individual are eliminated by aspirin/β-blockers, and fewer occurrences of MI ensue.

Immune Response

A final hypothesis proposes that psychological stress affects the immune response, which in turn may play a key role in the development and progression of arteriosclerosis and thus CHD. One study showed that natural killer (NK) activity is significantly higher in CHD patients compared with control subjects, and furthermore, NK activity was significantly elevated by the suppression of anger and negative emotions (Isihara et al. 2003). Future research should investigate the potential linkage between stress, hostility, and CHD development.

Implications for Treatment

Significant research attention is being paid to the negative impact of anger on CHD. Future research can add to our existing knowledge about the hostility–CHD link. The goal of such research is to improve the clinician's ability to predict who is most vulnerable to CHD. If physicians can identify those most at risk, they can then proceed to employ beneficial primary and secondary prevention measures. It follows that treatment interventions (whether by medication or behavior therapy) should also be studied and proven to improve cardiac health. Indeed, some studies have already shown that behavioral modification can improve hostility scores as well as general health and quality of life (Gidron and Davidson 1996; Lavid et al. 2000)

ANXIETY, PANIC DISORDER, AND CARDIAC DISEASE

Much attention has been focused on the interplay between depression and cardiac disease, and research continues to elucidate the mechanisms by which each may affect the pathogenesis and treatment of the other. Just as anxiety is increasingly being shown to play a significant role in depression, panic and other anxiety disorders are proving to be contributors to cardiac disease. They may each play a part as mediators of depressive illness (Watkins et al. 1999) or function as independent contributors to cardiac morbidity and mortality. Efforts are under way to differentiate between causative and associative relationships.

The onset of cardiac disease is in itself an anxiety-provoking event. Many cardiac conditions, including MI, arrhythmia, and the shortness of breath associated with congestive heart failure, provoke patients to feel anxious or fearful, sometimes even as the initial complaint. Considering that half of the diagnostic criteria for panic disorder are physiologic symptoms that are potentially cardiac complaints, it is not surprising that physicians and patients alike have difficulty elucidating which signs and symptoms are cardiac or psychiatric in origin. This can lead to costly workups that carry their own risks and, even in the event of no identifiable cardiac disease, do little to quell the anxiety of the patient (Katon et al. 1995).

Some research has suggested that patients with anxiety disorders have greater likelihood of medical illness, but this hypothesis has often been confounded by the question of whether these patients simply seek medical care more frequently out of anxiety. Harter et al. (2003) found, in a comparison of 169 patients with an anxiety disorder and 93 control subjects with no evidence of anxiety disorder, that the patients with psychiatric comorbidity exhibited a 4.6 odds ratio for cardiac disorders and a 2.6 odds ratio for hypertension. This study controlled for gender, comorbid substance abuse and dependence, and depression and made efforts to minimize bias related to patients' level of treatment-seeking behavior. Research is ongoing not only to replicate such findings but to clarify the mechanisms by which these patients are placed at increased risk. When cardiac events do occur in patients with panic or anxiety disorders, outcomes are generally poorer on measures of self-care, maintaining exercise and appropriate dietary changes, and postinfarct return to previous levels of activity (Huffman et al. 2002; Strik et al. 2003).

Assessing the Risk

In a recent attempt to assess whether anxiety and depression are predictors of incomplete recovery after a first MI, Strik et al. (2003) followed 318 men with self-reported symptoms of depression, anxiety, and/or hostility after a first MI. After following these patients for between 1 and 70 months (average 3.4 years), 25 new cardiac events occurred. Although symptoms of both depression and anxiety were positively correlated with recurrence of a cardiac event (hazard ratio for depression 2.32, for anxiety 3.01), multivariate analysis showed that it was the presence of anxiety that actually accounted for the relationship between cardiac events and depression (Strik et al. 2003). This finding suggests that future research should perhaps focus on depression as a mediator of anxiety's effects on cardiac disease, rather than the reverse. Furthermore, of the three parameters of anxiety, depression, and hostility, anxiety alone (odds ratio=2.0) was a predictor of rehospitalization and frequent outpatient visits.

In a prospective study of 39,999 male health professionals ages 40–75 years, Kawachi et al. (1994a) examined the risk of CHD in phobic anxiety. Using patient responses to the previously validated Crown-Crisp Index (Birtchnell et al. 1988; Crown and Crisp 1956) within 1 month of a first MI, the authors examined the outcomes of nonfatal MI and fatal CHD, which they further classified as sudden and nonsudden death. End points were evaluated with a survey 2 years later, tallying cardiac events and death (response rate 96%, including use of medical records and family and autopsy reports). The data were analyzed both including and excluding respondents who had any diagnosis of cardiac disease prior to the 2-year window. Although no association was found between nonfatal MI and phobic anxiety, the risk of fatal CHD was increased threefold in men scoring highest for phobic anxiety, and this risk was weighted heavily toward the occurrence of sudden death. The authors explore how phobic anxiety and panic disorder might relate so specifically to sudden death, with potential mechanisms including hyperventilation (known to be a causative factor in coronary spasm), arrhythmia, and the psychological factors leading to these events.

The same hypothesis was tested using data from the Normative Aging Study in a nested case–control design involving over 1,800 male subjects ages 21–80 (Kawachi et al. 1994b). The same results were seen—men reporting higher levels of anxiety as compared with subjects reporting minimal or no anxiety had an increased risk of fatal CHD and particularly sudden death, whereas nonfatal MI and angina were not found to pose such a risk. The levels of risk were of similar magnitude to the Health Professional Study, although the authors noted in this case that while the specificity of the findings that relate to sudden death have now been corroborated by multiple studies, their own estimates of risk may be somewhat imprecise due to small numbers of sudden death. Although the findings from these studies cannot be applied to the general or female population, in both cases the authors acknowledged the need for study replication, especially in light of the disproportionate number of women diagnosed with panic disorder.

Aside from the phobic components of anxiety, research has also focused on the issue of worry as a component of anxiety, again drawing on data from the Normative Aging Study (Kubzansky et al. 1997). In the case of one prospective look at 1,759 men, those with the highest level of chronic worrying were found to have relative risk for nonfatal MI of 2.41 and for total CHD of 1.48 (including nonfatal MI and fatal CHD). Taken with the other studies, this suggests a pattern of morbidity that may differentiate between panic disorder and more generalized anxiety—that is, the cardiac risk associated with panic mimics the nature of the panic episode, sudden and acute. This research also raises the point that the presence of anxiety creates patterns of behavior that indirectly increase cardiac risk. Specifically, those participants scoring higher on measures of anxiety were also more likely to be smokers and to drink two or more alcoholic drinks per day. One strength of this study was to subdivide worry into categories (i.e., health, financial, social conditions); by elucidating the relative cardiac concerns for patients voicing different types of worry, it allows health care providers to better focus interventions (i.e., medical, social support) to the patients most at risk for repeat events.

Clinical Problems and Presentation

Myriad cardiac problems have been associated with panic and other anxiety disorders, including tachycardia and arrhythmia, cardiomyopathy (Kahn et al. 1990), stroke, and hypertension. Perhaps the most studied of these in the past has been mitral valve prolapse (MVP). Since the late 1970s, research addressed the question of whether MVP could explain the presence of panic attacks in many patients or whether anxiety disorders played some causative role in prolapse itself. Although findings varied significantly, in part due to differing approaches to defining MVP, the general consensus maintains that a significant number of patients with panic disorder do have MVP. Furthermore, there is ultimately no significant difference in clinical outcomes or treatment approaches on either psychiatric or cardiac parameters if panic disorder with MVP and panic disorder without MVP are seen as two discrete entities (Fyer et al. 1995). Treatment of anxiety may reduce the incidence of prolapse, but the assumption is that anxiety should be treated whether prolapse is present or not. Another complaint often associated with anxiety and panic, equally familiar to every medical and psychiatric intern in the hospital setting, is chest pain. The occurrence of chest pain in the context of anxiety can be explained by mechanisms including coronary vasospasm, increased sympathetic tone of cardiac microvasculature, and various effects of hyperventilation, all with the common underlying theme of ischemia (Huffman et al. 2002). One recent review (Katerndahl 2004) looked at lipid abnormalities in panic and anxiety, summarizing that although findings of whether hyperlipidemia occurs in panic disorder have been variable, multiple studies support a relationship between elevated cholesterol and increased levels of catecholamines (Hayward et al. 1989; Peter et al. 2002; Shioiri et al. 2000).

Perhaps the most interesting current research in this area focuses on several heart rate and reactivity parameters as they relate to panic and anxiety. HRV can be used as a measurement of the normal physiologic cardiac response to a stressor, and patients with reduced HRV have been identified as a group at high risk for sudden cardiac death (Dreifus et al. 1993; Routledge et al. 2002). In patients with phobic anxiety, this decreased HRV manifests as a higher resting heart rate or lower vagal tone (Kawachi et al. 1995). When such individuals are faced with a stressor, any increase in heart rate over an *already elevated level* will amount to a narrower range in fluctuation than in a nonanxious subject with a lower resting heart rate. In a prospective study using data from the Normative Aging Study, Kawachi et al. (1995) established a pattern of decreased HRV in men with phobic anxiety and built a case for this being the factor linking phobic anxiety with risk for sudden death.

Another study by Shapiro et al. (1996) reiterated the supremacy of vagal innervation as a regulator of cardiac stress response. The authors matched cardiac transplant recipients (all of whom have necessarily undergone a disruption of vagal innervation to the heart) with age- and gender-matched control subjects who had not undergone heart transplant. When faced with a stressful mental arithmetic task, posttransplant subjects showed a blunted response to the stressor as compared with normal control subjects as well as a delayed return to baseline heart rate when the stressor was removed. Because transplant would have no effect on circulating catecholamines, this suggests a far greater contribution of sympathetic and parasympathetic input to normal HRV than that of circulating neurohormones.

Implications for Treatment and Future Questions

The ultimate relevance of these findings will depend on whether treatment of panic and other anxiety disorders improves morbidity and mortality of comorbid cardiac disease. One study (Tucker et al. 1997) specifically addressed the aforementioned issue of autonomic input on HRV. In a comparison of patients with panic disorder both before and after treatment with paroxetine (17 patients, 4-week treatment at 20 mg/day), not only was an increase found in total parasympathetic activity after medication, but abnormalities in patients' baseline baroreflex function (i.e., increased sympathetic response to orthostasis) were normalized.

In another relatively small study both HRV and QT interval variability were examined in panic patients before and after treatment with cognitive behavioral therapy with or without an SSRI. An increase in QT interval variability as measured on electrocardiogram, like a decrease in HRV, can be predictive of risk for sudden cardiac death and is exacerbated by hyperventilation. When patients simulated panic attack by hyperventilation, the variance of the combined measures of the QT_c interval was reduced after treatment as compared with pretreatment levels (Sullivan et al. 2004). Although many details of how anxiety and panic may amplify the presence and progression of cardiac disease are still to be clarified, evidence is becoming more compelling that treatment of these disorders should be prioritized for both cardiac and psychiatric health.

In summary, much exciting work has been done to explore the interrelationships between our moods or emotional states and the functioning of our hearts. These interrelationships appear to be complex and to involve many systems with many possible mediators. The research done to date suggests many additional areas of exploration. The promise for enhanced understanding of the intricacies of mind–body interactions, accompanied by the possibility of novel modes of treatment, makes this truly one of the most exciting areas of modern medical scientific research.

REFERENCES

Agelink MW, Boz C, Ulrich H, et al: Relationship between major depression and heart rate variability: clinical consequences and implications for antidepressant treatment. Psychiatry Res 113:139–149, 2002

Alexopolous GS, Meyers BS, Young RC, et al: Vascular depression hypothesis. Arch Gen Psychiatry VOL:PAGES, 1997

Anda R, Williamson D, Jones D, et al: Depressed affect, hopelessness, and the risk of ischemic heart disease in a cohort of U.S. adults. Epidemiology 4:285–294, 1993

Balogh S, Fitzpatrick DF, Hendrick SE, et al: Increased heart rate variability with successful treatment in patients with major depression. Psychopharmacol Bull 29:201–206, 1993

Barefoot JC, Schroll M: Symptoms of depression, acute myocardial infarction, and total mortality in a community sample. Circulation 93:1976–1980, 1996

Barefoot JC, Larsen S, von der Lieth L, et al: Hostility, incidence of acute myocardial infarction, and mortality in a sample of older Danish men and women. Am J Epidemiol 142:477–484, 1995

Barefoot JC, Helms MJ, Mark DB, et al: Depression and long-term mortality risk in patients with coronary artery disease. Am J Cardiol 78:613–617, 1996

Berkman LF, Blumenthal J, Burg M, et al: Effects of treating depression and low perceived social support on clinical events after myocardial infarction: the Enhancing Recovery in Coronary Heart Disease Patients (ENRICHD) Randomized Trial. JAMA 289:3106–3116, 2003

Birtchnell J, Evans C, Kennard J: The total score of the Crown-Crisp Experiential Index: a useful and valid measure of psychoneurotic pathology. Br J Med Psychol 61:255–266, 1988

Carels RA, Sherwood A, Babyak M, et al: Emotional responsivity and transient myocardial ischemia. J Consult Clin Psychol 67:605–610, 1999

Carney RM, Freedland KE, Rich MW, et al: Ventricular tachycardia and psychiatric depression in patients with coronary artery disease. Am J Med 95:23–28, 1993

Carney RM, Blumenthal JA, Freedland KE, et al: Depression and late mortality after myocardial infarction in the Enhancing Recovery in Coronary Heart Disease (ENRICHD) Study. Psychosom Med 66:466–474, 2004

Chang PP, Ford DE, Meoni LA, et al: Anger in young men and subsequent premature cardiovascular disease: the precursors study. Arch Intern Med 162:901–906, 2002

Chaput LA, Adams SH, Simon JA, et al: Hostility predicts recurrent events among postmenopausal women with coronary heart disease. Am J Epidemiol 156:1092–1099, 2002

Connerney I, Shapiro PA, McLaughlin JS, et al: Survival free of recurrent cardiac events after CABG for patients with and without major depressive disorder. Lancet 358:1766–1771, 2001

Crown S, Crisp AH: A short clinical diagnostic self-rating scale for psychoneurotic patients: the Middlesex Hospital questionnaire. Br J Psychiatry 112:9171, 1956

Delisi SM, Konopka LM, O'Connor FL, et al: Platelet cytosolic calcium responses to serotonin in depressed patients and controls: relationship to symptomatology and medication. Biol Psychiatry 43:327–334, 1998

Dreifus LS, Agarwal JB, Botvinick EH, et al: Heart rate variability for risk stratification of life-threatening arrhythmias. American College of Cardiology Cardiovascular Technology Assessment Committee. J Am Coll Cardiol 22:948–950, 1993

Eckart A, Gann H, Riemann D, et al: Elevated intracellular calcium levels after 5-HT_2 stimulation in platelets of depressed patients. Biol Psychiatry 34:565–568, 1993

Eng PM, Fitzmaurice G, Kubzansky L, et al: Anger expression and risk of stroke and coronary heart disease among male health professionals. Psychosom Med 65:100–110, 2003

Everson SA, Goldberg DE, Kaplan GA, et al: Anger expression and incident hypertension. Psychosom Med 60:730–735, 1998

Ferketich AK, Schwartzbaum JA, Frid DJ, et al: Depression as an antecedent to heart disease among women and men in the NHANES I study. National Health and Nutrition Examination Survey. Arch Intern Med 160:1261–1268, 2000

Ford DE, Mead LA, Chang PP, et al: Depression is a risk factor for coronary artery disease in men: the precursors study. Arch Intern Med 158:1422–1426, 1998

Frasure-Smith N: The Montreal Heart Attack Readjustment Trial. J Cardiopulm Rehabil 15:103–106, 1995

Frasure-Smith N, Lesperance F, Talajic M: Depression following myocardial infarction: impact on 6-month survival JAMA 270:999–1005, 1993

Frasure-Smith N, Lesperance F, Talajic M: Depression and 18-month prognosis after myocardial infarction. Circulation 91:999–1005, 1995

Frasure-Smith N, Lesperance F, Prince RH, et al: Randomized trial of home-based nursing intervention for patients recovering from myocardial infarction. Lancet 350:473–479, 1997

Fyer AJ, Mannuza S, Coplan JD: Panic disorders and agoraphobia, in Comprehensive Textbook of Psychiatry, 5th Edition. Edited by Kaplan VA, Sadock BJ. Baltimore, MD, Williams & Wilkins, 1995, pp 1191–1204

Gidron Y, Davidson K: Development and preliminary testing of a brief intervention for modifying CHD-predictive hostility components. J Behav Med 19:203–220, 1996

Glassman AH, O'Connor CM, Califf RM, et al: Sertraline treatment of major depression in patients with acute MI or unstable angina. JAMA 288:701–709, 2002

Goodman M, Quigley J, Moran G, et al: Hostility predicts restenosis after percutaneous transluminal coronary angioplasty. Mayo Clin Proc 72:487, 1997

Gorman JM, Sloan RP: Heart rate variability in depressive and anxiety disorders. Am Heart J 140(suppl):77–83, 2000

Greenwald BS, Kramer-Ginsberg E, Krishnan RR, et al: MRI signal hyperintensities in geriatric depression. Am J Psychiatry 153:1212–1215, 1996

Haft JI: Cardiovascular injury induced by sympathetic catecholamines. Prog Cardiovasc Dis 17:73–86, 1974

Haft JI: Catecholamines, stress, platelets and coronary artery disease, in Platelets and Prostaglandins in Cardiovascular Disease. Edited by Mehta J, Mehta P. New York, Futura Publishing, 1981, pp 265–277

Hagerup LM: Coronary heart disease risk factors in men and women. From the population study in Glostrup, Denmark. Acta Med Scand Suppl 557:1–116, 1974

Hance M, Carney RM, Freedland KE, et al: Depression in patients with coronary heart disease: a 12-month follow-up. Gen Hosp Psychiatry 18:61–65, 1996

Harburg E, Gleiberman L, Russell M, et al: Anger coping styles and blood pressure in blacks and whites. Psychosom Med 53:153–164, 1991

Harter MC, Conway KP, Merikangas KR: Associations between anxiety disorders and physical illness. Eur Arch Psychiatry Clin Neurosci 253:313–320, 2003

Hayward C, Taylor CB, Roth WT, et al: Plasma lipid levels in patients with panic disorder or agoraphobia. Am J Psychiatry 146:917–919, 1989

Huffman JC, Pollack MH, Stern TA: Panic disorder and chest pain: mechanisms, morbidity, and management. Prim Care Companion J Clin Psychiatry 4:54–62, 2002

Ishihara S, Makita S, Imai M, et al: Relationship between natural killer activity and anger expression in patients with coronary heart disease. Heart Vessels 18:85–92, 2003

Jern C, Eriksson E, Tengborn L, et al: Changes of plasma coagulation and fibrinolysis in response to mental stress. Thromb Haemost 62:767–771, 1989

Kahn JP, Gorman JM, King DL, et al: Cardiac left ventricular hypertrophy and chamber dilatation in panic disorder patients: implications for idiopathic dilated cardiomyopathy. Psychiatry Res 321:55–61, 1990

Katerndahl D: Panic and plaques: panic disorder and coronary artery disease in patients with chest pain. J Am Board Fam Pract 17:114–126, 2004

Katon W, Sullivan M, Clark M: Cardiovascular disorders, in Comprehensive Textbook of Psychiatry, 5th Edition. Edited by Kaplan VA, Sadock BJ. Baltimore, MD, Williams & Wilkins, 1995, pp 1491–1501

Kawachi I, Colditz GA, Ascherio A, et al: Coronary heart disease/myocardial infarction: prospective study of phobic anxiety and risk of coronary heart disease in men. Circulation 89:1992–1997, 1994a

Kawachi I, Sparrow D, Vokonas PS, et al: Coronary heart disease/myocardial infarction: symptoms of anxiety and risk of coronary heart disease. The Normative Aging Study. Circulation 90:2225–2229, 1994b

Kawachi I, Sparrow D, Vokonas PS, et al: Decreased heart rate variability in men with phobic anxiety (data from the Normative Aging Study). Am J Cardiol 75:882–885, 1995

Knox SS, Siegmund KD, Weidner G, et al: Hostility, social support, and coronary heart disease in the National Heart, Lung, and Blood Institute Family Heart Study. Am J Cardiol 82:1192–1196, 1998

Konopka LM, Cooper R, Crayton JW: Serotonin-induced increases in platelet cytosolic calcium concentration in depressed, schizophrenic, and substance abuse patients. Biol Psychiatry 39:708–713, 1996

Koskenkuo M, Kaprio J, Rose RJ, et al: Hostility as a risk factor for mortality and ischemic heart disease in men. Psychosom Med 50:153–164, 1988

Kubzansky LD, Kawachi I, Spiro A, et al: Is worrying bad for your heart? Circulation 95:818–824, 1997

Kusumi I, Koyoma T, Yamashita I: Serotonin-stimulated Ca^{2+} response is increased in the blood platelets of depressed patients. Biol Psychiatry 30:310–312, 1991

Kusumi I, Koyoma T, Yamashita I: Serotonin-induced platelet intracellular calcium mobilization in depressed patients. Psychopharmacol (Berl) 113:322–327, 1994

Ladwig KH, Kieser M, Konig J, et al: Affective disorders and survival after acute myocardial infarction: results from the Post-Infarction Late Potential Study. Eur Heart J 12:959–964, 1991

Laghrissi-Thode F, Wagner WR, Pollock BG, et al: Elevated platelet factor 4 and B-thromboglobulin plasma levels in depressed patients with ischemic heart disease. Biol Psychiatry 42:290–295, 1997

Lavid CJ, Milani RV: Effects of cardiac rehabilitation and exercise training programs on coronary patients with high levels of hostility. Mayo Clin Proc 75:315–316, 2000

Leiker M, Hailey BJ: A link between hostility and disease: poor health habits? Behav Med 14:129–133, 1988

Lesperance F, Frasure-Smith N, Juneau M, et al: Depression and 1-year prognosis in unstable angina. Arch Intern Med 160:1354–1360, 2000

Malzberg B: Mortality among patients with involution melancholia. Am J Psychiatry 93:1231–1238, 1937

Markovitz JH: Hostility is associated with increased platelet activation in coronary heart disease. Psychosom Med 60:586–591, 1998

McFarlane A, Kamath MV, Fallen EL, et al: Effect of sertraline on the recovery rate of cardiac autonomic function in depressed patients after acute myocardial infarction. Am Heart J 142:617–623, 2001

Mendelson S: The current status of the platelet 5-HT$_{2A}$ receptor in depression. J Affect Disord 57:13–24, 2000

Mittleman MA, Maclure M, Sherwood JB, et al: Triggering of acute myocardial infarction onset by episodes of anger: Determinants of Myocardial Infarction Onset investigators. Circulation 92:1720–1725, 1995

Murphy JM, Neff RK, Sobol AM, et al: Computer diagnosis of depression and anxiety: the Stirling County Study. Psychol Med 15:99–112, 1985

Murphy JM, Monson RR, Olivier DC, et al: Affective disorders and mortality. Arch Gen Psychiatry 44:473–480, 1987

Musselman DL, Tomer A, Manatunga AK, et al: Exaggerated platelet reactivity in major depression. Am J Psychiatry 153:1313–1317, 1996

Musselman DL, Evans DL, Nemeroff CB: The relationship of depression to cardiovascular disease: epidemiology, biology, and treatment. Arch Gen Psychiatry 55:580–592, 1998

Musselman DL, Marzec UM, Manatunga A, et al: Platelet reactivity in depressed patients treated with paroxetine: preliminary findings. Arch Gen Psychiatry 57:875–882, 2000

Nashoni E, Aizenberg D, Sigler M, et al: Heart rate variability in elderly patients before and after electroconvulsive therapy. Am J Geriatr Psychiatry 9:255–260, 2001

Nashoni E, Aravot D, Aizenberg D, et al: Heart rate variability in patients with major depression. Psychosomatics 45:129–134, 2004

Nemeroff CB, Musselman D: Are platelets the link between depression and ischemic heart disease? Am Heart J 140:557–562, 2000

Nemeroff CB, Musselman DL, Evans DL: Depression and cardiac disease. Depress Anxiety 8 (suppl 1):71–79, 1998

Otte C, Marmar CR, Pipkin SS, et al: Depression and 24-hour urinary cortisol in medical outpatients with coronary heart disease: the heart and soul study. Biol Psychiatry 56:241–247, 2004

Owens MJ, Nemeroff CB: Role of serotonin in the pathophysiology of depression: focus on the serotonin transporter. Clin Chem 40:288–295, 1994

Penninx BW, Beekman AT, Honig A, et al: Depression and cardiac mortality: results from a community-based longitudinal study. Arch Gen Psychiatry 58:221–227, 2001

Peter H, Hand I, Hohagen F, et al: Serum cholesterol level comparison: control subjects, anxiety disorder patients, and obsessive-compulsive disorder patients. Can J Psychiatry 47:557–561, 2002

Pollock BG, Lagghrissi-Thode F, Wagner WR: Evaluation of platelet activation in depressed patients with ischemic heart disease after paroxetine or nortriptyline treatment. J Clin Psychopharmacol 20:137–140, 2000

Pratt LA, Ford DE, Crum RM, et al: Depression, psychotropic medication, and risk of myocardial infarction: prospective data from the Baltimore ECA follow-up. Circulation 94:3123–3129, 1996

Rajagapalan R, Brook R, Rubenfire M, et al: Abnormal brachial artery flow-mediated vasodilation in young adults with major depression. Am J Cardiol 88:196–198, 2001

Rapp MA, Dahlman K, Sano M, et al: Neuropsychological differences between late-onset and recurrent geriatric major depression. Am J Psychiatry 1624:691–698, 2005

Rosenman RH, Brand RJ, Jenkins CD, et al: Final follow-up experience of 8 1/2 years. JAMA 233:872–877, 1975

Routledge HC, Chowdhary S, Townend JN: Heart rate variability: a therapeutic target? J Clin Pharmacol Ther 27:85–92, 2002

Schins A, Honig A, Crijns H, et al: Increased coronary events in depressed cardiovascular patients: 5-HT$_{2A}$ receptor as missing link? Psychosom Med 65:729–737, 2003

Schulz R, Beach SR, Ives DG, et al: Association between depression and mortality in older adults: the Cardiovascular Health Study. Arch Intern Med 60:1761–1768, 2000

Shapiro PA, Sloan RP, Horn EM, et al: Effect of innervation on heart rate response to mental stress. Arch Gen Psychiatry 50:275–279, 1993

Shapiro PA, Sloan RP, Bigger JT Jr, et al: Cardiac denervation and cardiovascular reactivity to psychological stress. Am J Psychiatry 151:1140–1147, 1994

Shapiro PA, Sloan RP, Bagiella E, et al: Heart rate reactivity and heart period variability throughout the first year after heart transplantation. Psychophysiology 33:54–62, 1996

Shimbo D, Child J, Davidson K, et al: Exaggerated serotonin-mediated platelet reactivity as a possible link in depression and acute coronary syndromes. Am J Cardiol 89:331–333, 2002

Shioiri T, Fujii K, Someya T, et al: Serum cholesterol levels and panic symptoms in patients with panic disorder. J Affect Dis 58:167–170, 2000

Siegman AW, Anderson RA, Herbst J, et al: Dimensions of anger-hostility and cardiovascular reactivity in provoked and angered men. J Behav Med 15:257–272, 1992

Sloan RP, Shapiro PA, Bigger JT Jr, et al: Cardiac autonomic control and hostility in healthy subjects. Am J Cardiol 74:298–300, 1994

Strik JJMH, Denollet J, Lousberg R, et al: Comparing symptoms of depression and anxiety as predictors of cardiac events and increased health care consumption after myocardial infarction. J Am Coll Cardiol 42:1801–1807, 2003

Suarez EC, Williams RB: The relationships between dimensions of hostility and cardiovascular reactivity as a function of task characteristics. Psychosom Med 52:558–570, 1990

Sullivan GM, Kent JM, Kleber M, et al: Effects of hyperventilation on heart rate and QT variability in panic disorder pre- and posttreatment. Psychiatry Res 125:29–39, 2004

Thoresen CE, Friedman M, Gill JK, et al: The recurrent coronary prevention project: some preliminary findings. Acta Med Scand Suppl 660:172–192, 1982

Tucker P, Adamson P, Miranda R Jr, et al: Paroxetine increases heart rate variability in panic disorder. J Clin Psychopharmacol 17:370–376, 1997

Verrier RL, Mittleman MA: Life-threatening cardiovascular consequences of anger in patients with coronary heart disease. Cardiol Clin 14:289–307, 1996

Vitaliano PP, Russo J, Bailey SL, et al: Psychosocial factors associated with cardiovascular reactivity in older adults. Psychosom Med 55:164–177, 1993

Watkins LL, Grossman P, Krishnan R, et al: Anxiety reduces baroreflex cardiac control in older adults with major depression. Psychosom Med 61:334–340, 1999

Welin C: Independent importance of psychosocial factors for prognosis after myocardial infarction. J Intern Med 247:629–639, 2000

Welin CL, Rosengren A, Wilhelmsen LW: Behavioural characteristics in patients with myocardial infarction: a case-control study. J Cardiovasc Risk 2:247–254, 1995

Williams JE, Paton CC, Siegler IC, et al: Anger proneness predicts coronary heart disease risk. Circulation 101:200–234, 2000

Yeung AC, Vekshtein VI, Krantz DS, et al: The effect of atherosclerosis on the vasomotor response of coronary arteries to mental stress. N Engl J Med 325:1579–1580, 1991

Zellweger MJ, Osterwalder RH, Langewitz W, et al: Coronary artery disease and depression. Eur Heart J 25:3–9, 2004

Depression

A Major, Unrecognized Risk Factor for Osteoporosis?

Giovanni Cizza, M.D., Ph.D., MH.Sc.

DEPRESSION IS A common disorder affecting 5%–9% of women and 1%–2% of men (Robins et al. 1984). It carries a considerable risk of morbidity and is associated with a two- to threefold increase in all-cause, non-suicide-related mortality, especially in men (Zheng et al. 1997). Hypercortisolism, a frequent finding in depressed patients (Steckler et al. 1999), may possibly contribute to some of the somatic consequences of depression, including bone loss, possibly periodontitis, and alterations in body composition (Bjorntorp and Rosmond 2000; Chrousos and Gold 1998; Genco et al. 1999; Rosmond and Bjorntorp 1998).

Osteoporosis is a condition characterized by bone fragility and increased risk of bone fracture (Consensus Development Conference Diagnosis 1993). Prevention of this common disorder should be reserved for subjects at risk; however, there is debate regarding which risk factors warrant further evaluation by measurements of bone mineral density (BMD). Evidence suggests that the diagnosis of osteoporosis should be considered when one or more of the accepted risk factors are present (i.e., personal history or family history of prior fracture, thinness, or current smoking). The identification of unrecognized risk factors for osteoporosis is therefore central in the diagnosis of osteoporosis and has not only scientific interest but also considerable clinical consequences.

As recently reviewed, decreased BMD is more frequently seen in depressed subjects than in the general population (Cizza et al. 2001); since this review was published, the number of studies on this topic has doubled. Because low BMD is one of the most important risk factors for having an osteoporotic fracture (Ross et al. 1990), these studies suggest that depression may be a significant but ignored risk factor for osteoporosis. The purpose of this chapter is to summarize the most recent evidence of depression as a risk factor for osteoporosis and to balance this relevance of depression against currently established risk factors for osteoporosis. To accomplish this, we review the published studies on the association between depression and osteoporosis. The endocrine and immune factors potentially responsible for the bone loss observed in subjects with depression, such as hypercortisolism, hypogonadism, and growth hormone (GH) deficiency, are discussed in further detail.

DEPRESSION AND OSTEOPOROSIS

Depression, Bone Mineral Density, and Fractures

A database search was conducted on "osteoporosis and depression." The most important studies regarding this relationship are summarized in Table 7–1.

In the study by Schweiger et al. (1994), trabecular bone density, assessed by a single-energy quantitative computed tomography (CT) scan at the lumbar spine, was approximately 15% lower in 80 depressed men and women older than 40 years compared with 57 nondepressed men and women (Schweiger et al. 1994). Important factors with the potential to influence bone loss, such as smoking, lifetime history of excessive or inadequate physical exercise, or a history of estrogen treatment, did not affect the regression model, suggesting indirectly that depression supposedly had an effect on bone mass. However, age of onset and total duration of depression did not reveal a significant influence on bone mass. As pointed out in a subsequent letter (Hay 1996), both female and male comparison subjects had similar lumbar BMD values, which raises the question of just how representative the comparison group was to the general population.

A follow-up study conducted in 18 depressed men and women with 21 comparison subjects from the original cohort indicated that the bone loss over a period of at least 24 months was 10%–15% greater in the depressed

TABLE 7–1. Summary of reports on depression and osteoporosis

Authors	Subjects	Bone and other measurements	Study design/ setting	Evaluation of depression	Findings
Amsterdam and Hooper 1998	6 depressed patients (3 men, 3 women; mean age 41 years) 5 healthy control subjects (mean age 38 years)	Spine BMD by DEXA 24-hour urinary free cortisol	Cross-sectional	DSM-III-R; Hamilton Depression Scale score >20	No differences in BMD
Coelho et al. 1999	102 women, randomly selected (mean age 58 years)	BMD at the spine and hip by DEXA	Cross-sectional Population-based	Beck Depression Inventory Hopkins Symptom Checklist–90	25%–35% higher scores of depressive symptoms and depression in women with osteoporosis
Forsén et al. 1999	18,612 Norwegian women (50–101 years; mean age 66 years)	Hip fractures	Prospective (3 years of follow-up), population-based study of association between mental distress and hip fractures	Mental distress index No specific evaluation for depression	Women in the highest (10%) mental distress category have a twofold increase in hip fractures (CI=1.15, 3.29) after adjustment for use of medications, smoking, BMI, physical activity, and other factors

TABLE 7–1. Summary of reports on depression and osteoporosis *(continued)*

Authors	Subjects	Bone and other measurements	Study design/ setting	Evaluation of depression	Findings
Greendale et al. 1999	684 men and women fracture-free at baseline (mean age 70–79 years) Part of the MacArthur Study of Successful Aging	Self-reported fractures 12-hour urinary free cortisol at baseline	Prospective study, 7-year follow-up	Depressive symptoms, Hopkins Symptom Checklist–90	70 fractures seen in 7 years with 684 participants Subjects in the highest quartile of the higher baseline urinary free cortisol are predictive of increased risk of fractures, more so in men (OR: women 2.08; men 5.19).
Herran et al. 2000	19 antidepressant-free women (mean age 45 years) with a single depressive episode 19 control subjects matched by age, BMI, and postmenopausal state	Osteocalcin, bone specific alkaline phosphatase, telopeptide, type I collagen propeptide, serum cortisol	Cross-sectional	Hamilton Depression Scale (mean score, 21)	Higher cortisol and increased bone turnover as indicated by increased bone formation (osteocalcin) Increased bone resorption (telopeptide and cross-laps) in depressed women

TABLE 7–1. Summary of reports on depression and osteoporosis *(continued)*

Authors	Subjects	Bone and other measurements	Study design/ setting	Evaluation of depression	Findings
Halbreich et al. 1995	33 women (mean age 44 years) 35 men (mean age 36 years) with various mental disorders 21 depressed subjects	BMD by DPA at the spine and hip Testosterone (in men), estradiol (in women), prolactin, cortisol	Observational study of hospitalized patients	DSM-III-R	Low BMD in depressed subjects, especially in depressed men Inverse correlation between plasma cortisol and BMD
Kavuncu et al. 2002	42 depressed women (mean age 35 years) 42 healthy control subjects matched by age	BMD by DEXA Biochemical markers of bone turnover	Cross-sectional	DSM-IV; Hamilton Depression Scale score >14	No difference in BMD between depressed women and control women Increased bone resorption in women with depression
Michelson et al. 1996	24 depressed women (mean age 41 years) 24 control women (mean age 41 years)	BMD by DEXA at the spine, hip, and radius Biochemical markers of bone turnover Cortisol, parathyroid hormone, vitamin D, insulinlike growth factor-1	Cross-sectional	DSM-III-R	6%–14% lower BMD at the spine and hip in depressed women

TABLE 7–1. Summary of reports on depression and osteoporosis *(continued)*

Authors	Subjects	Bone and other measurements	Study design/ setting	Evaluation of depression	Findings
Reginster et al. 1999	121 healthy postmenopausal women (mean age 63 years)	BMD by DEXA at the spine and hip	Cross-sectional study of screened patients at a clinic for osteoporosis	General health questionnaire	No association between depressive symptoms and BMD
Robbins et al. 2001	Random sampling of 1,566 patients (65 years or older) enrolled in the Cardiovascular Health Study	BMD by DEXA of the total hip	Cross-sectional evaluation of a large cohort of elderly persons	Center for Epidemiological Studies Depression Scale (CES-Dm)	16% of subjects were depressed (CES-Dm score >10) 25% of men and 13% of women were osteoporotic (*T* score lower than 2.5 SD) Depression negatively associated with total hip BMD (stronger association in women than in men) Depression scores predictive of bone loss 2 years later Hip BMD 5% lower in subjects with depression

TABLE 7–1. Summary of reports on depression and osteoporosis *(continued)*

Authors	Subjects	Bone and other measurements	Study design/ setting	Evaluation of depression	Findings
Schweiger et al. 1994	27 depressed men (mean age 58 years) 53 depressed women (mean age 62 years) 30 nondepressed men (mean age 63 years) 58 nondepressed women (mean age 58 years)	Spine BMD by single-energy computed tomography scan	Cross-sectional	DSM-III-R	15% lower spine BMD in depressed subjects
Schweiger et al. 2000	10 depressed men (mean age 57 years) 8 depressed women (mean age 61 years) 14 nondepressed men (mean age 65 years) 7 nondepressed women (mean age 63 years)	Same as Schweiger et al. 1994	Longitudinal, at least 24 months Follow-up on Schweiger et al. 1994	Same as Schweiger et al. 1994	10%–15% greater bone loss over at least 24 months in depressed subjects 6% greater bone loss in depressed men compared with depressed women

TABLE 7–1. Summary of reports on depression and osteoporosis *(continued)*

Authors	Subjects	Bone and other measurements	Study design/ setting	Evaluation of depression	Findings
Vrkljan et al. 2001	31 depressed subjects (19 men, 12 women; mean age 37 years) 17 healthy male control subjects (mean age 39 years)	BMD (skeletal site not specified), plasma cortisol, 24-hour urinary free cortisol, and 1 mg Dexamethasone Suppression Test	Cross-sectional	Unspecified	Negative correlation between *T* score and years of antidepressant therapy
Yazici et al. 2003	25 premenopausal women with depression (mean age 31 years; duration of illness 6 months; Hamilton Depression Scale score 23) 15 control women matched by age, BMI, calcium intake, physical activity, and socioeconomic status	BMD at the spine and hip by DEXA Bone chemical markers: alkaline phosphatase, osteocalcin, and urinary deoxypyridinoline	Cross-sectional	DSM-IV	11%–12% lower BMD at the total femur and spine in depressed women 50% increase in bone resorption No differences in plasma cortisol or bone formation Bone loss not related to clinical indices of depression

TABLE 7–1. Summary of reports on depression and osteoporosis *(continued)*

Authors	Subjects	Bone and other measurements	Study design/ setting	Evaluation of depression	Findings
Whooley et al. 1999	467 depressed women (mean age 75 years) 6,949 control subjects (mean age 73 years)	BMD by DEXA at the spine and hip; incidence of falls and fractures	Prospective cohort over 3.7 years	Geriatric Depression Scale	Greater incidence of falls (OR=1.6) and fractures (OR=2.3) but no difference in BMD between depressed and nondepressed women

Note. BMD=bone mineral density; BMI=body mass index; CI=confidence interval; DEXA= dual energy X-ray absorptiometry; DPA=dual photon absorptiometry.

subjects than in the comparison subjects (Schweiger et al. 2000). Interestingly, the bone loss was also about 6% greater in depressed men than in depressed women. The small number of subjects included in the follow-up study limited the statistical power of the study, and this made the matching of control subjects by gender, age, and body mass index (BMI) uncertain.

In the third study, BMD was measured by dual energy X-ray absorptiometry (DEXA) at the spine, hip, and radius in 22 pre- and 2 postmenopausal women with previous or current major depressive disorder (Michelson et al. 1996). The 24 control subjects were matched by age, menopausal status, race, and BMI. BMD was 6%–14% lower at the spine and hip in the depressed women as compared with the control subjects. In 10 of the depressed premenopausal women, the BMD was at least 2 standard deviations (SD) below the young normal mean value, which corresponds to having severe osteopenia (Consensus Development Conference Diagnosis 1993). By contrast, no premenopausal women in the control group had a deficit of any similar magnitude. Because the risk of fracture increased by a factor of 1.5–3 for each SD reduction in BMD (Schuit et al. 2004), a substantial lifetime risk of osteoporotic fractures related to depression was already established before menopause. Markers of bone turnover, serum osteocalcin, urinary deoxypyridinoline crosslinks, and urinary N-telopeptide crosslinks of type I collagen were about 15%–30% lower in depressed women as compared with the control subjects, which indicated a reduced bone turnover in depressed patients. Although still within the normal range in many of the patients, the urinary free cortisol excretion was about 40% higher in depressed women than in control subjects.

In a multicenter, prospective cohort study of 7,414 elderly women, the association among depression, BMD, falls, and risk of fracture was examined (Whooley et al. 1999). The study employed the Geriatric Depression Score, a 15-item validated checklist of symptoms designed to detect depression in the elderly. BMD was measured by DEXA at the spine and the hip. Incident vertebral fractures were documented by follow-up spine X-rays, and all self-reported falls were ascertained at follow-up visits. The prevalence of depression was found to be 6%, a consistent value reported by others (Robins et al. 1984). Depressed women were more likely to fall (70% versus 59%) and had a greater incidence of vertebral (11% versus 5%) and nonvertebral (28% versus 21%) fractures compared with the control subjects. In the tertile of women with the highest BMI (above 27.6 kg/m^2), the depressed women showed a 3%–5% lower BMD in the spine and hip. However, there were no differences shown in BMD in the depressed and nondepressed women in the any other BMI tertiles, nor in the cohort as a whole. Correction for a greater propensity to fall in depressed women partly explained the increased risk of fracture in this group. Adjustment for the use of antidepressants, sedatives, and hypnotics did not influence the association between depression and fractures. The authors proposed that the falls in depressed women may be related to nonspecific factors such as poor adjustment to old age, suggesting that the association between depression and low BMD might therefore be limited to younger women and/or to women with more severe, long-lasting depression. Degenerative bone changes are known to make BMD measurements less reliable in the elderly (Drinka et al. 1992), which may in part explain the vague association between BMD and fracture in this population. Nevertheless, this study underscores the importance of depression as a risk factor for osteoporotic fractures.

In a study of 35 men and 33 women consecutively hospitalized for mental disorders, BMD was measured by dual-photon densitometry at the spine and hip (Halbreich et al. 1995). The patients had depression, schizophrenia, mania, schizoaffective disorder, or adjustment disorders. Patients with depression or schizophrenia had significantly lower BMD than age- and gender-matched control subjects, and in general the bone loss was more severe in depressed men than in depressed women. A negative association between serum cortisol levels and BMD was observed in depressed subjects of both genders. In men there was a positive correlation between BMD and testosterone levels, whereas in women estradiol levels were not correlated with BMD.

The relationship between osteoporosis and indices of well-being or psychopathology was evaluated in a community sample of 105 ambulatory middle-aged women (Coelho et al. 1999). Depressive symptoms were evaluated by the Beck Depression Inventory, and BMD was measured by DEXA at the spine and hip. The prevalence of osteoporosis in this sample was 47%, which corresponds to reports from epidemiological studies (Melton et al. 1992). Depression was significantly more common in women with osteoporosis than in women without it (77% versus 54%), corresponding to an odds ratio of depression in women with osteoporosis of 2.9 (95% confidence interval=1.0, 7.6); women with osteoporosis had about 25%–35% higher depressive scores than women with normal bone mass. The association between depression and osteoporosis was independent of other risk factors for osteoporosis such as age or BMI. No differences were found in the general well-being scores, suggesting that depression was not a consequence of pain or physical distress in these asymptomatic women with a diagnosis of osteoporosis based on BMD determination.

Depressive symptomatology was assessed by the General Health Questionnaire in 121 postmenopausal women who spontaneously attended a screening visit for osteoporosis (Reginster et al. 1999). BMD was measured by DEXA at the spine and hip. Importantly, this study did not find any association between depressive symptoms or a depressive trait and low BMD, suggesting that only fully developed depression is a risk factor for osteoporosis.

Three small, cross-sectional studies recently conducted in Europe all reported that lower spine and hip BMD were associated with increased bone resorption in subjects with depression. In addition, there was a negative correlation between T scores and years of antidepressant usage (Vrkljan et al. 2001; Yazici et al. 2003). At the National Institutes of Health Clinical Center, we are currently conducting the Premenopausal, Osteoporosis, Women, Alendronate, Depression (POWER) Study, a prospective study of premenopausal women with major depression and matched control subjects. This study has enrolled more than 90 patients and 40 control subjects who have been followed for up to 24 months. The first findings from this study are now being published (Eskandari at al., in press). Women with MDD, in addition to having low bone mass, exhibited other somatic abnormalities. These include greater waist circumference and abdominal fat as well as significantly higher levels of the prothrombotic factors plasminogen activator inhibitor 1 (PAI-1) and factor VIII, which were independent of body weight. These alterations in prothrombotic factors may lead to hypercoagulability and subsequent cardiovascular diseases.

Primary hyperparathyroidism, a secondary cause of osteoporosis, has recently been associated with depression (Wilhelm et al. 2004). In a consecutive series of 360 subjects who underwent surgery for primary hyperparathyroidism, 35 subjects met criteria for major depression. Postoperatively, 90% of these subjects stated that depression no longer affected their ability to work or do daily activities, and many had stopped antidepressant medications. The mechanisms leading to depression in subjects with primary hyperparathyroidism are unclear but may possibly involve the effects of hypercalcemia on the central nervous system.

Not only is there a correlation with major depression and osteoporosis, but "stress" per se is also associated with osteoporosis and fractures. In a large, population-based prospective study conducted in Norway, women with the highest level of stress—defined by a composite index that included life satisfaction, nervousness, loneliness, and sleep disorders—were 50% more likely to have hip fractures after correcting for many factors including the use of medications (Forsén et al. 1999). Specifically, the 10% of women with the highest mental distress had a twofold increased risk of hip fracture as compared with the 10% of women with the lowest mental distress category. Therefore, the mental problems that led to the use of psychotropic medications may have had a direct effect on fracture risk, independent of the medication. The potential causes were not explored in this study; however, in another large study conducted in elderly subjects one of the potential causes for bone loss was thought to be an increase in cortisol level (Greendale et al. 1999). In 684 elderly subjects who were part of the Mac-Arthur Study of Successful Aging, higher urinary cortisol at baseline was predictive of the possibility of increased fractures. Interestingly, the predictive value was stronger for men than for women.

If depression is a cause for osteoporosis, one would expect in principle some kind of dose relationship between these two factors, with more severe depression being associated with greater bone loss. The existence of such a link should be apparent in large, prospective studies of long duration. The Cardiovascular Health Study is a population-based prospective study of more than 5,000 subjects. In a random subset of 1,566 elderly subjects, depression was negatively associated with hip BMD, and the clinical severity of depression was predictive of future bone loss 2 years later (Robbins et al. 2001).

For completeness, it should be noted that although the preponderance of reports on bone mineral density in women with major depression have found an association between these two conditions, this is not universally the case. In a well-conducted cross-sectional study of 42 premenopausal women with major depressive disorder and 42 closely matched control subjects, there were no differences in BMD between the groups; however, bone resorption was increased in women with major depression (Kavuncu et al. 2002). In another small study with six depressed and five control subjects, no differences in BMD were observed (Amsterdam and Hooper 1998).

Psychotropic Medications, Falls, and Fractures

The use of antidepressants, sedatives, and hypnotics is associated with a greater incidence of falls and fractures, especially in the elderly (Leipzig et al. 1999). These medications can increase the risk of falling by various mechanisms, such as inducing orthostatic hypotension and syncope, dizziness, vertigo, blurred vision, ataxia, or somnolence. The association between hip fractures, falls, and the use of two commonly prescribed classes of antidepressants—tricyclic antidepressants (TCAs) and selective serotonin reuptake inhibitors (SSRIs)—was investigated in a case–control study (Liu et al. 1998). Each of the 8,239 elderly men and women treated in a hospital setting for hip fractures within a 12-month period was matched by age and gender to five control subjects. Hospital records determined comorbidity and risk of falls during the 3 years preceding the hip fracture. Most of the subjects were women (78%), and a large proportion of these women were older than 85 years (40%). Depression was approximately threefold more common in patients with hip fracture compared with control subjects (14.9% versus 5.7%). Of the patients with hip fracture, 6.6% had been exposed to SSRIs, 2.6% to secondary TCAs, and 9.0% to tertiary TCAs. After adjusting for confounding variables, the odds ratio for hip fracture was 1.5 in patients exposed to tertiary TCA and 2.4 in patients exposed to SSRI. Consistently, current users of antidepressants were at higher risk than former users, and there was no relationship between dosage of anti-depressants and the risk of hip fracture. Because BMD was not measured in this study, it was not possible to establish whether the increased risk of fracture observed in depressed subjects reflected an underlying association between low BMD and depression. In addition, the study design did not allow for conclusions on cause-relationship, resulting in the remaining possibility that depression was in part the result of a debilitating fracture.

In another case–control study of elderly residents of a long-term facility, the incidence of falls was correlated to the general health of the residents and their use of medications (Granek et al. 1987). Falls and use of medications were significantly related, and in general this association was more related to the prescribed drug than to the underlying condition that initially required the prescription. In addition, the use of three or more drugs increased the risk of falling. Only depression and osteoarthritis were consistently associated with an increase risk of falling across the 12 therapeutic classes of drugs, which suggests an independent effect of these two medical conditions.

In addition to potentially impairing arousal and balance and thereby increasing the risk of falls, many of the drugs prescribed for depression have an effect on calcium metabolism and possibly on BMD. It is, however, unclear whether this effect contributes to the fractures resulting from drug-related falls. Lithium carbonate, a drug primarily used for bi- and unipolar affective disorders, potentiates the calcium-induced inhibition of parathyroid hormone secretion (Brown 1981). Use of this drug has been associated with secondary hyperparathyroidism (Bendz et al. 1996; Mak et al. 1998). In a small cross-sectional study, BMD at the hip and spine, plasma calcium, and parathyroid hormone levels were all found to be normal in 23 patients (5 men and 18 women) treated with lithium for various affective disorders over a period of 0.6–9.9 years (Cohen et al. 1998). Thyroid stimulating hormone–suppressive dosages of thyroxine treatment have been found to have a negative effect on BMD (Greenspan and Greenspan 1999). Both thyroxine and triiodothyronine are sometimes used in dosages sufficient enough to suppress thyroid stimulating hormone as adjunct treatment to antidepressive therapy in patients with major depression or rapid-cycling bipolar disorders; however, little is known about the effects of this treatment on BMD. A small cross-sectional study evaluated the BMD in 10 (9 pre- and 1 postmenopausal) women with bipolar disorder treated with thyroxine for at least 18 months (Gyulai et al. 1997). In this small series of patients, the use of thyroxine was not associated with a decrease in BMD at any site. A similar study conducted in 26 women with affective disorders followed for a period of 12 months or longer reached similar conclusions (Gyulai et al. 2001).

Carbamazepine, phenytoin, and other anticonvulsants are sometimes used in certain forms of severe and psychotic depression, especially in elderly subjects. A large prospective study of elderly, community-dwelling women reported a greater rate of decline at the calcaneus and hip levels in continuous phenytoin users. Such a decline would increase the risk of hip fractures by 29% over 5 years among women 65 years and older (Ensrud et al. 2004).

Glucocorticoid-Induced Osteoporosis

Osteoporosis is a known consequence of chronic steroid usage. The mechanism of bone loss in glucocorticoid-induced osteoporosis is similar to that observed in endogenous Cushing's syndrome, and it has relevance to depression-related osteoporosis because hypercortisolism is commonly observed in depressed subjects (Cizza et al. 2001).

Bone Loss in Endogenous Cushing's Syndrome

Bone loss induced by hypercortisolism seems to be primarily caused by decreased bone formation (Ziegler and Kasperk 1998), whereas the relative contribution of increased bone resorption is unknown. Bone loss is more pronounced in trabecular than in cortical bone, and it more frequently leads to fractures (Hermus et al. 1995). The degree of bone loss correlates with the severity and the duration rather than the underlying cause of the condition (Ziegler and Kasperk 1998). This includes the factitious and drug-related form (Cizza et al. 1996). Bone mass is only partially regained once the disease is cured, and this process may take many years (Ziegler and Kasperk 1998).

In a series of 20 consecutive patients with Cushing's syndrome, the majority had a bone loss at the spine and femoral neck of similar magnitude (Hermus et al. 1995). Most patients did not fully regain BMD for up to 60 months after the correction of hypercortisolism. About 3 months after curative surgery, the level of osteocalcin and deoxypyridinoline increased, thus suggesting a reactivation of both osteoblastic and osteoclastic activity. Interestingly, depressed women experienced a more pronounced bone loss at the hip than was observed in subjects with Cushing's syndrome. This suggests that other biological factors in addition to hypercortisolism may contribute to bone loss in depressed subjects (Cizza et al. 2001).

Endogenous hypercortisolism is particularly deleterious to bone during growth. This was demonstrated in a longitudinal study of two identical twin girls, one of whom was diagnosed at 14 years of age with an adrenocorticotropic hormone–secreting pituitary adenoma (Leong et al. 1996). The affected twin had a spine BMD of –3.2 SD as compared with her age-matched control twin's mean value and a decrease in osteocalcin and deoxypyridinoline levels. Surgical cure led to increased bone formation as indicated by osteocalcin levels. However, more than 2 years after surgery, the BMD had only improved to a level of –1.9 SD. Additionally, the affected twin was 21 cm shorter, had a delayed puberty with suppressed gonadotropin and estradiol secretion, and exhibited a decrease in lean mass with an increase in fat mass.

Bone loss in Cushing's syndrome can be restored by specific anti-osteoporotic treatments. Bisphosphonates inhibit osteoclast-related resorption of bone (Fleisch 1998). In a prospective, open-label study, treatment with the bisphosphonate alendronate increased BMD at the hip and spine in patients with Cushing's syndrome (Di Somma et al. 1998). Thirty-nine consecutive patients with Cushing's disease (18 women and 21 men, ages 29–51 years) underwent selective adenomectomy. Cured patients ($n=21$) were randomly allocated for either treatment with alendronate (10 mg/day) or for no treatment. Noncured patients ($n=18$) were randomly assigned either to treatment with ketoconazole (200–600 mg/day [$n=8$]), which is an inhibitor of adrenal steroidogenesis, or to treatment with ketoconazole plus alendronate (10 mg/day [$n=10$]). BMD was lower at the hip and spine in all patients with Cushing's syndrome as compared with the healthy control subjects matched for age and BMI. Nine patients with Cushing's syndrome had osteoporosis, and 20 patients had osteopenia. Treatment with alendronate for 12 months increased BMD both in the cured patients and in the patients with active disease by 1.7%–2.4% at the spine and by 1.2%–1.8% at the hip. No improvements in BMD were observed in patients with the active disease who received only ketoconazole.

Bone loss is common in patients who receive long-term glucocorticoid therapy (Ziegler and Kasperk 1998). A 48-week, randomized, double-blind, placebo-controlled study of alendronate in 477 men and women (ages 17–83 years), all of whom received glucocorticoid therapy for various diseases, was recently published (Saag et al. 1998). Patients requiring long-term therapy (at least 1 year) with a daily dosage of at least 7.5 mg of prednisolone or its equivalent were followed for 48 weeks after randomization for daily placebo or alendronate treatment. All patients also received a daily supplement of 800–1,000 mg calcium and 250–500 IU of vitamin D. At baseline, 32% of the patients had osteoporosis and 16% had asymptomatic vertebral fractures. After 48 weeks of treatment with 10 mg/day alendronate, the BMD of these patients had increased by 2.9% at the spine, whereas the placebo group experienced a decrease of 0.4%. Similar results were obtained in a study of 141 subjects with glucocorticoid-induced osteoporosis who were treated with bisphosphonate etidronate (Adachi et al. 1997).

Hypercortisolism may affect the calcium metabolism by various mechanisms: decreased calcium absorption, increased calcium excretion, or transient hypocalcemia, all of which may trigger secondary hyperparathyroidism (Ziegler and Kasperk 1998). The conversion of vitamin D to its active metabolites is also affected by hypercortisolemia, resulting in further impairment of intestinal calcium absorption (Chan et al. 1984). Treatment with calcium and vitamin D are effective preventive treatments of glucocorticoid-induced osteoporosis (Sambrook et al. 1993). A total of 103 patients starting corticosteroid therapy were randomly assigned to receive 1,000 mg calcium per day and either oral calcitriol (0.5–1.0 g/day) plus intranasal salmon calcitonin (400 IU/day), calcitriol plus a placebo nasal spray, or a double placebo for 1 year (Sambrook et al. 1993). Treatment with calcitriol with or without calcitonin prevented spinal bone loss more effectively than did calcium alone. However, bone loss at the femoral neck and distal radius was not significantly affected by any of the treatments.

Potential Mechanisms of Bone Loss in Depression

One of the mechanisms by which depression may induce bone loss is hypercortisolism. Osteoporosis is in fact one known consequence of hypercortisolism, usually seen in the form of endogenous Cushing's syndrome or in chronic steroidal use. Bone loss in Cushing's syndrome seems to be primarily caused by decreased bone formation (Ziegler and Kasperk 1998), whereas the relative contribution of increased bone resorption is unknown. Bone loss is more pronounced in trabecular rather than in cortical bone, and it frequently leads to fractures (Hermus et al. 1995). The degree of bone loss correlates with the severity and the duration of this condition rather than with the underlying cause (Ziegler and Kasperk 1998). This includes the factitious and drug-related forms (Cizza et al. 1996). Bone mass is only partially regained once the disease is cured, and this process may take many years (Ziegler and Kasperk 1998). Depression does seem to be associated, in any case, with increased bone turnover, as indicated by a small cross-sectional study in 19 women with a moderate single depressive episode who reportedly had both increased markers of bone formation and turnover (Herran et al. 2000).

Hypercortisolism, a well-known biological correlate of depression, may be the consequence of a dysregulation of the corticotropin-releasing hormone (CRH) system and the hypothalamic-pituitary-adrenal axis (Chrousos and Gold 1992; see Figure 7–1). CRH hypersecretion and hypercortisolism in turn lead to inhibition of the reproductive axis and hypogonadism. The latter is an established risk factor for bone loss in both genders (Harper and Weber 1998). In addition, CRH hypersecretion and hypercortisolism tend to decrease the activity of the GH/insulinlike growth factor-1 axis, an important enhancer of bone formation (Chrousos and Gold 1992). In depression, a dysregulation of several inflammatory mediators, including interleukin-6 (IL-6), has been reported (Cizza et al. 2004a). This cytokine may also be implicated in some of the other medical consequences of major depression, such as cardiovascular disease and insulin resistance (Licinio and Wong 1999; Papanicolaou et al. 1998). IL-6, a major mediator of bone resorption, is elevated in depressed subjects, especially at an older age (Dentino et al. 1999). Increased sympathetic activity, often observed in depressed subjects (Wong et al. 2000), also tends to increase IL-6 secretion. As recently reviewed (Young and Korszun 2002), the reproductive axis is altered in women with major depression; however, no clear hormonal abnormalities have been documented in this axis in women with major depression. More studies are needed to evaluate the influence of depression on the age at menarche, menopause, the actual levels of circulating hormones, and on the proper rhythmicity of these hormones in women. When this reliable information on both the clinical characteristics and the length of the menstrual cycle in women with major depression is prospectively collected, it will serve to be very useful.

It recently has been reported that leptin, a hormone secreted by the white adipose tissue, inhibits bone formation through a central mechanism involving a hypothalamic relay (Ducy et al. 2000; Takeda et al. 2002). Intracerebroventricular administration of leptin to leptin-deficient (ob/ob) mice, a strain characterized by abnormally elevated bone mass, not only caused a marked decrease in food intake, an increase in energy expenditure, and a decrease weight loss, but it also induced bone loss. This effect is centrally mediated at the level of the hypothalamus and does not involve any direct effect of circulating leptin on the bone cells, for no leptin receptors are present on any osteoblasts or on any other bone cells. Because the secretion of leptin is increased at night in depressed subjects (Antonijevic et al. 1998), we hypothesize that an additional potential mechanism of bone loss in major depression may include central inhibition of bone formation by leptin. We have recently also speculated that seasonal changes in leptin levels may also be implicated in preserving bone mass during the winter in hibernating animals (Cizza et al. 2004b). Interestingly, the phenotype of the ob/ob mice also includes hypercortisolism and hypogonadism, two features also commonly seen in depressed subjects. Finally, both major depression and osteoporosis are likely to be associated with multiple genes, perhaps involved in the regulation of phospholipids (Horrobin and Bennett 1999). Whether depression and osteoporosis share a common genetic predisposition or are mediated by a common genetic setup remains to be determined.

The nature of the relationship between depression and osteoporosis has therefore been discussed based upon the novel perspective that depression may induce bone loss via all the potential biological mechanisms discussed earlier. Osteoporosis may be a silent disease and as such may go undiagnosed for quite a long time—that is, until pathological fractures ensue. Several of the studies reviewed have reported subjects with major depression in whom bone loss had gone asymptomatic and undiagnosed. It would be very difficult to sustain the notion that osteoporosis, a largely asymptomatic condition that the subject is not aware of having, could induce depressive symptoms. However, bone loss does eventually cause fractures, and if these fractures are present at the hip site, they could cause a very serious and disabling condition. For example, the quality of life is profoundly threatened by falls and hip fractures among elderly women (Salkeld et al. 2000). In this scenario, it is conceivable that clinical osteoporosis, especially if causing pain and physical disability, may induce reactive depressive symptoms. Whether such depressive symptoms are in turn followed by changes in cortisol and other hormones remains to be determined. In summary, the relationship between depression and osteoporosis, similarly to other clinical situations such as stroke, rheumatoid arthritis, and any other debilitating conditions in which depression coexists with a medical condition, should be seen as a bidirectional one, with the two conditions influencing each other in a vicious circle.

CONCLUSION

The studies outlined in this chapter found a consistent association between depression and osteoporosis, thus suggesting that depression is a substantial yet previously unrecognized risk factor for osteoporosis similar to other well-established risk factors such as low BMI (Ravn et al. 1999), smoking, or a family history of osteoporosis (Lindsay and Meunier 1998). Despite the evidence presented, the nature of the relationship between these two conditions is so far only partly elucidated. It is therefore important to note some of the limitations of the literature reviewed. To begin with, most studies were cross-sectional and were, by design, only able to indicate associations, not causal links. Furthermore, different diagnostic systems were used to diagnose and estimate the severity of depression. These differences may have contributed to the wide range of the prevalence of depression reported in subjects affected by osteoporosis. In several studies of bone loss, actively depressed subjects were pooled with subjects who only carried a historical diagnosis of depression. It is problematic to not know whether the impact of bone loss in those with current depression is equivalent to those who had a past history of depression. Retrospective evaluation of depression certainly has limited reliability, because it is solely based upon subject recollection. In addition, many of these studies were small, with heterogeneous patients. It is also important to note that those studies that used the diagnosis of major depression as the "threshold" for severity of depression, a far more severe condition than depressive symptomatology, found a clear association between depression and osteoporosis.

Finally, it should be noted that any review of the literature of this kind may have an inherent selective publication bias due to the fact that studies that fail to prove the original hypothesis, either because of lack of statistical power or because the hypothesis proved to be untrue, are three or more times less likely not to be published than positive studies, a phenomenon known as the "file drawer problem" (Thornton and Lee 2000). Therefore, it is possible that there may be unpublished studies of which we are unaware that may have failed to find an association between depression and osteoporosis or may have proven that there is no association between these two terms. To reduce the possibility of such bias, some researchers are now advocating that their institution use a registry listing of all the clinical studies started on a given research topic.

Within these limitations, all of the studies discussed raise questions that should be addressed in the future. The existence of a causal link between depression and osteoporosis as well as whether bone loss only occurs when a patient is actively depressed should be determined. Additionally, it should be established whether successful treatments of depression and/or use of antidepressants have any important impact on bone turnover. The prevalence of osteoporosis in depressed subjects should be further investigated as well as whether there exists a particular subgroup of these depressed subjects that are more at risk of becoming osteoporotic, because many may be candidates for treatment. Moreover, additional research is needed to understand the putative role of depression in male osteoporosis, because this condition is poorly understood and until recently has been relatively neglected, being labeled as "idiopathic" in approximately one-third of the subjects (Ebeling 1998; Orwoll et al. 2000). At a mechanistic level, it is crucial to understand the specific roles of the endocrine and paracrine factors responsible for the bone loss in depression and their relative contribution to the bone loss of decreased bone formation and of increased bone resorption.

Only prospective, long-term studies with sufficient statistical power will be able to answer these questions and allow the needed insight into the pathogenesis of bone loss in depression. In conclusion, the clinical evaluation of subjects with idiopathic bone loss, especially in premenopausal women and in young/middle-aged men, should also include an assessment of depression. Conversely, a history of nontraumatic fractures in a depressed subject should alert the physician to the possibility of undiagnosed osteoporosis.

REFERENCES

Adachi JD, Bell MJ, Bensen WG, et al: Intermittent etidronate therapy to prevent corticosteroid-induced osteoporosis. N Engl J Med 337:382–387, 1997

Amsterdam JD, Hooper MB: Bone density measurement in major depression. Prog Neuropsychopharmacol Biol Psychiatry 22:267–277, 1998

Antonijevic IA, Murck H, Friebos RM, et al: Elevated nocturnal profiles of serum leptin in patients with depression. J Psychiatr Res 32:403–410, 1998

Bendz H, Sjodin I, Toss G, et al: Hyperparathyroidism and long-term lithium therapy—a cross-sectional study and the effect of lithium withdrawal. J Intern Med 240:357–365, 1996

Bjorntorp P, Rosmond R: The metabolic syndrome—a neuroendocrine disorder? Br J Nutr 83 (suppl):S49–S57, 2000

Brown EM: Lithium induces abnormal calcium-regulated PTH release in dispersed bovine parathyroid cells. J Clin Endocrinol Metab 52:1046–1048, 1981

Chan SD, Chiu DK, Atkins D: Mechanism of the regulation of the 1 alpha, 25-dihydroxyvitamin D3 receptor in the rat jejunum by glucocorticoids. J Endocrinol 103:295–300, 1984

Chrousos GP, Gold PW: The concepts of stress and stress system disorders: overview of physical and behavioral homeostasis. JAMA 267:1244–1252, 1992

Chrousos GP, Gold PW: A healthy body in a healthy mind—and vice versa—the damaging power of "uncontrollable" stress. J Clin Endocrinol Metab 83:1842–1845, 1998

Cizza G, Nieman LK, Doppman JL, et al: Factitious Cushing syndrome. J Clin Endocrinol Metab 81:3573–3577, 1996

Cizza G, Ravn P, Chrousos GP, et al: Depression: a major, unrecognized risk factor for osteoporosis? Trends Endocrinol Metab 12:198–203, 2001

Cizza G, Mistry S, Eskandari F, et al: A group of 21 to 45 year old women with major depression exhibits greater plasma proinflammatory and lower anti-inflammatory cytokines: potential implications for depression-induced osteoporosis and other medical consequences of depression. Paper presented at the annual meeting of the Endocrine Society, New Orleans, LA, June 2004a

Cizza G, Mistry S, Phillips T: Serum markers of bone metabolism show bone loss in hibernating bears. Clin Orthop 422:281–283, 2004b

Coelho R, Silva C, Maia A, et al: Bone mineral density and depression: a community study in women. J Psychosom Res 46:29–35, 1999

Cohen O, Rais T, Lepkifker E, et al: Lithium carbonate therapy is not a risk factor for osteoporosis. Horm Metab Res 30:594–597, 1998

Consensus Development Conference Diagnosis: Prophylaxis and treatment of osteoporosis. Am J Med 94:636–638, 1993

Dentino AN, Pieper CF, Rao MK, et al: Association of interleukin-6 and other biological variables with depression in older people living in the community. J Am Geriatr Soc 47:6–11, 1999

Di Somma C, Colao A, Pivonello R, et al: Effectiveness of chronic treatment with alendronate in the osteoporosis of Cushing's disease. Clin Endocrinol (Oxf) 48:655–662, 1998

Drinka PJ, DeSmet AA, Bauwens SF, et al: The effect of overlying calcification on lumbar bone densitometry. Calcif Tissue Int 50:507–510, 1992

Ducy P, Amling M, Takeda S, et al: Leptin inhibits bone formation through a hypothalamic relay: a central control of bone mass. Cell 100:197–207, 2000

Ebeling PR: Osteoporosis in men: new insights into aetiology, pathogenesis, prevention and management. Drugs Aging 13:421–434, 1998

Ensrud KE, Walczak TS, Blackwell T, et al: Antiepileptic drug use increases rates of bone loss in older women: a prospective study. Neurology 62:2051–2057, 2004

Eskandari F, Mistry S, Martinez PE, Torvik S, Kotila C, Sebring N, Drinkard BI, Levy C, Reynold JC, Csako G, Gold PW, Horne M, Cizza G: Younger, premenopausal women with major depressive disorder have more abdominal fat and increased serum levels of pro-thrombotic factors: implications for greater cardiovascular risk. The P.O.W.E.R. Study. Metabolism (in press)

Fleisch H: Bisphosphonates: mechanism of action. Endocr Rev 19:80–100, 1998

Forsén L, Meyer HE, Sogaard AJ, et al: Mental distress and risk of hip fracture: do broken hearts lead to broken bones? J Epidemiol Community Health 53:343–347, 1999

Genco RJ, Ho AW, Grossi SG, et al: Relationship of stress, distress and inadequate coping behaviors to periodontal disease. J Periodontol 70:711–723, 1999

Granek E, Baker SP, Abbey H, et al: Medications and diagnoses in relation to falls in a long-term care facility. J Am Geriatr Soc 35:503–511, 1987

Greendale GA, Unger JB, Rowe JW, et al: The relation between cortisol excretion and fractures in healthy older people: results from the MacArthur studies. J Am Geriatr Soc 47:799–803, 1999

Greenspan SL, Greenspan FS: The effect of thyroid hormone on skeletal integrity. Ann Intern Med 130:750–758, 1999

Gyulai L, Jaggi J, Bauer MS, et al: Bone mineral density and L-thyroxine treatment in rapidly cycling bipolar disorder. Biol Psychiatry 41:503–506, 1997

Gyulai L, Bauer M, Garcia-Espana F, et al: Bone mineral density in pre-and post-menopausal women with affective disorder treated with long-term L-thyroxine augmentation. J Affect Disord 66:185–191, 2001

Halbreich U, Rojansky N, Palter S, et al: Decreased bone mineral density in medicated psychiatric patients. Psychosom Med 57:485–491, 1995

Harper KD, Weber TJ: Secondary osteoporosis: diagnostic considerations. Endocrinol Metab Clin North Am 27:325–348, 1998

Hay P: Treatable risk factor for osteoporosis? Am J Psychiatry 153:140, 1996

Hermus AR, Smals AG, Swinkels LM, et al: Bone mineral density and bone turnover before and after surgical cure of Cushing's syndrome. J Clin Endocrinol Metab 80:2859–2865, 1995

Herran A, Amado JA, Garcia-Unzueta MT, et al: Increased bone remodeling in first-episode major depressive disorder. Psychosom Med 62:779–782, 2000

Horrobin DF, Bennett CN: Depression and bipolar disorder: relationships to impaired fatty acid and phospholipids metabolism and to diabetes, cardiovascular disease, immunological abnormalities, cancer ageing, and osteoporosis. Possible candidate genes. Prostaglandins Leukot Essent Fatty Acids 60:217–34, 1999

Kavuncu V, Kuloglu M, Kaya A, et al: Bone metabolism and bone mineral density in premenopausal women with mild depression. Yonsei Med J 43:101–108, 2002

Leipzig RM, Cumming RG, Tinetti ME: Drugs and falls in older people: a systematic review and meta-analysis, I: psychotropic drugs. J Am Geriatr Soc 47:30–39, 1999

Leong GM, Mercado-Asis LB, Reynolds JC, et al: The effect of Cushing's syndrome on bone mineral density, body composition, growth, and puberty: a report of an identical adolescent twin pair. J Clin Endocrinol Metab 81:1905–1911, 1996

Licinio J, Wong ML: The role of inflammatory mediators in the biology of major depression: central nervous system cytokines modulate the biological substrate of depressive symptoms, regulate stress-responsive systems, and contribute to neurotoxicity and neuroprotection. Mol Psychiatry 4:317–327, 1999

Lindsay R, Meunier P: Osteoporosis: Review of the evidence for prevention, diagnosis and treatment and cost-effectiveness analysis. Osteoporos Int 8:11–21, 1998

Liu B, Anderson G, Mittmann N, et al: Use of selective serotonin reuptake inhibitors or tricyclic antidepressants and risk of hip fractures in elderly people. Lancet 351:1303–1307, 1998

Mak TW, Shek CC, Chow CC, et al: Effects of lithium therapy on bone mineral metabolism: a two-year prospective longitudinal study. J Clin Endocrinol Metab 83:3857–3859, 1998

Melton LJ III, Chrischilles EA, Cooper C, et al: Perspective: how many women have osteoporosis? J Bone Miner Res 7:1005–1010, 1992

Michelson D, Stratakis C, Hill L, et al: Bone mineral density in women with depression. N Engl J Med 335:1176–1181, 1996

Orwoll E, Ettinger M, Weiss S, et al: Alendronate for the treatment of osteoporosis in men. N Engl J Med 343:604–610, 2000

Papanicolaou DA, Wilder RL, Manolagas SC, et al: The pathophysiological roles of interleukin-6 in human disease. Ann Intern Med 128:127–137, 1998

Ravn P, Cizza G, Bjamason NH, et al: Low body mass index is an important risk factor for low bone mass and increased bone loss in early postmenopausal women: Early Postmenopausal Intervention Cohort (EPIC) study group. J Bone Miner Res 14:1622–1627, 1999

Reginster JY, Deroisy R, Paul I, et al: Depressive vulnerability is not an independent risk factor for osteoporosis in postmenopausal women. Maturitas 33:133–137, 1999

Robins LN, Helzer JE, Weissman MM, et al: Lifetime prevalence of specific psychiatry disorders in three sites. Arch Gen Psychiatry 41:949–958, 1984

Robbins J, Hirsch C, Whitmer R, et al: The association of bone mineral density and depression in an older population. J Am Geriatr Soc 49:732–736, 2001

Rosmond R, Bjorntorp P: Endocrine and metabolic aberrations in men with abdominal obesity in relation to anxio-depressive infirmity. Metabolism 10:187–193, 1998

Ross PD, Davis JW, Vogel JM, et al: A critical review of bone mass and the risk of fractures in osteoporosis. Calcif Tissue Int 46:149–161, 1990

Saag KG, Emkey R, Schnitzer TJ, et al: Alendronate for the prevention and treatment of glucocorticoid-induced osteoporosis. Glucocorticoid-Induced Osteoporosis Intervention Study Group. N Engl J Med 339:292–299, 1998

Salkeld G, Cameron ID, Cummin RG, et al: Quality of life related to fear of falling and hip fracture in older women: a time trade off study BMJ 320:241–246, 2000

Sambrook P, Birmingham J, Kelly P, et al: Prevention of corticosteroid osteoporosis: a comparison of calcium, calcitriol, and calcitonin. N Engl J Med 328:1747–1752, 1993

Schuit SC, van der Klift M, Weel AE, et al: Fracture incidence and association with bone mineral density in elderly men and women: the Rotterdam Study. Bone 34:195–202, 2004

Schweiger U, Deuschle M, Korner A: Low lumbar bone mineral density in patients with major depression. Am J Psychiatry 151:1691–1693, 1994

Schweiger U, Weber B, Deuschle M, et al: Lumbar bone mineral density in patients with major depression: evidence of increased bone loss at follow-up. Am J Psychiatry 157:118–120, 2000

Steckler T, Holsboer F, Reul JM: Glucocorticoids and depression. Baillieres Best Pract Res Clin Endocrinol Metab 4:597–614, 1999

Takeda S, Elefteriou F, Levasseur R, et al: Leptin regulates bone formation via the sympathetic nervous system. Cell 111:305–317, 2002

Thornton A, Lee P: Publication bias in meta-analysis: its causes and consequences. J Clin Epidemiol 53:207–216, 2000

Vrkljan M, Thaller V, Lovricevic I, et al: Depressive disorder as possible risk factor of osteoporosis. Coll Antropol 25:485–492, 2001

Wilhelm SM, Lee J, Prinz RA: Major depression due to primary hyperparathyroidism: a frequent and correctable disorder. Am Surg 70:175–180, 2004

Whooley MA, Kip KE, Cauley JA, et al: Depression, falls and risk of fracture in older women: Study of Osteoporotic Fractures Research Group. Arch Intern Med 159:484–490, 1999

Wong ML, Kling MA, Munson PJ, et al: Pronounced and sustained central hypernoradrenergic function in major depression with melancholic features: relation to hypercortisolism and corticotropin-releasing hormone. Proc Natl Acad Sci 97:325–30, 2000

Yazici KM, Akinci A, Sutcu A, et al: Bone mineral density in premenopausal women with major depressive disorder. Psychiatry Res 117:271–275, 2003

Young EA, Korszun A: The hypothalamic-pituitary-gonadal axis in mood disorders. Endocrinol Metab Clin North Am 31:63–78, 2002

Zheng D, Ferguson JE, Macera CA, et al: Major depression and all-cause mortality among white adults in the United States. Ann Epidemiol 7:213–218, 1997

Ziegler R, Kasperk C: Glucocorticoid-induced osteoporosis: prevention and treatment. Steroids 63:344–348, 1998

CHAPTER

8

Cognitive Impairment and the Phenomenology and Course of Geriatric Depression

George S. Alexopoulos, M.D.

THE U.S. SURGEON GENERAL'S (1999) Report on Mental Health noted that "The relationship between somatic illness and mental disorders is likely to be reciprocal, but the mechanisms are far from understood" (p. 350). Indeed, geriatric depression is more common in medical settings than in the community (Alexopoulos 1996). Aging is associated with lesions or other brain changes that may contribute to depression (Alexopoulos 1990; Coffey et al. 1990). For this reason, late life can function as a laboratory of nature. The findings on the interaction between medical illnesses and geriatric depression have been used to generate pathogenetic hypotheses both on the mechanisms of depression and the pathophysiology of treatment response.

This work was supported by National Institute of Mental Health grants RO1 MH65653, RO1 MH42819, RO1 MH51842, and P30 MH68638 and by the Sanchez Foundation.

THE LATE-ONSET DEPRESSION HYPOTHESIS

Depression first occurring in late life has been an initial early focus of research seeking to understand the relationship between depression and aging-related medical and neurological disorders. It was hypothesized that late-onset depression is a heterogeneous syndrome that includes patients with cognitive impairment and neurological stigmata that may or may not be clinically evident when the depression first appears (Alexopoulos 1990). Although some disagreement exists (Conwell et al. 1989; Greenwald et al. 1988; Herrmann et al. 1989), elderly patients with late-onset depression have been found to have more cognitive (Alexopoulos et al. 1993a, 1993b) and neuroradiological abnormalities (Alexopoulos et al. 1992; Coffey et al. 1990; Jacoby and Levy 1980), more neurosensory hearing impairment (Kalayam et al. 1995), greater disability (Alexopoulos et al. 1996a), a lower familial prevalence of mood disorders (Baron et al. 1981), and less person-ality dysfunction (Abrams et al. 1994) than elderly patients with early-onset depression.

Late-onset depressive symptoms or syndromes often are a prodrome of cognitive decline. In elderly community-residing women, depressive symp-toms were associated with poorer cognitive function at baseline and with cognitive decline over a 4-year period (Yaffe et al. 1999). Depressive symp-toms, and depressed mood in particular, predicted cognitive decline 3 years later (Bassuk et al. 1998). Among community-residing elders, depressed mood was a predictor of dementia 5 years later (Devanand et al. 1996). In individuals with subclinical cognitive dysfunction, those who developed dementia 3 years later had more depressive symptoms (Ritchie et al. 1999). Recent history of depression is associated with increased incidence of Alz-heimer's disease (Jorm 2001; Jorm et al. 1991; Kokmen et al. 1991; Speck et al. 1995). Among elderly twins, those without an *ApoEε4* allele and late-onset depression had 2.95 times higher risk for Alzheimer's disease than those without history of depression (Steffens et al. 1997). Individuals with late-life depression and transient cognitive impairment frequently develop either Alzheimer's disease or vascular dementia within a few years after the onset of depression (Alexopoulos et al. 1993a, 1993b; Kral and Emery 1989; Reding et al. 1985). Taken together, these observations suggest that some late-life depressive syndromes often are early manifestations of dementing disorders.

There is some evidence that age and late-onset of first episode influence the course of geriatric depression. Among depressed elderly patients, age, age at onset, and chronicity of the index episode predicted time to recovery;

the strongest predictor of slow recovery was late age at onset. However, age at onset may not be a predictor of recovery in younger adults (Alexopoulos et al. 1996b). Finally, advanced age appears to be risk factor for recurrence of geriatric depression (Mueller et al. 2004).

The late-onset hypothesis has several limitations. On a methodological level, onset of depression may be difficult to identify, especially when the first episode of depression is of mild severity (Wiener et al. 2001). On a substance level, two concerns originate from the assumptions of homogeneity and independence of successive depressive episodes. The assumption of homogeneity is unfounded, because some depressive episodes during the early life of an individual (e.g., postpartum depression) may have different mechanisms than episodes occurring in late life of the same individual (e.g., depression following a silent brain infarct). Equally unfounded is the assumption that episodes of depression occurring across the life span of an individual are independent. It can be argued that early-onset, recurrent depression not only fails to protect from brain events associated with late-onset depression but may even predispose to such events. For example, recurrent depression has been associated with reduced volume of the hippocampus and the amygdala structures (Sheline 2003; Sheline et al. 1996, 1999). Abnormalities in these structures may increase vulnerability and, when other aging-related abnormalities occur, lead to the clinical expression of a depressive episode. Similar interactions between depression-induced changes and other brain pathology have been proposed in the dementia literature, where early-onset depression appears to predispose to dementing disorders (Jorm 2001; Jorm et al. 1991; Speck et al. 1995; van Duijn et al. 1994). These methodological and substantive limitations of the late-onset hypothesis may explain some of the negative findings in studies comparing the clinical manifestations and outcomes of late-onset and early-onset geriatric depression (Conwell et al. 1989; Greenwald et al. 1988; Herrmann et al. 1989).

Although the late-onset hypothesis did not propose a mechanistic theory for depression, it provided a conceptual step for identifying more homogeneous groups of geriatric depression. Research in this area focused on cognitive impairment as well as the course of illness.

TOWARD A MODEL OF GERIATRIC DEPRESSION

Studies related to the late-onset hypothesis used neurological comorbidity as a research window into the brain. However, it has been clear that single lesions are unlikely to be the direct cause of depression. There are several reasons for the absence of a direct lesion–depressive syndrome relationship. Brain abnormalities associated with depression affect high-level redundant and interactive neural systems. Redundancy, interaction with other neural networks, and plasticity may explain why individuals with almost identical brain lesions do not all develop depressive syndromes and those who develop depressive syndromes have heterogeneous clinical presentation as other centers can assume some of the functions of the lesioned circuitry. Another reason for the lack of a direct brain lesion–depression relationship is the contribution of peripheral medical illnesses that both directly and through the resultant disability facilitate the development of psychopathology. Moreover, the individual's coping skills may facilitate or protect from depression when a brain insult occurs. Late life is full of adversity that challenges the individual's coping mechanisms. A person with a history of successful adaptation may be less likely to develop depression than a passive person with limited coping resources easily overwhelmed by stressors. Finally, personal or family history of psychiatric disorders may be an additional contributing factor. This is the case in stroke, where personal and family history of a depressive disorder has been shown to increase the likelihood to develop poststroke depression at least as much as the site of lesion (Morris et al. 1992).

The complexity of geriatric depression suggests that the search for understanding its biology should focus on brain abnormalities predisposing to depression rather than lesions directly leading to depression. Such brain abnormalities may be caused by diverse processes commonly occurring in late life, including vascular, inflammatory (cytokine hypothesis), autoimmune, and endocrine processes. Brain abnormalities predisposing to depression may facilitate the development of the state-dependent brain changes transiently occurring during depressive episodes—that is, hypermetabolism in ventral limbic structures and hypometabolism of dorsal neocortical structures (Mayberg 2001). Moreover, predisposing brain abnormalities may influence the clinical presentation, treatment response, and course of geriatric depression.

Brain abnormalities predisposing to depression need not be limited to a single brain region. Abnormalities in one region may influence other functionally connected regions. Moreover, elderly patients may have abnormalities in more than one brain region, creating complex interactions predisposing to depression. Abnormalities in frontostriatal structures, the amygdala, and the hippocampus have been identified in patients with depressive disorders. These abnormalities may predispose to depression and facilitate its expression, especially when psychosocial and/or nonspecific medical contributors are also present.

ROLE OF COGNITIVE IMPAIRMENT
- -

Our work on abnormalities predisposing to depression was guided by clinical observations of associations between geriatric depression and cognitive impairment. For heuristic reasons, we assumed that brain abnormalities underlying the cognitive impairment of geriatric depression may predispose to the syndrome and influence its clinical presentation and course.

Cognitive deficits often are part of the clinical presentation of late-life depression. The combination of impaired cognition and depressive symptoms doubles in frequency at each 5-year interval after the age of 70 in community residents (Arve et al. 1999); combined depression and cognitive dysfunction is present in 25% of 85-year-old subjects. Geriatric depression has been associated with impairment in short-term memory (Hart et al. 1987), visuospatial skills (Boone et al. 1995; Lesser et al. 1996), and psychomotor functioning (Nebes et al. 2001; van Ojen et al. 1995). Recent studies of geriatric patients with major depression have documented disturbances in executive functioning, including impaired planning, organizing, initiating, sequencing, and shifting (Butters et al. 2000; Goodwin 1997). Specifically, severely depressed older adults present impairments in attentional set-shifting, verbal fluency, psychomotor speed, recognition memory, and planning on the Cambridge Neuropsychological Test Automated Battery (CANTAB; Beats et al. 1996). On the same battery, moderately depressed middle-aged patients have demonstrated deficits in planning, strategy development, spatial working memory, and verbal fluency despite exhibiting intact set-shifting abilities and psychomotor speed (Elliott et al. 1996). In yet another study, severely depressed patients displayed set-shifting deficits but intact verbal fluency (Jones et al. 1988). Approximately 42% of elderly subjects with major depression also have abnormal initiation/perseveration scores, an aspect of executive dysfunction (Alexopoulos et al. 2002a).

In an attempt to dissect and describe specific executive dysfunctions of geriatric depression, we compared cognitive functions of elders with major depression with those of younger depressed patients as well as those of older and younger normal control subjects (Lockwood et al. 2002). Relative to their depressed younger counterparts and to the nondepressed elderly group, depressed elderly subjects had disproportionately poorer scores on neuropsychological tasks associated with frontal lobe functioning. In particular, depressed elders had greater impairment in response initiation and inhibition, active switching, processing speed, and complex mental manipulation, all executive functions of the inhibitory control and focused effort domains (Lockwood et al. 2002). In contrast, depressed younger patients presented isolated difficulties in maintaining their level of performance over time as well as mild weaknesses in perceptual sensitivity (i.e., auditory and visual signal detection) relative to the nondepressed younger group. This finding is in keeping with mild impairment in selective attention. Older age, regardless of mood state, was associated with mild difficulties in selective and sustained attention.

Executive dysfunction may influence the clinical presentation of the depressive syndrome. Patients with the depression and executive dysfunction have more psychomotor retardation, reduced interest in activities, and more pronounced disability but a less prominent vegetative syndrome compared with depressed elderly patients without significant executive dysfunction (Alexopoulos et al. 2002b; Krishnan et al. 1997). The neuropsychological deficits of these patients consisted of impaired verbal fluency and visual naming as well as poor performance on tasks of initiation and perseveration. Depressive ideation, psychomotor retardation, and executive dysfunction were associated with compromised instrumental activities of daily living (Alexopoulos et al. 1996a; Kiosses et al. 2000, 2001). Although a frontal lobe syndrome can exist independently of depression, patients of this study met criteria for both major depression and executive dysfunction and had sad mood, hopelessness, helplessness, and worthlessness of similar severity to patients with major depression without impairment in executive performance. These observations suggest that depressive symptoms and executive impairment originate from related brain dysfunctions in at least a subgroup of elderly patients.

Treatment studies of late-life depression indicate that a substantial number of patients continue to experience neuropsychological deficits even after improvement of mood-related symptoms (Butters et al. 2000; Murphy and Alexopoulos 2003; Nebes et al. 2003). This observation is consistent with the view that the brain abnormalities underlying executive impairment predispose to depression rather than being state-dependent changes.

The mechanisms underlying executive dysfunction in geriatric depression are not well understood. A potential mechanism may involve the cortico-striatal-pallido-thalamo-cortical (CSPTC) pathways, because these networks are implicated in the development of spontaneous performance strategies demanded by executive tasks. In particular, response initiation and inhibition are mediated by the orbitofrontal pathway; the anterior cingulate is critical to response inhibition, focused attention, detection of error, and consistency of response; and response sequencing, focusing, and active switching are influenced by the dorsolateral frontal cortex (Cohen et al. 1998). Subcortical systems, including the thalamic nuclei, serve a gatekeeping function for incoming sensory information through which motor control signals processed in the basal ganglia are relayed by the thalamus to frontal and supplementary motor areas, while motor response selection is reliant on the caudate nucleus (Cohen et al. 1998). Along with functional relationships of the CSPTC pathways to executive task performance, clinical observations, structural and functional neuroimaging, and neuropathology studies implicate CSPTC dysfunction in depression.

Neurological disorders compromising CSPTC circuitry are often complicated by depression (Alexopoulos 2002). Stroke of the basal ganglia and their frontal projections (Starkstein and Robinson 1993) often lead to both depression and executive dysfunction. Stroke of the caudate head is the location most likely to be complicated by depression (Starkstein et al. 1988). A large percentage of depressed patients with silent cerebral infarction have lesions in the perforating arteries territory (Fujikawa et al. 1993), which supply the basal ganglia and their frontal connections. Subcortical dementing disorders, including vascular dementia, Parkinson's disease, and Huntington's disease, are more likely to result in depression than cortical dementias (Sobin and Sackeim 1997). Similarly, Alzheimer's patients with subcortical atrophy are more likely to develop depression than are Alzheimer's patients with less-impaired cortical structures (Reichman and Coyne 1995; Starkstein et al. 1995).

In addition to these clinical observations, structural neuroimaging and neuropathology studies suggest that abnormalities of subcortical structures, part of the CSPTC networks, are associated with depression and executive dysfunction (Alexopoulos 2002). Low volumes of the subgenual anterior cingulate have been reported in younger depressed subjects compared with control subjects (Drevets et al. 1997). Reduction in glia of the subgenual prelimbic anterior cingulate gyrus has been demonstrated in unipolar depressed patients (Rajkowska et al. 1999). Geriatric studies report similar findings. Reduced volumes of the white and gray matter of the anterior cingulate and the orbitofrontal cortex have been observed in depressed elderly patients compared with nondepressed elderly subjects (Ballmaier et al. 2004). Others have reported bilateral reduction in orbitofrontal cortex volume in depressed elderly patients compared with control subjects (Lai et al. 2000). Smaller volumes of the caudate head (Krishnan et al. 1992) and putamen (Husain et al. 1991) have been reported in depressed younger patients compared with control subjects. Bilateral white matter hyperintensities are prevalent in geriatric depression and mainly occur in subcortical structures and their frontal projections (Coffey et al. 1998; Kumar et al. 2000; Steffens et al. 1999), especially the medial orbitofrontal cortex (MacFall et al. 2000). Subcortical white matter hyperintensities have been associated with executive dysfunction (Boone et al. 1992; Lesser et al. 1996) and disability (Steffens et al. 2002b). Autopsy studies in depressed patients have demonstrated abnormalities in neurons of the dorsolateral prefrontal cortex (Ongur et al. 1998), an area participating in the performance of executive tasks.

In addition to subcortical abnormalities, depressed patients have reduced volumes of limbic and paralimbic structures. The amygdala volume was found to be enlarged in first episode of major depression (Frodl et al. 2002), whereas reduction of the amygdala volume has been reported with increased duration of depression (Sheline et al. 1999). Reduced hippocampal volume has been found in depressed elderly (Steffens et al. 2001, 2002a) and younger adults (Sheline 2000). In younger adults, hippocampal volume was not low during the first episode but declined over several years despite administration of antidepressant treatment (MacQueen et al. 2003). Small left hippocampal volume in geriatric depression was associated with later development of dementia (Steffens et al. 2002a).

Functional neuroimaging studies suggest that depressed states are accompanied by increased metabolism in limbic structures and reduced metabolism of dorsal neocortical structures. Increased metabolism has been documented in the amygdala (Drevets 1999, 2000; Wu et al. 1992), the pregenual and subgenual anterior cingulate (Drevets and Raichle 1998), and the posterior orbital cortex (Drevets et al. 1992; Ebert et al. 1991) of depressed younger adults as well as the posterior cingulate and the medial cerebellum (Bench et al. 1992; Buchsbaum et al. 1997). Unlike limbic structures, the dorsal anterior cingulate, the lateral and dorsolateral prefrontal cortex, and the caudate nucleus have reduced metabolism during depression (Drevets 2000; Liotti and Mayberg 2001; Mayberg 2001). Metabolic increases have been observed in the subgenual cingulate and ventral and mid-posterior insula, and decreases have been observed in the right prefrontal dorsal, dorsal anterior cingulate, posterior cingulate, and inferior parietal regions (Goldapple et al. 2004; Mayberg 2001).

Some of the functional neuroimaging abnormalities observed during depressive states may mediate aspects of cognitive and mood symptoms occurring during depression (Alexopoulos 2002). During an executive function task, depressed younger adults failed to activate the striatum and the cingulate and only weakly activated other prefrontal and posterior cortical areas compared with control subjects (Elliott et al. 1997). Reduced bilateral activation of the dorsal anterior cingulate and the hippocampus was recently reported in severely depressed, nondemented elderly patients performing a word activation task (de Asis et al. 2001). Cognitive impairment was shown to be correlated with decreased activity in the left medial prefrontal region, whereas psychomotor retardation was correlated with decreased activity in the left anterolateral cortex in depressed cognitive impaired patients (Dolan et al. 1992). Anxiety occurring in the context of depression of younger adults was associated with increased activity in the right posterior cingulate and bilateral inferior parietal areas (Bench et al. 1992). These observations suggest that some depressive symptoms are associated with rather specific functional brain abnormalities.

Most of the structures subserving mood regulation and executive processing are interconnected. Reciprocal pathways link midline limbic structures with brainstem, striatal, paralimbic, and neocortical sites (Carmichael and Price 1995; Pandya and Yeterian 1996; Rolls 1990). Limbic structures participate in evaluating the emotional value (reward-related significance) of stimuli and in organizing aspects of stress response (Rolls 1990). Neocortical structures such as the dorsal anterior cingulate are activated during tasks requiring discriminative attention and selection of action, and the lateral and dorsolateral prefrontal cortex is activated when visual or visuospatial activation is maintained in working memory and processed (Drevets and Raichle 1998). Besides neuroanatomical evidence of connections among limbic and neocortical structures, treatment studies of depression suggest that reciprocal changes occur in these structures when depressed states are brought to remission. Following antidepressant treatment, reduced metabolism of limbic structures occurs and is accompanied by changes in neocortical structures (Goldapple et al. 2004; Mayberg et al. 1999).

On a clinical level, depressive symptoms can be reduced by cognitive therapy, which has a "top-down" cortical influence on limbic pathways (Mayberg et al. 1999), as well as with pharmacological therapies, which have a "bottom-up" (or combined bottom-up and top-down) effect because their principal sites of action are the dorsal raphe and the locus coeruleus (Chaput et al. 1991; Hyman and Nestler 1996). Based on these observations, it has been proposed that abnormalities in the reciprocal relationship between ventral limbic and dorsal cortical neural systems is a critical physiological disturbance in depression (Drevets 2000; Mayberg 2001; McEwen 2003). Microstructural white matter abnormalities compromising connections between limbic and dorsal cortical structures may interfere with limbic–dorsal balance and lead to chronic depressive syndromes.

FRONTOSTRIATAL-LIMBIC DYSFUNCTION AND THE COURSE OF GERIATRIC DEPRESSION

The studies we have described identified an association between clinical, neuroanatomical, and functional aspects of frontostriatal-limbic pathways and geriatric depression. However, cross-sectional comparisons of depressed elders with control subjects, by themselves, are insufficient to demonstrate that frontostriatal-limbic dysfunction is a predisposing factor to geriatric depression. Such an argument could only be supported by demonstrating a relationship between indices of frontostriatal-limbic dysfunction and a biological parameter serving as the validating "gold rule" for geriatric depression. In the absence of such a "gold rule," course of illness may function as an alternative.

A series of studies suggest that executive dysfunction, the clinical expression of frontostriatal abnormalities, influences adversely the course of geriatric depression (Alexopoulos 2003). In an early study, we investigated the relationship of clinical, neuropsychological, and electrophysiological measures of frontostriatal dysfunction to treatment response of geriatric depression (Kalayam and Alexopoulos 1999). Subjects were examined prior to and after receiving 6 weeks of adequate antidepressant treatment and were compared with elderly control subjects with no history or presence of psychiatric disorders. In this study, abnormal initiation/perseveration score on the Mattis Dementia Scale (Mattis 1989), psychomotor retardation, and long latency of the P300 auditory-evoked potential predicted 58% of the variance in change in depression scores from baseline to 6 weeks. Depressed patients who remained symptomatic after antidepressant treatment had more abnormal initiation/perseveration scores and longer P300 latency than depressed patients who achieved remission with antidepressant treatment and healthy control subjects.

Limitations of the study included the small number of subjects, the use of multiple antidepressants (albeit at adequate dosages), and the limited assessment of executive dysfunction. For this reason, we pursued a replication of the original findings in a new and larger group of elders with major depression treated with a target dosage of citalopram 40 mg/day and assessed with both the Mattis Dementia Scale and the Stroop Color-Word test (Golden 1978). Survival analysis showed that abnormal scores in both the initiation-perseveration domain of the Mattis Dementia Rating Scale and the Stroop Color-Word test each predicted a poor remission rate of citalopram-treated elders with major depression over the 8-week period of the study (Alexopoulos et al. 2004). These relationships were rather specific, because impairment in other cognitive domains of the Mattis Dementia Rating Scale were not associated with remission. Functional neuroimaging studies suggest that tasks of the initiation-perseveration test and the Stroop Color-Word test depend on integrity of primarily the anterior cingulate (Bush et al. 2000; Davidson et al. 2002; Jueptner et al. 1997) and to some extent the dorsolateral prefrontal cortex (Frith et al. 1991). For this reason, subsequent studies focused on the relationship of structural and functional abnormalities of the anterior cingulate to treatment response of geriatric depression.

Executive dysfunction has been associated with white matter hyperintensities, abnormalities frequently found in geriatric depression. Theoretically, compromise in white matter can cause a disconnection state resulting in impaired cingulate function, clinically expressed as executive dysfunction predisposing to poor response to antidepressant treatment. Functional neuroimaging findings suggest that treatment resistance and increased risk for relapse are associated with hypermetabolism of ventral limbic structures (amygdala, subgenual cingulate, and posterior orbital cortex) and hypometabolism of cortical dorsal structures (lateral and dorsolateral cortex, dorsal anterior cingulate, and caudate nucleus) (Drevets 2000; Goldapple et al. 2004; Mayberg 2001; Mayberg et al. 1997). Based on these observations, we hypothesized that microstructural white matter abnormalities interfering with the interaction of dorsal cortical and ventral limbic structures may inhibit response to antidepressant drug treatment (Alexopoulos et al. 2002b). This hypothesis was tested in a preliminary study of small number of older patients with major depression treated with a citalopram target daily dosage of 40 mg for 12 weeks. The integrity of white matter was assessed using fractional anisotropy, a measure derived from diffusion tensor magnetic resonance imaging. Regions of interest were placed on white matter lateral to the anterior cingulate at 15 mm, 10 mm, 5 mm, 0 mm, and –5 mm above the anterior commissure–posterior commissure (AC-PC) line. Survival analysis showed that abnormal fractional anisotropy 15 mm above the AC-PC line was associated with poor remission rate to citalopram. As in our earlier studies, depressed elders who remained depressed had more abnormal initiation-perseveration scores than patients who achieved remission of depression. Moreover, fractional anisotropy at 15 mm above the AC-PC line was correlated with initiation-perseveration scores. This preliminary study requires replication. Nonetheless, its findings suggest that microstructural white matter abnormalities lateral to the anterior cingulate are correlated with executive dysfunction requiring functional integrity of the anterior cingulate. Moreover, both white matter abnormalities lateral to the anterior cingulate and executive dysfunction were associated with poor remission rate following antidepressant treatment.

To further examine the role of anterior cingulate in antidepressant response, we studied the error negative waves (ERN) following the response inhibition task of the Stroop test (Kalayam and Alexopoulos 2003). Performance in the Stroop task is subserved by the anterior cingulate. ERN occur when errors are committed during the Stroop task and are thought to reflect cingulate activity (Liotti et al. 2000). This preliminary study observed that elders with major depression who remained symptomatic following treatment with citalopram at a target daily dosage of 40 mg for 8 weeks had a larger left frontal ERN during Stroop activation than patients who achieved remission. Moreover, large left frontal ERN was associated with Dementia Rating Scale—Initiation/Perseveration domain (DRS-IP) impairment, an abnormality also associated with poor antidepressant response. The lateralizing ERN effect to the left is consistent with left-sided abnormalities of the cingulate and other limbic regions in depression and depression-related states. Increased metabolism of the left anterior cingulate was found in younger depressed patients with poor treatment response (Drevets et al. 2002; Mayberg et al. 1997). Threat-related words activate the left posterior cingulate gyrus (Maddock and Buonocore 1997). Depressed mood and psychomotor retardation are associated with low metabolism of the left angular gyrus and the left dorsolateral cortex (Bench et al. 1993), structures connected with the cingulate and the amygdala. Finally, dysphoric stimuli activate the left more than the right amygdala, a structure reciprocally connected to the anterior cingulate (Schneider et al. 1997).

These studies suggest that executive dysfunction as well as structural and functional abnormalities of frontostriatal pathways, and of the anterior cingulate in particular, predict poor or slow response to antidepressant drug therapy. Based on these findings, we hypothesized that executive dysfunction influences not only the occurrence but also the stability of antidepressant response in elders who had been able to achieve remission of depression. To test this hypothesis, we investigated the relationship of executive and memory impairment to relapse, recurrence, and residual depressive symptoms (Alexopoulos et al. 2000). The subjects of this study were elderly patients who had remitted from major depression and received continuation treatment with nortriptyline (blood levels, 60–150 ng/mL) for 16 weeks. Those who remained well by the end of the continuation treatment phase were randomly assigned to either remain on nortriptyline or receive placebo for up to 2 years. Survival analysis demonstrated that abnormal initiation-perseveration scores of the Mattis Dementia Scale predicted relapse and recurrence of depression. Moreover, use of mixed effects models showed that abnormal initiation-perseveration scores were associated with fluctuations of depressive symptoms in the whole group and in the subjects who never relapsed during the follow-up period of the study. Disability, medical burden, memory impairment, social support, and history of previous episodes did not influence the outcomes of depression, thus suggesting a rather specific relationship of executive dysfunction to relapse and recurrence of late-life depression.

IMPLICATIONS FOR PHARMACOTHERAPY
- -

The association of slow, poor, and unstable response of depressed elderly persons to clinical (executive deficits), structural, and functional evidence of frontostriatal dysfunction offers the rationale for novel pharmacological research approaches (Alexopoulos 2003). Two strategies appear promising. The first strategy focuses on agents targeting some of the frontostriatal circuitry neurotransmitters such as dopamine, norepinephrine, acetylcholine, and endogenous opioids. Such agents may be studied in patients with depression and executive dysfunction to investigate their effect on depressive symptoms and cognition. There is already some evidence that the dopamine D_3 receptor agonist pramipexole has antidepressant properties (Corrigan and Evans 1997). Bupropion, an agent enhancing noradrenergic activity, is an antidepressant, and there is some evidence that cholinesterase inhibitors improve mood-related symptoms in Alzheimer's patients (Feldman et al. 2001). The antidepressant action of pramipexole, bupropion, and cholinesterase inhibitors may be even more pronounced in depressed elders with executive dysfunction because these patients are likely to have dopaminergic, noradrenergic, and cholinergic deficits.

The second pharmacological approach may rely on the observation that some depressive symptoms and sleep abnormalities such as insomnia, appetite disturbance, and short rapid eye movement sleep latency are associated with abnormal regulation of hypocretin 1 and 2 (also known as orexin A and B) in the hypothalamus (Alexopoulos 2003). Hypocretins are critical for maintaining normal wakefulness. Dysfunction of the hypocretin system leads to narcolepsy, a disorder with a high comorbidity of depression. Hypocretins appear to regulate monoaminergic and cholinergic components of the ascending reticular activating system (ARAS) as well as sleep- and wake-promoter neurons in the hypothalamus. The wake-promoter neurons project to the cortex using the neurotransmitter histamine to promote arousal, whereas sleep-promoter neurons use the neurotransmitters γ-aminobutyric acid (GABA) and galantin. Stimulated vigilance appears to be mediated by dopamine, monoamines, norepinephrine, serotonin, and acetylcholine via the ARAS; internal vigilance may be mediated by the ascending histaminergic neurons arising from the hypothalamus (Salin-Pascual et al. 2001; Saper et al. 2001). Stimulants (e.g., amphetamine) may be able to treat symptoms of depression associated with malfunctioning hypocretin signaling by activating both arousal systems, although their arousal of the external vigilance system may cause motor hyperactivity and jitteriness. Modafinil can selectively activate internal vigilance at the tuberomammillary nucleus level and potentially improve fatigue, executive function, and psychomotor retardation in elderly patients with depression without causing hyperarousal. Moreover, studies of young normal humans have shown a beneficial effect of modafinil on executive functions (Turner et al. 2003). These observations provide the rationale for studies of psychostimulants and modafinil in geriatric depression with executive dysfunction in which these drugs may be used either as single agents or as agents augmenting antidepressants.

IMPLICATIONS FOR BEHAVIORAL INTERVENTIONS

Behavioral interventions helping patients to develop coping strategies with which to remedy behavioral deficits resulting from depression and executive dysfunction may be effective in reducing depressive symptoms and disability. To this end, in collaboration with Patricia Arean, we modified problem-solving therapy to focus on behavioral abnormalities of depressed elders with executive dysfunction. In a preliminary study, we compared the efficacy of the modified therapy with that of supportive therapy in elders with major depression and abnormal scores in initiation-perseveration and response inhibition tests (Alexopoulos et al. 2003). Study results indicated that problem-solving therapy was more effective than supportive therapy in inducing remission and reducing residual depressive symptoms and disability. These beneficial effects occurred without a significant improvement in executive function tests. Nonpharmacological treatment may be an effective therapeutic alternative for patients with depression and executive dysfunction who respond poorly to antidepressant treatments.

CONCLUSION

Despite methodological and substantive limitations, studies on late-onset depression offered evidence that such late-life mood syndromes occur in the context of cognitive impairment and other neurological stigmata. Moreover, research on late-life depression as well as increasing knowledge of the functional neuroanatomy of depression suggest that single brain lesions may not function as the direct cause of depression. Instead, changes in specific brain structures—that is, frontostriatal networks, hippocampus, and amygdala—may confer vulnerability to depression. The causes of brain structure changes are likely heterogeneous and may include vascular, inflammatory, autoimmune, and endocrine processes. Brain abnormalities predisposing to depression may facilitate the development of the state-dependent brain changes transiently occurring during depressive episodes (i.e., increased metabolism in ventral limbic structures and decreased metabolism of dorsal neocortical structures. Moreover, predisposing brain abnormalities may influence the clinical presentation, treatment response, and course of geriatric depression.

These observations provide the rationale for novel treatment approaches. Agents optimizing the function of some of the frontostriatal circuitry neurotransmitters need to be studied in elders with depression and executive dysfunction. Similarly, monotherapy or augmentation therapy with agents likely to enhance internal vigilance and improve executive functions may be investigated in such patients. Finally, there is some evidence that psychosocial interventions targeting the behavioral deficits of depressed elders with executive dysfunction may be effective. Focusing on cognitive dysfunctions of late-life depression and on their underlying brain abnormalities may contribute to the development of brain mechanism-driven nosology and even guide the search for novel treatments for these difficult-to-treat patients.

Based on this model, several studies have attempted to characterize cognitive impairment accompanying late-life depression in an effort to identify a clinical window into brain abnormalities predisposing to this disorder. Executive dysfunction emerged as a common abnormality of late-life depression. Elders with depression and executive dysfunction are likely to present with psychomotor retardation, diminished interest in activities, limited insight, and pronounced behavioral disability, a presentation resembling a medial frontal lobe syndrome. Moreover, abnormal performance in some executive function tasks predicts slow, poor, and unstable response to classic antidepressant drugs. Preliminary studies suggest that structural and functional abnormalities of the anterior cingulate interfere with antidepressant response. These observations suggest that dysfunction of the anterior cingulate is one of the abnormalities predisposing to late-life depression and influencing its course.

REFERENCES

Abrams RC, Rosendahl E, Card C, et al: Personality disorder correlates of late- and early-onset depression. J Am Geriatr Soc 42:727–731, 1994

Alexopoulos GS: Clinical and biological findings in late-onset depression, in Review of Psychiatry, Vol 9. Edited by Tasman A, Goldfinger SM, Kaufman CA. Washington, DC, American Psychiatric Press, 1990, pp 249–262

Alexopoulos GS: Geriatric depression in primary care. Int J Geriatr Psychiatry 11:397–400, 1996

Alexopoulos GS: Frontostriatal and limbic dysfunction in late-life depression. Am J Geriatr Psychiatry 10:687–95, 2002

Alexopoulos GS: Role of executive function in late life depression. J Clin Psychiatry 64(suppl):18–23, 2003

Alexopoulos GS, Young RC, Shindledecker R: Brain computed tomography in geriatric depression and primary degenerative dementia. Biol Psychiatry 31:591–599, 1992

Alexopoulos GS, Meyers BS, Young RC, et al: The course of geriatric depression with "reversible dementia." Am J Psychiatry 150:1693–1699, 1993a

Alexopoulos GS, Young RC, Meyers BS: Geriatric depression: age of onset and dementia. Biol Psychiatry 34:141–145, 1993b

Alexopoulos GS, Vrontou C, Kakuma T, et al: Disability in geriatric depression. Am J Psychiatry 153: 877–885, 1996a

Alexopoulos GS, Meyers BS, Young RC, et al: Recovery in geriatric depression. Arch Gen Psychiatry 53: 305–312, 1996b

Alexopoulos GS, Meyers BS, Young RC, et al: Executive dysfunction and long-term outcomes of geriatric depression. Arch Gen Psychiatry 57:285–290, 2000

Alexopoulos GS, Kiosses DN, Klimstra S, et al: Clinical presentation of the "depression-executive dysfunction syndrome" of late life. Am J Geriatr Psychiatry 10:98–102, 2002a

Alexopoulos GS, Kiosses DM, Steven JC, et al: Frontal white matter microstructure and treatment response of late-life depression: a preliminary study. Am J Psychiatry 11:1929–1931, 2002b

Alexopoulos GS, Raue P, Arean P: Problem-solving therapy in geriatric depression with executive dysfunction. Am J Geriatr Psychiatry 11:46–52, 2003

Alexopoulos GS, Kiosses DN, Murphy C, et al: Executive dysfunction, heart disease burden, and remission of geriatric depression. Neuropsychopharmacology 29:2278–2284, 2004

Arve S, Tilvis RS, Lehtonen A, et al: Coexistence of lowered mood and cognitive impairment of elderly people in five birth cohorts. Aging 11:90–95, 1999

Ballmaier M, Toga AW, Blanton RE, et al: Anterior cingulate, gyrus rectus, and orbitofrontal abnormalities in elderly depressed patients: An MRI-based parcellation of the prefrontal cortex. Am J Psychiatry 161:99–108, 2004

Baron M, Mendlewicz J, Klotz J: Age-of-onset and genetic transmission in affective disorders. Acta Psychiatr Scand 64:373–380, 1981

Bassuk SS, Berkman LF, Wypij D: Depressive symptomatology and incident cognitive decline in an elderly community sample. Arch Gen Psychiatry 55:1073–1081, 1998

Beats BC, Sahakian BJ, Levy R: Cognitive performance in tests sensitive to frontal lobe dysfunction in the elderly depressed. Psychol Med 26:591–603, 1996

Bench CJ, Friston KJ, Brown RG, et al: The anatomy of melancholia: focal abnormalities of cerebral blood flow in major depression. Psychol Med 22:607–615, 1992

Bench CJ, Friston KJ, Brown RG, et al: Regional cerebral blood flow in depression measured by positron emission tomography: the relationship with clinical dimensions. Psychol Med 23:579–590, 1993

Boone KB, Miller BL, Lesser IM, et al: Neuropsychological correlates of white matter lesions in healthy elderly subjects. Arch Neurol 49:549–554, 1992

Boone KB, Lesser IM, Miller BL, et al: Cognitive functioning in older depressed outpatients: relationship of presence and severity of depression to neuropsychological test scores. Neuropsychology 9:390–398, 1995

Buchsbaum MS, Wu J, Siegel BV, et al: Effect of sertraline on regional metabolic rate in patients with affective disorder. Biol Psychiatry 41:15–22, 1997

Bush G, Luu P, Posner MI: Cognitive and emotional influences in anterior cingulate cortex. Trends Cogn Sci 4:215–222, 2000

Butters MA, Becker JT, Nebes RD, et al: Changes in cognitive functioning following treatment of late-life depression. Am J Psychiatry 157:1949–1954, 2000

Carmichael ST, Price JL: Limbic connections of the orbital and medial prefrontal cortex in macaque monkeys. J Comp Neurol 363:615–641, 1995

Chaput Y, deMontigny C, Blier P: Presynaptic and postsynaptic modifications of the serotonin system by long-term administration of antidepressant treatments: an in vitro electrophysiologic study in the rat. Neuropsychopharmacology 5:219–229, 1991

Coffey CE, Figiel GS, Djang WT, et al: Leukoencephalopathy in elderly depressed patients referred for ECT. Biol Psychiatry 24:143–161, 1988

Coffey CE, Figiel GS, Djang WT, et al: Subcortical hyperintensity in MRI: a comparison of normal and depressed elderly subjects. Am J Psychiatry 147:187–189, 1990

Cohen RA, Malloy P, Jenkins M: Disorders of attention, in Clinical Neuropsychology. Edited by Snyder PJ, Nussbaum PD. Washington, DC, American Psychological Association, 1998, pp 541–572

Conwell Y, Nelson JC, Kim KM, et al: Depression in late life: age of onset as marker of a subtype. J Affect Disord 17:189–195, 1989

Corrigan M, Evans D: Pramipexole, a dopamine agonist, in the treatment of major depression. Presented at the annual meeting of the American College of Neuropsychopharmacology, San Juan, Puerto Rico, December 1997

Davidson RJ, Pizzagalli D, Nitschke JB, et al: Depression: perspectives from affective neuroscience. Annu Rev Psychol 53:545–574, 2002

de Asis JM, Stern E, Alexopoulos GS, et al: Hippocampal and anterior cingulate activation deficits in patients with geriatric depression. Am J Psychiatry 158:1321–1323, 2001

Devanand DP, Sano M, Tang MX, et al: Depressed mood and the incidence of Alzheimer's disease in the elderly living in the community. Arch Gen Psychiatry 53:175–182, 1996

Dolan RJ, Bench CJ, Brown RG, et al: Regional cerebral blood flow abnormalities in depressed patients with cognitive impairment. J Neurol Neurosurg Psychiatry 55:768–773, 1992

Drevets WC: Prefrontal cortical-amygdalar metabolism in major depression. Ann NY Acad Sci 877:614–637, 1999

Drevets WC: Neuroimaging studies of mood disorders. Biol Psychiatry 49:813–819, 2000

Drevets WC, Raichle ME: Reciprocal suppression of regional cerebral blood flow during emotional versus higher cognitive processes: implications for interactions between emotion and cognition. Cogn Emotion 12:353–385, 1998

Drevets WC, Videen TO, Price JL, et al: A functional anatomical study of unipolar depression. J Neurosci 12:3628–3641, 1992

Drevets WC, Price JL, Simpson JR, et al: Subgenual prefrontal cortex abnormalities in mood disorders. Nature 386:824–827, 1997

Drevets WC, Bogers W, Raichle ME: Functional anatomical correlates of antidepressant drug treatment assessed using PET measures of regional glucose metabolism. Eur Neuropsychopharmacol 12:527–544, 2002

Ebert D, Feistel H, Barocka A: Effects of sleep deprivation on the limbic system and the frontal lobes in affective disorders: a study with Tc-99 m-HMPAO SPECT. Psychiatry Res 40:247–251, 1991

Elliot R, Sahakian BJ, McKay AP, et al: Neuropsychological impairments in unipolar depression: the influence of perceived failure on subsequent performance. Psychol Med 26:975–989, 1996

Elliott R, Baker SC, Rogers RD, et al: Prefrontal dysfunction in depressed patients performing a complex planning task: a study using positron emission tomography. Psychol Med 27:931–942, 1997

Feldman H, Gauthier S, Hecker J, et al: A 24-week randomized, double-blind study of donepezil in moderate to severe Alzheimer's disease. Neurology 57:613–620, 2001

Frith CD, Friston KJ, Liddle PF, et al: A PET study of word finding. Neuropsychologia 12:1137–1148, 1991

Frodl T, Meizenzhal E, Zetzsche T, et al: Enlargement of amygdala in patients with first episode major depression. Biol Psychiatry 51:708–714, 2002

Fujikawa T, Yamawaki S, Touhouda Y: Incidence of silent cerebral infarction in patients with major depression. Stroke 24:1631–1634, 1993

Goldapple K, Segal Z, Garson C, et al: Modulation of cortical-limbic pathways in major depression: treatment-specific effects of cognitive behavior therapy. Arch Gen Psychiatry 61:34–41, 2004

Golden CJ: The Stroop Color and Word Test (Manual). Chicago, IL, Stoetling, 1978

Goodwin GM: Neuropsychological and neuroimaging evidence for the involvement of the frontal lobes in depression. J Psychopharmacol 11:115–122, 1997

Greenwald BS, Kramer-Ginsberg E: Age of onset in geriatric depression: relationship to clinical variables. J Affect Disord 15:61–68, 1988

Hart RP, Kwentus JA, Taylor JR, et al: Rate of forgetting in dementia and depression. J Consult Clin Psychol 55:101–105, 1987

Herrmann N, Lieff S, Silberfeld M: The effect of age of onset on depression in the elderly. J Geriatr Psychiatry Neurol 2:182–187, 1989

Husain M, McDonald W, Doraiswamy P, et al: A magnetic resonance imaging study of putamen nuclei in major depression. Psychiatry Res 1:213–215, 1991

Hyman SE, Nestler EJ: Initiation and adaptation: a paradigm for understanding psychotropic drug action. Am J Psychiatry 153:151–162, 1996

Jacoby RJ, Levy R: Computed tomography in the elderly, 3: affective disorder. Br J Psychiatry 136:270–275, 1980

Jones B, Henderson M, Welch CA: Executive functions in unipolar depression before and after electroconvulsive therapy. Int J Neurosci 38:287–297, 1988

Jorm AF: History of depression as a risk factor for dementia: an updated review. Aust N Z J Psychiatry 35:776–781, 2001

Jorm AF, van Duijn CM, Chandra V, et al: Psychiatric history and related exposures as risk factors for Alzheimer's disease: A collaborative re-analysis of case-control studies. Int J Epidemiol 20 (suppl 2):S43–47, 1991

Jueptner M, Stephan KM, Frith CD, et al: Anatomy of motor learning, I: frontal cortex and attention to action. J Neurophysiol 77:1313–1324, 1997

Kalayam B, Alexopoulos GS: Prefrontal dysfunction and treatment response in geriatric depression. Arch Gen Psychiatry 56:713–718, 1999

Kalayam B, Alexopoulos GS: Left frontal error negativity and symptom improvement in geriatric depression: a preliminary study. Am J Psychiatry 160:2054–2056, 2003

Kalayam B, Meyers BS, Kakuma T, et al: Age of onset of geriatric depression and sensorimotor hearing deficits. Biol Psychiatry 38:649–658, 1995

Kiosses DN, Alexopoulos GS, Murphy C: Symptoms of striatofrontal dysfunction contribute to disability in geriatric depression. Int J Geriatr Psychiatry 15:992–999, 2000

Kiosses DN, Klimstra S, Murphy C, et al: Executive dysfunction and disability in elderly patients with major depression. Am J Geriatr Psychiatry 9:269–274, 2001

Kokmen E, Beard CM, Chandra V, et al: Clinical risk factors for Alzheimer's disease: a population-based case-control study. Neurology 41:1393–1397, 1991

Kral VA, Emery OB: Long-term follow-up of depressive pseudodementia of the aged. Can J Psychiatry 34:445–446, 1989

Krishnan KRR, McDonald W, Escalona R, et al: Magnetic resonance imaging of the caudate nuclei in depression. Arch Gen Psychiatry 49:553–557, 1992

Krishnan KRR, Hays JC, Blazer DG: MRI-defined vascular depression. Am J Psychiatry 154:497–500, 1997

Kumar A, Bilker W, Jin Z, et al: Atrophy and high intensity lesions: complementary neurobiological mechanisms in late-life depression. Neuropsychopharmacology 22:264–174, 2000

Lai T, Payne ME, Byrum CE, et al: Reduction of orbital frontal cortex volume in geriatric depression. Biol Psychiatry 48:971–975, 2000

Lesser I, Boone KB, Mehringer CM, et al: Cognition and white matter hyperintensities in older depressed adults. Am J Psychiatry 153:1280–1287, 1996

Liotti M, Mayberg HS: The role of functional neuroimaging in the neuropsychology of depression. J Clin Exp Neuropsychol 23:121–136, 2001

Liotti M, Woldorff MG, Perez R, et al: An ERP study of the temporal course of the Stroop Color-Word Interference Test. Neuropsychologia 38:701–711, 2000

Lockwood CA, Alexopoulos GS, van Gorp WG: Executive dysfunction in geriatric depression. Am J Psychiatry 159:1119–1126, 2002

MacFall JR, Payne ME, Provenzale JE, et al: Medial orbital frontal lesions in late-onset depression. Biol Psychiatry 49:803–806, 2000

MacQueen GM, Campbell S, Macdonald K, et al: Course of illness, hippocampal function and hippocampal volume in major depression. Proc Natl Acad Sci USA 100:1387–1392, 2003

Maddock RJ, Buonocore MH: Activation of left posterior cingulate gyrus by the auditory presentation of threat-related words: an fMRI study. Psychiatry Res 75:1–4, 1997

Mattis S: Dementia Rating Scale. Odessa, FL, Psychological Assessment Resources, 1989

Mayberg HS: Depression and frontal-subcortical circuits: focus on prefrontal-limbic interactions, in Frontal-Subcortical Circuits in Psychiatric and Neurological Disorders. Edited by Lichter DC, Cummings JL. New York, Guilford, 2001, pp 177–206

Mayberg HS, Brannan SK, Mahurin RK, et al: Cingulate function in depression: a potential predictor of treatment response. Neuroreport 8:1057–1061, 1997

Mayberg HS, Liotti M, Brannan SK, et al: Reciprocal limbic-cortical function and negative mood: converging PET findings in depression and normal sadness. Am J Psychiatry 156:675–682, 1999

McEwen BS: Mood disorders and allostatic load. Biol Psychiatry 54:200–207, 2003

Morris PL, Robinson RG, Raphael B, et al: The relationship between risk factors for affective disorder and poststroke depression in hospitalised stroke patients. Aust N Z J Psychiatry 26:208–217, 1992

Mueller TI, Kohn R, Leventhal N, et al: The course of depression in elderly patients. Am J Geriatr Psychiatry 12:22–29, 2004

Murphy CF, Alexopoulos GS: Longitudinal association of initiation/perseveration and severity of geriatric depression. Am J Geriatr Psychiatry 11:1–7, 2003

Nebes RD, Butters MA, Houck PR, et al: Dual-task performance in depressed geriatric patients. Psychiatry Res 102:139–151, 2001

Nebes RD, Pollock BG, Houck PR, et al: Persistence of cognitive impairment in geriatric patients following antidepressant treatment: a randomized, double-blind clinical trial with nortriptyline and paroxetine. J Psychiatr Res 37:99–108, 2003

Ongur D, Drevets WC, Price JL: Glial reduction in the prefrontal cortex in mood disorders. Proc Natl Acad Sci USA 95:13290–13295, 1998

Pandya DN, Yeterian EH: Comparison of prefrontal architecture and connections. Philos Trans R Soc Lond B Biol Sci 351:1423–1432, 1996

Rajkowska G, Miguel-Hidalgo LL, Wei J: Morphometric evidence for neuronal and glial prefrontal cell pathology in major depression. Biol Psychiatry 45:1085–1098, 1999

Reding M, Haycox J, Blass J: Depression in patients referred to a dementia clinic: a three-year prospective study. Arch Neurol 42: 894–896, 1985

Reichman WE, Coyne AC: Depressive symptoms in Alzheimer's disease and multi-infarct dementia. J Geriatr Psychiatry Neurol 8:96–99, 1995

Ritchie K, Gilman C, Ledesert B, et al: Depressive illness, depressive symptomatology, and regional cerebral blood flow in elderly people with subclinical cognitive impairment. Age Ageing 28:385–391, 1999

Rolls ET: A theory of emotion, and its application to understanding the neural basis of emotion. Cognition and Emotion 4:161–190, 1990

Salin-Pascual R, Gerashchenko D, Greco M, et al: Hypothalamic regulation of sleep. Neuropsychopharmacology 25(suppl):S21–S27, 2001

Saper CB, Chou TC, Scammell TE: The sleep switch: hypothalamic control of sleep and wakefulness. Trends Neurosci 24:726–731, 2001

Schneider F, Grodd W, Weiss U, et al: Functional MRI reveals left amygdala activation during emotion. Psychiatry Res 76:75–82, 1997

Sheline YI: 3D MRI studies of neuroanatomical changes in unipolar major depression: the role of stress and medical comorbidity. Biol Psychiatry 48:791–800, 2000

Sheline YI: Neuroimaging studies of mood disorder effects on the brain: Biol Psychiatry 54:338–352, 2003

Sheline YI, Wang PW, Gado MH, et al: Hippocampal atrophy in recurrent major depression. Proc Natl Acad Sci USA 93:3908–3913, 1996

Sheline YI, Sanghavi M, Mintun MA, et al: Depression duration but not age predicts hippocampal volume loss in medically healthy women with recurrent major depression. J Neurosci 19:5034–5043, 1999

Sobin C, Sackeim HA: Psychomotor symptoms of depression. Am J Psychiatry 154:4–17, 1997

Speck CE, Kukull WA, Brenner DE, et al: History of depression as a risk factor for Alzheimer's disease. Epidemiology 6:366–369, 1995

Starkstein SE, Robinson RG: Depression in cerebrovascular disease, in Depression in Neurological Disease. Edited by Starkstein SE, Robinson RG. Baltimore, MD, Johns Hopkins University Press, 1993, pp 28–49

Starkstein SE, Robinson RG, Berthier ML, et al: Differential mood changes following basal ganglia vs thalamic lesions. Arch Neurol 45:725–730, 1988

Starkstein SE, Migliorelli R, Teson A, et al: Prevalence and clinical correlates of pathological affective display in Alzheimer's disease. J Neurol Neurosurg Psychiatry 59:55–60, 1995

Steffens DC, Plassman BL, Helms MJ, et al: A twin study of late-onset depression and apolipoprotein E epsilon 4 as risk factors for Alzheimer's disease. Biol Psychiatry 41:851–856, 1997

Steffens DC, Helms MJ, Krishnan KR, et al: Cerebrovascular disease and depression symptoms in the cardiovascular health study. Stroke 30:2159–2166, 1999

Steffens DC, Byrum CE, McQuaid DR, et al: Hippocampal volume in geriatric depression. Biol Psychiatry 50:68–69, 2001

Steffens DC, Payne ME, Greenberg DL, et al: Hippocampal volume and incident dementia in geriatric depression. Am J Geriatr Psychiatry 10:62–71, 2002a

Steffens DC, Bosworth HB, Provenzale JM, et al: Subcortical white matter lesions and functional impairment in geriatric depression. Depress Anxiety 15:23–28, 2002b

Turner DC, Robbins TW, Clark L, et al: Cognitive enhancing effects of modafinil in healthy volunteers. Psychopharmacology 165:260–269, 2003

U.S. Surgeon General: Mental Health: A Report of the Surgeon General. Washington, DC, U.S. Department of Health and Human Services, 1999

van Duijn CM, Clayton DG, Chandra V, et al: Interaction between genetic and environmental risk factors for Alzheimer's disease: a reanalysis of case-control studies. Genet Epidemiol 11:539–551, 1994

van Ojen R, Hooijer C, Bezemer D, et al: Late-life depressive disorder in the community, I: the relationship between MMSE score and depression in subjects with and without psychiatric history. Br J Psychiatry 166:311–319, 1995

Wiener PK, Kiosses DN, Klimstra S, et al: A short-term inpatient program for agitated demented nursing home residents. Int J Geriatr Psychiatry 16:866–872, 2001

Wu J, Gillin C, Buchsbaum MS, et al: Effect of sleep deprivation on brain metabolism of depressed patients. Am J Psychiatry 149:538–543, 1992

Yaffe K, Blackwell T, Gore R, et al: Depressive symptoms and cognitive decline in nondemented elderly women: a prospective study. Arch Gen Psychiatry 56:425–430, 1999

Emotions and Health

Allostasis and Allostatic Load Over the Life Course

Teresa E. Seeman, Ph.D.

Tara L. Gruenewald, Ph.D.

IN THIS CHAPTER, we review the concepts of *allostasis* and *allostatic load* and examine evidence indicating that there is population variation in the accumulation of allostatic load related to differences in age and exposure to stressful life experiences. The concept of allostasis (i.e., stability through change), first introduced by Sterling and Eyer (1988), refers to the idea that parameters of most physiological regulatory systems change to accommodate environmental demands. In contrast to *homeostasis*, which refers to negative feedback systems in the body that serve to maintain a given physiological parameter at a certain setpoint or within a narrow range (McEwen 1998; McEwen and Wingfield 2003; Sterling and Eyer 1988), *allostasis* refers to processes of one or more physiological systems that vary more broadly to adapt to internal or external challenges such as infection, fleeing a predator, or an argument with one's spouse. As highlighted by Sterling and Eyer, the complex brain–body processes of allostasis manifested across the body's multiple regulatory systems allow for a fine-tuning of physiological resources, including tuning as a function of anticipation and experience, to meet the demands of life's events.

Although allostatic processes are critical for adaptive functioning, chronic or repeated activation of physiological systems in response to life's challenges are hypothesized to exact a toll on such systems. This hypothesis is reflected in the concept of allostatic load, which was proposed by McEwen and Stellar (1993). *Allostatic load* refers to the idea that biological regulatory systems may begin to exhibit cumulative patterns of dysregulation (i.e., "wear and tear") over time as a consequence of ongoing efforts to adapt to life demands. An adaptive allostatic response can be thought to represent a dynamic response of any of a variety of biological parameters to some stimulus, such as an elevation in the level and activity of a physiological parameter in response to the stimulus and then a return to initial level. Evidence of allostatic load might be reflected in a physiological system that is no longer able to maintain a "normal" basal level under unstimulated conditions and/or a system that exhibits a prolonged period of activity (i.e., less efficient return to basal level) when challenged. Although this example characterizes allostasis in the form of elevation of a physiological parameter and allostatic load in terms of excessive or heightened physiological activity, allostatic processes encompass other forms of adaptive change (e.g., decreased level or activity of a physiological parameter), and patterns of dysregulation can also be characterized by low levels or hyporesponsivity of a physiological parameter.

A number of physiological systems are believed to carry out allostatic processes, including the sympathetic nervous system, the hypothalamic-pituitary-adrenal (HPA) system, hormones, neurostransmitters, and chemical messengers of the cardiovascular, metabolic, and immune systems, among others. Adaptive responses of these physiological systems as a result of exposure to environmental demands (allostasis) are also hypothesized to be moderated by individual difference factors. The combination of individual characteristics and individual exposure to life experiences that require allostasis can in turn affect patterns of physiological response and possible dysregulation. Allostatic load can be thought to represent the cumulative physiological toll that occurs across time and across physiological systems as a result of such characteristics and experiences. Although allostatic load can be reflected in dysregulation in only a single physiological system, the complex interconnections between physiological mediators of allostasis often result in patterns of dysregulation across multiple physiological systems. Thus, one heuristic value of allostatic load is its conception of a multi-systems view of the physiological price paid by the body to meet life's challenges, a price that is likely to vary across individuals and time. As we document here, cumulative physiological toll as reflected in allostatic load appears to vary as a function of age, socioeconomic status, and psychosocial factors such as the quantity and quality of social relationships. Evidence presented here is not meant to be comprehensive; rather, we have selected illustrative examples, largely from our own research with data from several large population-based cohort studies.

OPERATIONALIZATION OF ALLOSTATIC LOAD

Our initial work on allostatic load was based on secondary analyses of available data from the MacArthur Study of Successful Aging (Seeman et al. 2004). This study is a longitudinal investigation of older men and women sampled from three community-based cohorts from the Established Populations for Epidemiological Studies of the Elderly (EPESE) on the basis of age (70–79 years of age) and high levels of physical and cognitive functioning (eligible participants had to score in the top third of their age group on four physical and two cognitive functioning measures) (Berkman et al. 1993). Of 4,030 age-eligible participants in the EPESE, 1,313 met screening criteria and 1,189 agreed to participate in the MacArthur Study of Successful Aging. Subjects participated in a face-to-face interview and provided physiological samples (e.g., blood, overnight urine, blood pressure measurements) during a baseline period of data collection (1988–1989) and at follow-up assessments in 1991 and 1996.

The biological measures from this study that we utilized in our initial analyses of allostatic load are listed in Table 9–1. We assessed 10 biological indicators of the HPA axis and of the cardiovascular, metabolic, and sympathetic nervous systems. As an initial approach to a cumulative index of allostatic load, we simply calculated for each subject the total number of these different parameters for which they had a value that placed them in the highest-risk quartile (highest or lowest quartile depending on parameter; see Table 9–1). Individuals with larger summary scores (i.e., who had values on biological parameters in many high-risk quartiles) were taken to exhibit evidence of greater allostatic load.

Using this summary of allostatic load, we have shown that higher scores predict subsequent health outcomes in terms of risks for cognitive and physical decline, incident cardiovascular disease, and mortality (Seeman et al. 1997, 2001) Higher levels of allostatic load were associated with greater levels of physical and cognitive decline and greater incidence of cardiovascular events assessed during both the 2.5-year and 7-year follow-ups. Perhaps most important, increasing levels of allostatic load were associated with increasing levels of mortality risk assessed at each follow-up. For example, compared with those showing no evidence of allostatic load at the baseline survey, individuals showing evidence of allostatic load dysregulation on three or four of the physiological parameters evidenced almost

TABLE 9–1.   Biological indicators assessed in allostatic load index

		High-risk quartile
Biological indicators assessed in original index		
Cardiovascular system	Systolic blood pressure (resting)	Top
	Diastolic blood pressure (resting)	Top
Hypothalamic-pituitary-adrenal axis	Urinary cortisol (12-hour overnight)	Top
	Dehydroepiandrosterone sulfate	Bottom
Sympathetic nervous system	Urinary epinephrine (12-hour overnight)	Top
	Urinary norepinephrine (12-hour overnight)	Top
Metabolism	Glycosylated hemoglobin	Top
	High-density lipoprotein	Bottom
	Ratio total/high-density lipoprotein cholesterol	Top
	Waist/hip ratio	Top
Additional biological indicators assessed		
Inflammation	Interleukin-6	Top
	Fibrinogen	Top
	Albumin	Bottom
Lung function	Peak flow rate	Bottom
Renal function	Creatinine clearance	Bottom

2.5 times greater mortality risk over the 7-year follow-up, whereas those showing dysregulation on seven or more parameters showed greater than six times the mortality risk of those showing no evidence of allostatic load (see Seeman et al. 2001).

Although these initial findings are certainly consistent with the idea that cumulative burdens of dysregulation are consequential with respect to subsequent health outcomes, there are a number of reasons why this initial index of allostatic load should not be seen as the "gold standard" measure for this new concept. First, this initial operationalization of allostatic load was based on available physiological measurements in a study that was not designed to assess allostatic load, limiting the comprehensiveness of the assessment of multisystem dysregulation. Second, our summary scoring method for this initial assessment was deliberately simple and straightfor-

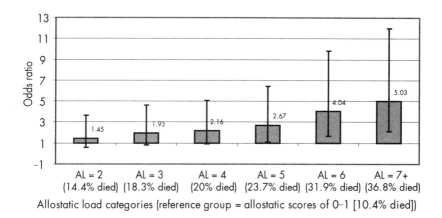

FIGURE 9–1. Odds (±95% confidence intervals) of mortality over 7-year follow-up with increasing levels of allostatic load (AL) for participants: MacArthur Study of Successful Aging.

Note.   Allostatic load score for reference group=0. Linear trend $P<0.0001$.

ward (i.e., a simple definition of "relatively more dysregulation" based on score location in the cohort distribution and a simple count of parameters for which the individual had a "higher risk" score). As discussed later, we have since expanded the range of biological indicators included in the measurement of allostatic load and explored alternative operational scoring systems.

In more recent analyses, we have been able to augment the initial measure of allostatic load with markers of inflammation and lung and renal function (peak flow and creatinine clearance, respectively; see lower portion of Table 9–1). Analyses including these additional parameters in our summary measure of allostatic load replicated earlier findings of increasing risk of mortality during the 7-year follow-up period with increasing levels of allostatic load assessed during the baseline period (Seeman et al. 2004). As shown in Figure 9–1, there is a positive relationship between increasing allostatic load and increasing mortality risk, controlling for standard sociodemographic characteristics (age, gender, socioeconomic status) and baseline health status and health behaviors. As shown, relative to those with the lowest allostatic load scores (i.e., scores of 0–1), the odds of mortality increase with increasing allostatic load scores.

As noted, our original and revised measures of allostatic load are potent predictors of mortality. However, one concern that can be raised is whether

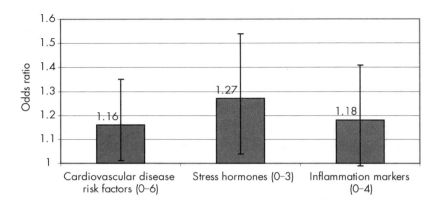

FIGURE 9–2.   Odds (±95% confidence intervals) of mortality over 7-year follow-up per unit increase in subcomponents of allostatic load index: MacArthur Study of Successful Aging.

Note.   Allostatic load subcomponent scores for reference group=0.

our summary index of allostatic load predicts mortality simply because it is a proxy for cardiovascular risk, given that a number of the physiological parameters that compose the allostatic load index are traditional cardiovascular disease risk factors. In other words, the relative contribution of dysregulation in other systems in the allostatic load index—such as the HPA axis, the sympathetic nervous system, or inflammatory variables—to mortality risk may be minimal.

To address this concern, we decomposed the overall allostatic load index into three major subcomponents by grouping physiological indicators into cardiovascular disease risk factors, stress hormones, and markers of inflammation. As illustrated in Figure 9–2, each of these subcomponents contributes significantly and independently to mortality risk. Although the increases in mortality risk per unit increase in each subcomponent are not large, comparisons of those scoring highest versus lowest on each of these subcomponents indicate that the relative risks are greater than 2 for the cardiovascular disease risk factors and stress hormones subcomponents and greater than 3 for the inflammation markers subcomponent. These findings provide support for the contribution of multiple physiological systems to mortality risk and point to the value of a multisystems index of pathophysiology as captured in measures of allostatic load in assessing risk for negative health outcomes.

We have also examined alternative methods of scoring allostatic load. One such approach used canonical correlation analyses to develop summary scores reflecting the optimal linear combinations of the biological parameters that were maximally correlated with summary measures of cognitive and physical functioning decline (Karlamangla et al. 2002). Such canonical correlation analyses produced a set of canonical weights for each biological parameter in our allostatic load index, which were then used to compute an overall allostatic load score. Whereas the original scoring system simply counted the total number of the 10 biological parameters for which a participant's score on a given parameter fell into the highest risk quartile or not, the scoring method based on canonical correlation analysis used the full range of raw scores for each parameter and allowed for unequal contribution (weighting) of the different parameters to the overall score.

Figure 9–3 illustrates the variation in the canonical weights for each biological parameter in the allostatic load index obtained from two analyses, one examining relationships to a summary measure of decline in physical functioning and the second examining relationships to a summary measure of cognitive decline over the 7-year follow-up. The weights depicted for each biological parameter for each of the two functional decline measures represent those obtained from the final model in each analysis, which allowed for biological parameters that did not contribute significantly from the model to be removed. As can be seen in Figure 9–3, not only did the biological variables that contributed significantly to the outcomes vary across the cognitive and physical outcomes but the canonical weights obtained from each analysis also varied across the biological parameters, indicating that the biological variables differed in the significance and magnitude of their contribution to the cognitive and physical decline outcomes. This is not surprising given the complexity of biological regulation and the interconnections among these systems as well as the differential pathophysiology that likely underlies these different functional outcomes. Notably, however, and consistent with allostatic load's hypothesized multisystems conceptualization of biological risk, for each outcome, biological parameters found to contribute to risk for decline include multiple markers of different major regulatory systems.

When we compare our original and canonical-based methods of scoring allostatic load with respect to their ability to predict cognitive and physical function decline, we find that the allostatic load scores derived from the canonical correlation analyses are more highly correlated with both outcomes (Figure 9–4). This would be expected given that the canonical correlation method reflects the "optimal" linear combination of the 10 biological parameters for predicting each outcome. Notably, however, as can be seen in Figure 9–4, the original scoring system yields results that are only modestly weaker. This suggests that our initial and relatively straightfor-

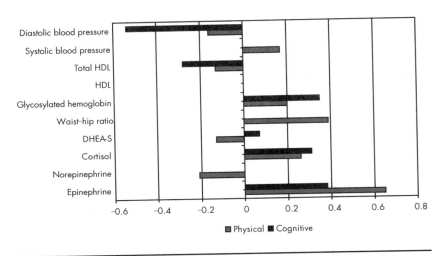

FIGURE 9–3. Canonical weights for 7-year change in physical and cognitive performance: MacArthur Study of Successful Aging.

Note. DHEA-S = dehydroepiandrosterone sulfate; HDL = high-density lipoprotein.

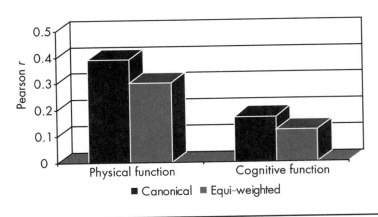

FIGURE 9–4. Correlation of canonical-based versus equi-weighted allostatic load scores with 7-year decline in physical and cognitive function scores: MacArthur Study of Successful Aging.

ward method of assessing allostatic load captures much of the significant information in terms of predicting subsequent health outcomes.

POPULATION VARIATION IN ALLOSTATIC LOAD

Because allostatic load is thought to be a function of cumulative life experiences requiring physiological adaptation (allostasis), population variation in the levels of pathophysiological burden captured in measures of allostatic load would be expected as a function of factors thought to influence life experience, such as age and socioeconomic status. Furthermore, psychosocial and environmental characteristics should also interact with life events to moderate the accumulation of allostatic load, with such individual difference factors serving protective or risk-inducing effects.

Age

Recently, in collaboration with Dr. Eileen Crimmins, we have begun to examine data from the National Health and Nutrition Examination Survey (NHANES III), which is a nationally representative sample of noninstitutionalized adults ages 20 years and older. More than 18,000 individuals were surveyed and examined during the period from 1988 to 1994 for NHANES III (see Crimmins et al. 2003 for detailed description). Data from NHANES III can provide evidence of levels of allostatic load across a wide age range of individuals, with a large number of participants in each age bracket allowing for good estimates of allostatic load. The biological parameters available in the NHANES database that we have included as an index of allostatic load are provided in Table 9–2. For some of these parameters there are _existing clinical "high-risk" criteria established in the biomedical literature, and we used such established cutpoints to define "high risk" groups for each parameter. For those parameters in which no standard clinical risk criteria existed, "high risk" quartiles were defined according to empirical cutpoints derived from the top or bottom quartile (depending on parameter) of the distribution for the full NHANES sample (all ages combined).

As described, a summary allostatic load score was computed by simply counting the total number of the available biological parameters for which individuals had scores that placed them into the high-risk categories. As can be seen in Figure 9–5, scores on this measure of allostatic load show a linear increase with age in the NHANES III sample. This pattern is consistent with the hypothesis that those of greater ages have experienced a greater level of life experiences that required physiological adaptation (allostasis),

TABLE 9–2. Biological indicators in National Health and Nutrition Examination Survey III allostatic load index

Cardiovascular system	Systolic blood pressure (resting)
	Diastolic blood pressure (resting)
Metabolism	Glycosylated hemoglobin
	High-density lipoprotein
	Total cholesterol
	Triglycerides
	Body mass index
Inflammation	C-reactive protein
	Fibrinogen
	Albumin
Lung function	Peak flow rate
Renal function	Creatinine clearance
	Homocysteine

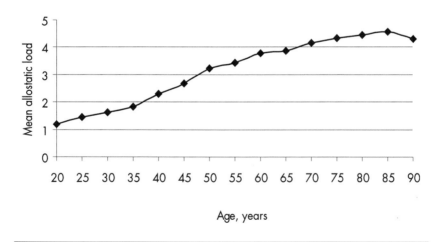

FIGURE 9–5. Mean allostatic load scores, by age: National Health and Nutrition Examination Survey III.

resulting in increased levels of pathophysiological burden (as reflected in our allostatic load index). Further inspection of various individual biological parameters included in the allostatic load measure indicated that this trend of increased allostatic load with increased age was evident across nearly all of the parameters.

Socioeconomic Status

Strong and consistent associations between socioeconomic status (SES) and morbidity for a wide array of diseases, as well as disease-specific and all-cause mortality, have been exhibited in many investigations (Adler et al. 1994; Crimmins et al. 2004; MacIntyre 1997; Pincus and Callahan 1995). Variations in exposure to life stressors that are associated with different levels of SES have been proposed as one plausible pathway in SES–health relationships. The general hypothesis is that those of lower SES experience higher levels of unpleasant and trying life demands in the context of fewer resources with which to cope with these demands. Thus we might expect that such greater exposure will be reflected in higher levels of allostatic load, with levels of allostatic load decreasing as SES increases and exposure to life stressors presumably decreases.

As hypothesized, evidence from several studies reveals the hypothesized inverse association between indices of SES and levels of allostatic load. The relationship between level of educational attainment and allostatic load in older adults from the MacArthur Study of Successful Aging is shown in Figure 9–6. It is notable that education levels (which are generally established early in adulthood) were associated with levels of biological dysregulation late in life, suggesting that education is apparently associated with patterns of life experience affecting allostatic processes over the course of life.

Similar findings have also been reported by Singer and Ryff (1999) based on data from the Wisconsin Longitudinal Study (WLS), a longitudinal investigation of men and women who graduated from Wisconsin high schools in 1957 and who were surveyed in 1957, 1975, and 1992–1993. Biological measures paralleling the 10 parameters used in the initial analyses of allostatic load in the MacArthur Successful Aging Study were gathered for a subset of WLS participants in 1996 when they were in their late 50s or early 60s (approximately a decade younger than the MacArthur Aging Study cohort). A summary allostatic load index based on the total count of parameters for which participants had scores in high-risk quartiles was used.

One benefit of the WLS is that information on both current adult and childhood SES is available for study participants. To examine associations between allostatic load level and the combination of childhood and adult SES, participants were grouped into those who reported low or high SES at both time periods, or a differing combination of childhood and adult SES levels. Low SES at both time points was defined as household income below the median household income for the state of Wisconsin (in 1957 for childhood SES when participants were 18 years of age and in 1992–1993 for

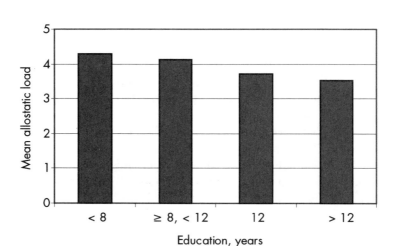

FIGURE 9–6. Mean allostatic load scores, by level of educational attainment: MacArthur Study of Successful Aging.

Source. Reprinted from Seeman TE, Crimmins E, Singer B, et al: "Cumulative Biological Risk and Socio-Economic Differences in Mortality: MacArthur Studies of Successful Aging." *Social Science and Medicine* 58:1985–1997, 2004. Copyright 2004, Elsevier. Used with permission.

adult SES). Figure 9–7 depicts the percentage of the sample with high levels of allostatic load (defined as those with allostatic load scores of 3 or above) by SES group. Participants who reported low levels of both childhood and adult SES had the greatest prevalence of high allostatic load, whereas those reporting high levels of SES at both timepoints had the lowest prevalence of high allostatic load. Those who experienced downward mobility (i.e., having high childhood but low adult SES) were the second highest in prevalence of high allostatic load, whereas those who experienced upward mobility in SES had somewhat lower prevalence levels. These results suggest that both childhood and adult economic adversity contribute to cumulation of allostatic load and that the experience of economic adversity at both life stages is associated with the highest levels of pathophysiological burden in later adulthood.

Recent analyses of data from the NHANES III provide a picture of allostatic load across combinations of SES and age. Levels of allostatic load by SES across groups ranging in age from the 20s to the 90s are depicted in Figure 9–8. In this analysis, SES groupings were defined on the basis of a poverty income ratio representing the ratio of household income to the federal poverty threshold; thus higher values indicate higher household

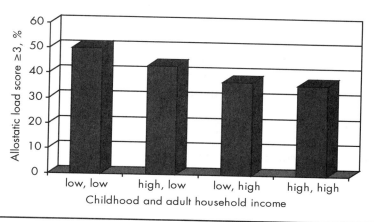

FIGURE 9–7. Economic adversity and prevalence of high levels of allostatic load (score of 3 or greater): Wisconsin Longitudinal Study.

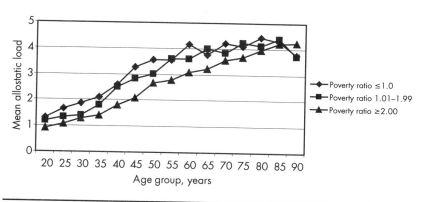

FIGURE 9–8. Mean allostatic load scores, by age and poverty ratio: National Health and Nutrition Examination Survey III.

Note. The numerator of the poverty income ratio was the midpoint of the observed family income category, and the denominator was composed of a combination of the age of the family reference person, the calendar year in which the family was interviewed, and the federal poverty threshold for that year. Persons who reported having no income were assigned a value of zero.

income. As can be seen in the figure, all income groups show the expected age-related increase in allostatic load. However, those with higher income levels (poverty ratio of 2 or higher) show lower levels of allostatic load than the other two income groups at each age up to age 80 years. Those in the lowest income category show the highest levels of allostatic load in many of the age categories, although age-specific levels of allostatic load for the low- and middle-income categories overlap considerably. It should be noted that variations in allostatic load by SES are greatest in middle to early old age, indicating that the pathophysiological burden associated with economic adversity may be most apparent in this age range.

Social Factors

There is also accumulating evidence for systematic variations in allostatic load as a function of differences in social environment. Specifically, evidence indicates that differences in allostatic load are related to levels of social integration as well as to more qualitative aspects of one's social relationships and that these relationships can be seen in both younger and older adults.

We found a negative relationship between social integration, measured in terms of reported number of ties with close family and friends, and allostatic load in the MacArthur Successful Aging Study (Figure 9–9; Seeman et al. 2002). For both men and women, a greater percentage of those reporting fewer social ties (i.e., 0–2 ties) had high levels of allostatic load (defined as a score of 5 or greater on the allostatic load index) as compared with those individuals reporting three or more close ties.

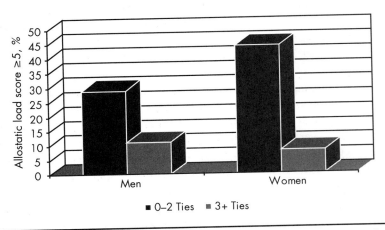

FIGURE 9–9.   Social integration and prevalence of high allostatic load (score of 5 or greater): MacArthur Study of Successful Aging.

Negative relationships between allostatic load levels and the *quality* of social relationships for individuals in the WLS have also been found (Seeman et al. 2002; Singer and Ryff 1999). Because the WLS has information on the quality of social relationships in childhood with parents and in adulthood with a partner, a history of social relationship experiences can be examined. Specifically, a measure of parental bonding is available that assessed participants' experience of affection, warmth, and attention with each parent during childhood, and another measure assessed emotional, sexual, intellectual, and recreational intimacy with spouses in adulthood (see Singer and Ryff 1999 for more detailed description).

Childhood and adulthood relationship experiences were combined to produce negative or positive relationship histories. Individuals reporting a lack of parental warmth or affection from both parents in childhood and/or lack of intimacy on combined emotional-sexual and intellectual-recreational adult intimacy measures were designated as having a negative relationship pathway. Individuals reporting parental warmth from at least one parent and a positive score on at least one of the two emotional-sexual or intellectual-recreational spousal intimacy measures were assigned to the positive relationship pathway. As shown in Figure 9–10, a greater percentage of male and female WLS respondents with negative relationship pathways had high levels of allostatic load in midlife (defined as scores of 3 or more) compared with those with more positive relationship histories (Seeman et al. 2002).

In addition to associations between high levels of allostatic load and impoverished social conditions (e.g., low levels of social integration or lack of emotionally supportive social relationships), there is also evidence of an association between actual negative social interactions and increased levels of allostatic load. In the MacArthur Successful Aging Study, we have found that higher reported frequency of conflict with—and/or excessive demands from—one's spouse, children, or close friends and relatives is associated with increased odds for high levels of allostatic load (scores of 5 or greater) in both men and women (Figure 9–11). There are also gender differences in the association between high levels of allostatic load and the category of social others for whom individuals report negative social interactions. As shown in Figure 9–11, negative spousal interactions are associated with much higher odds of high allostatic load in men as compared with women: men reporting frequent conflict and/or excessive demands from their wife are five times more likely to have high allostatic load scores. By contrast, it appears that negative interactions with children are most consequential for women, followed by negative interactions with close friends or relatives. Although the relative importance of different categories of individuals with whom one experiences negative interactions may differ for men and women

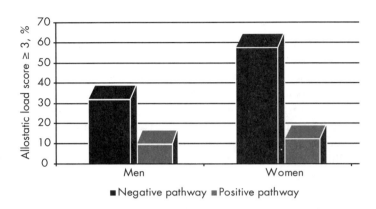

FIGURE 9–10. Social relationship history and prevalence of high allostatic load (score of 3 or greater): Wisconsin Longitudinal Study.

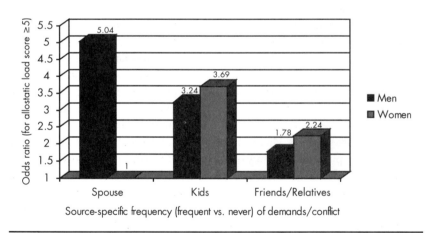

FIGURE 9–11. Frequency of social demands/conflicts and odds of high allostatic load (score of 5 or greater): MacArthur Study of Successful Aging.

in terms of odds of high allostatic load, the common theme is that greater experience of negative social interactions within important social relationships is associated with a greater likelihood of high levels of allostatic load in both men and women.

CONCLUSION

The evidence reviewed here suggests that a multisystems view of physiological dysregulation (allostatic load) holds promise as a valuable research construct for understanding the wear and tear on important physiological regulatory systems as a function of life's demands. Measurement of multisystem physiological dysregulation may help elucidate important biological mechanisms through which life experience is associated with health outcomes. The evidence confirms that greater levels of cumulative physiological dysregulation as reflected in higher allostatic load scores have been found to predict declines in cognitive and physical functioning, the incidence of cardiovascular disease, and mortality in older adults.

Support for hypothesized contributions of life stress to more rapid accumulation of such multisystem physiological dysregulation is provided by evidence that population variation in allostatic load is associated with variation in age, SES, and the quantity and quality of social ties. Assessment of allostatic load may be a very useful measure of the physiological price paid by the body in its attempts to adapt to life's demands. This price appears to vary in a predictable way according to individual characteristics and experience, being higher for those who are older and who are characterized by impoverished socioeconomic and social conditions. Although more research will be need to ascertain the best methods for measuring this multisystem index of physiological burden, research to date indicates that assessment of allostatic load may prove fruitful to our understanding of how life experience gets under the skin to affect health and well-being.

REFERENCES

Adler NE, Boyce T, Chesney MA, et al: Socioeconomic status and health: the challenge of the gradient. Am Psychol 49:15–24, 1994

Berkman LF, Seeman TE, Albert M, et al: High, usual and impaired functioning in community-dwelling older men and women: findings from the MacArthur Foundation Research Network on Successful Aging. J Clin Epidemiol 46:1129–1140, 1993

Crimmins EM, Johnston M, Hayward M, et al: Age differences in allostatic load: an index of physiological dysregulation. Exp Gerontol 38:731–734, 2003

Crimmins EM, Hayward MD, Seeman TE: Race/ethnicity, socioeconomic status and health, in Critical Perspectives on Racial and Ethnic Differences in Health in Late Life. Edited by Anderson NB, Bulatao RA, Cohen B. Washington, DC, National Research Council of the National Academies, 2004, pp 310–352

Karlamangla AS, Singer BH, McEwen BS, et al: Allostatic load as a predictor of functional decline: MacArthur studies of successful aging. J Clin Epidemiol 55:696–710, 2002

Macintyre S: The Black Report and beyond: what are the issues? Soc Sci Med 44:723–745, 1997

McEwen BS: Stress, adaptation, and disease: allostasis and allostatic load. Ann N Y Acad Sci 840:33–44, 1998

McEwen BS, Stellar E: Stress and the individual: mechanisms leading to disease (comment). Arch Intern Med 153:2093–2101, 1993

McEwen BS, Wingfield JC: The concept of allostasis in biology and biomedicine. Horm Behav 43:2–15, 2003

Pincus T, Callahan LF: What explains the association between socioeconomic status and health: primarily access to medical care or mind-body variables? ADVANCES: Journal of Mind–Body Health 11:4–36, 1995

Seeman TE, Singer BH, Rowe JW, et al: Price of adaptation: allostatic load and its health consequences. MacArthur Studies of Successful Aging. Arch Intern Med 157:2259–2268, 1997

Seeman TE, McEwen BS, Rowe JW, et al: Allostatic load as a marker of cumulative biological risk: MacArthur Studies of Successful Aging. Proc Natl Acad Sci USA 98:4770–4775, 2001

Seeman TE, Singer BH, Ryff CD, et al: Social relationships, gender, and allostatic load across two age cohorts. Psychosom Med 64:395–406, 2002

Seeman TE, Crimmins E, Huang MH, et al: Cumulative biological risk and socioeconomic differences in mortality: MacArthur Studies of Successful Aging. Soc Sci Med 58:1985–1997, 2004

Singer B, Ryff CD: Hierarchies of life histories and associated health risks. Ann NY Acad Sci 896:96–115, 1999

Sterling P, Eyer J: Allostasis: A new paradigm to explain arousal pathology, in Handbook of Life Stress, Cognition and Health. Edited by Fisher S, Reason J. New York, John Wiley & Sons, 1988, pp 631–651

Emotions, Personality, and Health

Laura D. Kubzansky, Ph.D.

"This is Descartes' error: the abyssal separation between body
and mind…the separation of the most refined operations of mind
from the structure and operation of a biological organism."

Damasio 1994, pp. 249–250

DESPITE THE EMBRACE of Descartes' perspectives by Western medicine
(Damasio 1994), the notion that emotions are linked to physical health has
endured. Proponents of the idea that psychological factors can cause or
exacerbate disease-related processes in the body point to the intuitions of
many of the great physicians in medicine (e.g., Sir William Osler; Hippo-
crates) as well as to scientific research on the topic. Detractors argue that
studies of the relationship between mental states and disease are not scientifically sound and are therefore unconvincing (Angell 1985). In the past
several decades, methodologically sound epidemiological research has provided more compelling evidence of such linkages, with relative risk estimates that are comparable with known risk factors such as smoking.
Although the debate continues, the magnitude and weight of the evidence
demand continued consideration of the hypothesis.

There are a variety of ways in which emotion might be related to physical health. Generally, evidence for one type of association should not be taken as support for any other. Perhaps the most controversial hypothesis is that emotions are involved in the development or etiology of disease outcomes. For example, there has been a long-standing hypothesis that high levels of anger may initiate pathophysiological processes that lead to coronary heart disease (CHD) (Kawachi et al. 1996). Alternatively, emotions may exacerbate symptoms or trigger acute disease-related events. For example, anxiety may trigger an asthma episode (Wright et al. 1998). Relatedly, emotion may be involved in the progression of disease. For example, depression after an initial myocardial infarction (MI) has been associated with decreased survival time (Frasure-Smith et al. 1995). Emotions may also affect compliance with medical regimen and disease management. Of course, disease may also influence emotion states. For example, the concept of vascular depression grew out of research suggesting that physiological changes incurred by cerebrovascular incidents also cause a predisposition to late-onset depression in older adults (Hinkle 1974). It is beyond the scope of this chapter to evaluate fully the evidence for any of these types of relationships. Rather, I focus on the most controversial of them—the possible role of emotion in the etiology of disease. I first consider a general model of emotion and health and then consider methodologies that may provide reasonably compelling evidence of an association. Examples of studies using these methodologies are provided from my own work, and outstanding issues are discussed.

A MODEL OF EMOTION AND HEALTH

As illustrated in Figure 10–1, research on emotion and health has converged on a general model, with some slight differences in the details (Baum and Posleszny 1999; Cohen et al. 1995; Kiecolt-Glaser et al. 2002; Kubzansky and Kawachi 2000; Salovey et al. 2000). The model suggests that emotions are a product of the interaction between the individual and the environment. Because emotions depend on an individual's construal and evaluation of the environment, both the social environment and personality play an important role in shaping emotional experiences. Personality characteristics can affect how the social environment is experienced. For example, individuals may differ in the types of environments they tend to select or create, or different individuals exposed to the same environment may experience it, interpret it, and react to it differently (Kubzansky et al. 2004). Events in the environment are appraised in terms of whether they

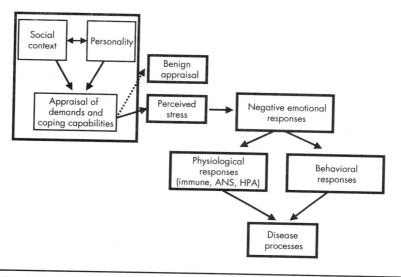

FIGURE 10–1.   A general model of emotion and health.
ANS = autonomic nervous system; HPA = hypothalamic-pituitary-adrenal axis.

are potentially harmful (e.g., associated with threat or loss) or beneficial (e.g., associated with actual or potential gain) (Frijda 1986; Lazarus 1991a). If demands are perceived to exceed one's coping capabilities, individuals experience a sense of stress and, subsequently, a negative emotional response. Emotions are hypothesized to influence health directly because they evoke physiological processes (e.g., activation of the hypothalamic-pituitary-adrenal axis) and indirectly because they influence health-related behaviors and other coping resources.

Emotion theorists have suggested that specific emotions are biologically based and mediate between continually changing situations and the individual's behavior (Arnold 1960; Frijda 1986; Lazarus 1968). The state of subjective feeling serves as a compelling signal that the individual is faced with a particular type of challenge, and it motivates the individual to respond to this fact (Frijda 1986). For example, fear motivates a person to escape danger, sadness motivates a person to disengage from loss, and so on (Lazarus 1991b). As such, emotions motivate individuals to respond to their environment and allow an adaptive flexibility of response not available to organisms that rely on instinct (Ellsworth and Smith 1988; Scherer 1982). Emotions also serve to communicate the individual's emotional state and likely behaviors to others in the social environment (Frijda 1986; Scherer 1982). Thus, emotions may be considered to be functionally appropriate processes that have dysfunctional consequences when the system is over-taxed (Frijda 1993).

Emotions are conceptualized as having identifiable cognitive, neurobiological, and behavioral components (Barlow 1988; Frijda 1986; Leventhal and Patrick-Miller 1993; Scherer 1982). The experience of most emotions occurs along a continuum. There is a range within which emotion levels are considered to be normal, but when they occur in inappropriate contexts and at high intensities, they may be identified as pathological (Frijda 1994). Thus, anxiety and depression are commonly experienced emotions that can also underlie clinical disorders. Criteria for diagnosing such disorders rely on the intensity, stability, consequences, and antecedents of the emotion (Lader and Marks 1973; Ohman 1993). Psychological research has suggested that pathological and normal emotion reactions essentially overlap in their cognitive, neurobiological, and behavioral components (Clark and Watson 1994; Frijda 1994). This is a critical issue for research on the role of emotion in physical health. The shared components of emotion at both ends of the spectrum suggest that their effects may occur all along the continuum—that is, before experiences are characterized as clinically relevant. If so, one might expect to see dose–response relationships between emotion and health outcomes, rather than threshold effects. As a result, research that looks only at presence or absence of clinically diagnosed disorders as a measure of emotion may be underestimating effects.

Most emotions may be seen either as transitory *states* brought on by specific situations or as *traits* that are stable and general dispositions to experience particular emotions (Lazarus 1994; Spielberger and Sarason 1978). Individuals high in trait anger, for example, experience the transitory state of anger more frequently and intensely than individuals low in trait anger. Thus, certain personality types are hypothesized to be vulnerable to disease partly because these individuals are predisposed to experience particular emotions. For example, hostility is considered a personality trait that predisposes individuals to experience frequent episodes of anger, suspicion, and cynicism (Smith and Frohm 1985). One recent study provided support for this idea, finding that hostile individuals were more likely to interpret ambiguous stimuli as more threatening relative to less hostile individuals (Chen and Matthews 2003). Such "predispositions" may also occur because hostile individuals are more likely to engage in cynical, mistrusting, aggressive behavior that contributes to maintaining a hostile environment.

Models of emotions and health generally hypothesize two types of effects. Short-term physiological changes may occur as a function of intense emotion experiences. For example, acute anxiety states may lead to hyperventilation, which may then trigger coronary vasospasm (Rasmussen et al. 1986). Such effects are not the focus of the current chapter but are reviewed elsewhere (Kamarck and Jennings 1991). Much of the work on emotion and health has hypothesized cumulative effects over time, whereby the repeated experience of specific emotions may subsequently set pathophysiological processes in motion. Such a hypothesis is only viable, however, if we can demonstrate long-standing patterns in emotion experience within individuals. As a result, the general model of emotion and health requires a life course perspective.

A variety of research suggests that continuity between personality and emotional functioning over time is likely (Caspi 2000; Gest 1997). Using data from the National Collaborative Perinatal Project, my colleagues and I recently examined this question directly. In this study, 694 children were followed for 30 years, and we tested whether childhood personality attributes were associated with specific patterns of adult emotional functioning (Kubzansky et al. 2004). At age 7 years, childhood personality was measured based on observer ratings of behavioral characteristics, and at age 35 years, individuals were asked to self-report emotional distress in various domains. Findings suggested that long-standing patterns of emotional experience do occur. For example, relative to children who were rated as low on distress proneness at age 7, children with high levels were at almost threefold risk of experiencing high levels of anger and hostility as adults (odds ratio=2.86; 95% confidence interval (CI)=1.31, 6.25). Unfortunately, repeated measures of emotional function over time were unavailable; further research demonstrating such patterns with repeated measures over time would confirm the epidemiological findings.

The general model of emotion and health proposes two primary pathways by which recurring emotion experience may cumulatively influence health and disease outcomes. Direct effects posit that emotions may alter biological systems. For example, negative emotions are associated with neuroendocrine and immune changes that may set in motion a cascade of physiological effects. These changes largely reflect catabolic activation whereby stored energy is converted to a usable resource and growth and repair functions are inhibited (see Baum et al. 1999 for a more extensive review). Different types of stress-related damage have been hypothesized, including damage due to repeated elevations of key hormones over long periods of time; failure to dampen physiological activation associated with negative emotion and stress; and inadequate hormonal response associated with stressful events that allows other systems to become overactive (McEwen 1998). Over time, such effects may set disease-related physiological processes in motion.

Negative emotions may also indirectly affect health through effects on health-related behaviors and coping resources. Data from the Stirling County Study suggest that individuals who become depressed are more likely to begin or continue smoking than those who never became depressed over 22 years of follow-up (Murphy et al. 2003). Negative emotions have also been linked to excessive alcohol consumption, greater body mass, and lower physical activity, and in turn these processes have been identified as risk factors for an array of diseases (Everson et al. 1997; Hayward 1995; Siegler 1994). Negative emotions may also disrupt social relationships, which are themselves associated with health outcomes. For example, in a study of social and interpersonal maladjustments, Paykel and Weissman (1973) compared changes in adjustment over 8 months of follow-up among 40 depressed women and 40 nondepressed women. Social functioning improved as symptoms improved, whereas greater symptomatology was associated with poorer social and interpersonal adjustments. However, interpersonal friction and inhibited communications were still evident in the depressed group, even when depressive symptoms improved. Thus, emotions may trigger cognitive, behavioral, or social processes that in turn affect health.

WHAT CONSTITUTES CAUSAL EVIDENCE?

One of the primary criticisms of studies of emotion and health has been methodological. Causality between emotion and health is bidirectional, and effects accumulate over a long period of time. Prior to 1985, most tests of the hypothesis were based on case-control or cross-sectional studies, which are particularly subject to recall and other biases. Because of the preservation of the temporal order of the link between emotion and disease onset, more compelling evidence is provided by prospective studies that measure emotions among initially disease-free individuals. Reports of such studies are becoming more commonplace, and many of these studies are able to control for an array of potential confounders (Kubzansky and Kawachi 2000). For example, using data from 1,759 men participating in the Normative Aging Study, we examined the relationship between CHD and worry, an important cognitive component of anxiety (Kubzansky et al. 1997). Worry was measured using a self-administered questionnaire that assessed five domains: social conditions, health, finances, self-definition, and aging. Participants were assessed by a physical examination every 3–5 years, and CHD was assessed using Framingham Heart Study criteria. Over 14 years of follow-up, compared with men reporting the lowest levels of worry about social conditions, those reporting the highest levels had a multivariate adjusted relative risk of 2.41 (95% CI, 1.40–4.13) for nonfatal MI, with a dose–response relationship between worry level and overall CHD risk. Some associations were also evident between the health and financial worries subscales and CHD (Kubzansky et al. 1997). Associations remained strong after controlling for known coronary risk factors.

General models of emotion and health have largely focused on effects of negative emotion and have failed to consider whether positive emotions (and related personality attributes) might also influence health. Zautra (2003) argued that positive and negative feeling states are not opposites, but rather, represent distinct emotional forces in our lives. Thus, a focus on negative emotions can only partially inform our understanding of the role emotions may play in health. Although theoretical models linking positive emotion and health are yet to be fully developed, empirical studies have begun to examine the question. Generally, positive emotions and attributes are hypothesized to have general systemic effects that may be seen across a spectrum of health outcomes rather than a one-to-one correspondence with any single outcome.

Two studies have explicitly examined effects of positive emotion and found them to be protective for several outcomes, including development of the common cold and premature mortality (Cohen et al. 2003; Danner et al. 2001). More work has considered optimism, a personality attribute considered to be linked with positive emotion. In separate studies, we recently examined the relationship between optimism and two health outcomes, CHD and pulmonary function, using data from the Normative Aging Study (Kubzansky et al. 2001, 2002). In both studies, an explanatory style measure of optimism was obtained that assesses optimism or pessimism based on how people explain routine events in their lives. An optimistic explanatory style is characterized by the belief that the future will be pleasant because one can control important outcomes (Peterson et al. 1998), whereas a pessimistic explanatory style has been linked to a sense of hopelessness and is marked by the view that problems are permanent and reflect one's shortcomings (Seligman 1991). Findings suggest a protective effect of optimism on the incidence of nonfatal and fatal CHD (relative risk=0.44; 95% CI=0.26, 0.74) among 1,306 men over the 10-year follow-up period (Kubzansky et al. 2001). Effects were maintained even after controlling for relevant coronary risk factors and possible confounding effects of negative emotions. Optimism was similarly protective in relation to lung function decline over 8 years of follow-up (Kubzansky et al. 2002). In this study, we considered whether an optimistic explanatory style would protect against rapid pulmonary decline, a risk factor for premature mortality, and other poor health outcomes. After controlling for initial levels of pulmonary function, weight, height, and smoking, we found optimists had a significantly slower rate of decline than pessimists. For example, pessimistic individuals declined approximately 43 cc's per year in forced expiratory volume over 1 second compared with more optimistic individuals, who declined 37 cc's. This difference in rate of decline is comparable to differences of 5–7 cc's per year reported between male current smokers versus never smokers in other studies (Griffith et al. 2001).

WHY DOES SOCIAL CONTEXT MATTER?

Models of emotion and health vary in their emphasis on the social context within which such relationships occur. However, although emotions may feel highly personal and unique, evidence suggests that they are conditioned to some extent by external social factors and in fact are socially patterned. Because many emotions are responses to power and status differentials embedded within social situations (Kemper 1993; Nolen-Hoeksema et al. 1999), the social context plays an important role in determining which emotions are likely to be experienced, how they are expressed, and what their consequences will be (Gross 1998; Kemper 1993). For example, data from the Stirling County Study indicated that the prevalence of depression was significantly and persistently higher in the group with low socioeconomic status (SES) relative to individuals at other socioeconomic levels (Murphy et al. 1991). Moreover, incidence of depression was also higher among those in the low SES group over the follow-up period. Further study in this sample suggested that low SES was causally related to poor emotional outcomes (although some downward social mobility due to depression also occurred). In our own work, we have similarly found that individuals with less education were significantly more likely to be pessimistic (Kubzansky et al. 2001). The social environment may also affect the degree to which individuals are susceptible to emotion–disease relationships. An explicit consideration of the social context will inform a more precise understanding of the emotion–health relationship.

ONGOING RESEARCH CHALLENGES

Many challenges remain for this work. Much of the research on emotions and health lies at the intersection between psychiatric epidemiology, social epidemiology, and psychology. Classification and measurement of emotion present thorny ongoing questions. Because of their ease of use, many epidemiological studies have relied on symptom measures of emotion (e.g., Center for Epidemiologic Studies Depression scale [CES-D]) that can provide only a snapshot of experience at any one time. Because they do not take account of lifetime experience, these studies cannot truly evaluate cumulative effects of emotion. For example, given the episodic nature of depression, it is possible that an individual reports few depressive symptoms on a questionnaire but has had several depressive episodes over the course of his or her lifetime. As a result, symptom measures may represent only the most anemic test of the hypothesis that emotions influence health. Thus, many questions remain as to the chronicity and severity of emotion experiences needed to trigger pathophysiological effects. Interestingly, epidemiological studies using symptom measures have not suggested a threshold at which effects are more likely to occur; rather, risk appears to increase with each additional symptom (Kubzansky and Kawachi 2000).

Measurement of emotions has other challenges as well, particularly when measures are derived from self-assessments. Few emotions occur in pure form. For example, anxiety and depressive symptoms frequently occur together, and clinical diagnoses of their disorders are highly comorbid. However, measurement approaches often fail to discriminate clearly between different emotions (Kubzansky and Kawachi 2000). Other investigators have argued that self-report data are problematic because they cannot distinguish between genuine mental well-being (i.e., low anxiety) and the façade of health created by psychological defenses (Shedler et al. 1993). Both repression (failure to attend to emotions) and suppression (conscious inhibition of the expression of emotion when emotionally aroused) have been linked with poor health outcomes as well, albeit inconsistently (Davison and Petrie 1997; Gross and Levenson 1993; Pennebaker and Beall 1986). What are appropriate measures for such experiences is still unclear, and empirical research evaluating links between repression or suppression and health remains limited.

Other methodological and conceptual issues also deserve consideration. Even supposing one could obtain accurate measures of each emotion, determine whether different emotions have specific disease-related effects, or determine whether emotions have similar and general systemic effects is a topic of some debate (McEwen 1998; Melnechuk 1988). Moreover, the focus on specific emotion effects may be somewhat limited. There is an emerging sense that the ability to regulate emotions or manage emotional complexity may play a critical role in both mental and physical health (Gross 1998; Pennebaker 1997; Zautra 2003). Appropriate regulation of emotions may rest on avoiding the extremes of inhibition and expression (Siegman 1994). A true measure of emotional health may consider one's ability both to regulate emotions in terms of the various forms of expression and also to manage emotions in terms of successfully integrating or balancing the experience of negative and positive experiences (Zautra 2003). Levels of any specific emotion may give some insight into regulatory capability. For example, individuals who consistently experience high anxiety levels are unlikely to have effective regulatory strategies. However, a better measure of risk may be to evaluate emotional health directly.

DO EMOTIONS INFLUENCE HEALTH?

These challenges notwithstanding, taken in its totality the research to date is strongly suggestive of a causal relationship between emotions and health. However, despite methodological improvements in recent research, there continues to be a deep and abiding skepticism for this proposition. Although many skeptics agree that anecdotal evidence is striking, they argue that the correlation is illusory, or that causality runs from disease to emotion, or that there is some underlying factor (i.e., genetics) driving both emotion and disease states. Skeptics argue that the notion that emotions may influence health goes against known laws of physics and that no objective or credible evidence exists when the research is held to standards that should be applied for all biomedical research (Relman 2000). Investigators who support the hypothesis argue that this research is held to a higher standard than more traditional biomedical research (Williams et al. 2002).

This raises the question of what kind of evidence could be considered credible. There is no perfect study design—all have their flaws. Studies of emotion in the etiology of disease are particularly difficult to bring into an randomized, controlled setting, the gold standard for studies in human populations. Prospective studies in healthy individuals are largely infeasible. Most randomized trials work with individuals who are already ill, and it is entirely plausible that effects of emotion differ depending on whether biological systems are healthy at the outset or are already damaged. Moreover, such designs, powerful though they may be, are still flawed. Because of the nature of the variables under study, serious questions can be raised about who is willing to participate in trials addressing these issues, heterogeneity in reasons for which individuals are willing to participate in the trial, and difficulty in assembling a control group who could not also access treatment (Ryff and Singer 1998). By definition, interpretation of findings and quality of the evidence almost becomes an article of faith, depending on whether one focuses on design limitations or the strength of the findings despite the real-world constraints imposed by the nature of the question.

Where does that leave us in evaluating the hypothesis that emotions influence health outcomes? This question is not dissimilar to the initial debate on whether smoking is causally related to CHD risk. Yet in the absence of randomized clinical trials, such a conclusion is now largely uncontested (Hennekens and Buring 1987). In some ways, the role of smoking in disease etiology is easier to examine, because conceptualization and measurement of smoking are more straightforward relative to emotion. The smoking model is informative nonetheless. Epidemiologists have argued that evidence may be judged to support a cause/effect relationship when numerous studies are conducted by different investigators at various times, and all show generally similar results (Hennekens and Buring 1987). Studies should use a range of methodologies in diverse geographic or cultural settings and among different populations. To evaluate a causal role of emotion in disease processes, we need to use a similar strategy. Informative research will include a range of study designs, such as prospective observational studies, experimental work in human populations that may examine short-term outcomes (e.g., immediate effects of anxiety on heart rate variability), and experimental work in animal populations. Because much of the research to date grows out of different disciplines and secondary analyses, additional steps should be taken to improve our ability to evaluate research across methods and disciplines in terms of standardizing measures and designing studies explicitly for the purpose of testing a possible etiological role of emotion in health. By triangulating our methods, we can then examine the weight of the evidence in total. Although results from every study may not be consistent, we should expect to see trends either in support of or against the hypothesis. What is needed is both a conscious understanding of the challenges in bringing this question under scientific study and clear guidelines on what evidence will be considered credible, derived from investigators on both sides of the issue. Then we might take this question out of the realm of faith and into the realm of science.

REFERENCES

Angell M: Disease as a reflection of the psyche. N Engl J Med 312:1570–1572, 1985
Arnold MB: Emotion and Personality. New York, Columbia University Press, 1960
Barlow DH: Anxiety and Its Disorders. New York, Guilford, 1988
Baum A, Posleszny DM: Health psychology: mapping biobehavioral contributions to health and illness. Annu Rev Psychol 50:137–163, 1999
Caspi A: The child is father of the man: personality continuities from childhood to adulthood. J Pers Soc Psychol 78:158–172, 2000

Chen E, Matthews KA: Development of the Cognitive Appraisal and Understanding of Social Events (CAUSE) videos. Health Psychol 22:106–110, 2003

Clark LA, Watson D: Distinguishing functional from dysfunctional affective responses, in The Nature of Emotion. Edited by Ekman P, Davidson RJ. New York, Oxford University Press, 1994, pp 131–137

Cohen S, Kessler RC, Gordon LU: Measuring Stress: A Guide for Health and Social Scientists. New York, Oxford University Press, 1995

Cohen S, Doyle WJ, Turner RB, et al: Emotional style and susceptibility to the common cold. Psychosom Med 65:652–657, 2003

Damasio AR: Descartes' Error. New York, Avon Books, 1994

Danner DD, Snowdon DA, Friesen WV: Positive emotions in early life and longevity: findings from the Nun Study. J Pers Soc Psychol 80:804–813, 2001

Davison K, Petrie K: Emotional expression and health, in Cambridge Handbook of Psychology, Health, and Medicine. Edited by Baum A, Newman S, Weinman J, et al. Cambridge, Cambridge University Press, 1997, pp 103–106

Ellsworth PC, Smith CA: From appraisal to emotion: differences among unpleasant feelings. Motivation and Emotion 12:271–302, 1988

Everson SA, Kauhanen J, Kaplan GA, et al: Hostility and increased risk of mortality and acute myocardial infarction: the mediating role of behavioral risk factors. Am J Epidemiol 146:142–152, 1997

Frasure-Smith N, Lesperance F, Talajic M: Depression and 18-month prognosis after myocardial infarction (comment). Circulation 91:999–1005, 1995

Frijda NH: The Emotions. Cambridge, Cambridge University Press, 1986

Frijda NH: Moods, emotions episodes, and emotions, in Handbook of Emotions. Edited by Lewis M, Haviland JM. New York, Guilford, 1993, pp 381–405

Frijda NH: Emotions are functional, most of the time, in The Nature of Emotion. Edited by Ekman P, Davidson RJ. New York, Oxford University Press, 1994, pp 112–122

Gest SD: Behavioral inhibition: stability and associations with adaptation from childhood to early adulthood. J Pers Soc Psychol 72:467–475, 1997

Griffith KA, Sherrill DL, Siegel EM, et al: Predictors of loss of lung function in the elderly: The Cardiovascular Health Study. Am J Respir Crit Care Med 163:61–68, 2001

Gross JJ: The emerging field of emotion regulation: an integrative review. Rev Gen Psychol 2:271–299, 1998

Gross JJ, Levenson RW: Emotional suppression: physiology, self-report, and expressive behavior. J Pers Soc Psychol 64:970–986, 1993

Hayward C: Psychiatric illness and cardiovascular disease risk. Epidemiol Rev 17:129–138, 1995

Hennekens CH, Buring JE: Epidemiology in Medicine. Boston, MA, Little, Brown, 1987

Hinkle LE: The effect of exposure to culture change, social change, and changes in interpersonal relationships on health, in Stressful Life Events: Their Nature and Effects. Edited by Dohrenwend BS, Dohrenwend BP. New York, John Wiley and Sons, 1974, pp 9–44

Kamarck T, Jennings JR: Biobehavioral factors in sudden cardiac death. Psychol Bull 109:42–75, 1991

Kawachi I, Sparrow D, Spiro A, et al: A prospective study of anger and coronary heart disease. The Normative Aging Study. Circulation 94:2090–2095, 1996

Kemper TD: Sociological models in the explanation of emotions, in Handbook of Emotions. Edited by Lewis M, Haviland JM. New York, Guilford, 1993, pp 41–52

Kiecolt-Glaser JK, McGuire L, Robles TF, et al: Emotions, morbidity, and mortality: new perspectives from psychoneuroimmunology. Annu Rev Psychol 53:83–107, 2002

Kubzansky LD, Kawachi I: Going to the heart of the matter: do negative emotions cause coronary heart disease? J Psychosom Res 48:323–337, 2000

Kubzansky LD, Kawachi I, Spiro A III, et al: Is worrying bad for your heart? A prospective study of worry and coronary heart disease in the Normative Aging Study. Circulation 95:818–824, 1997

Kubzansky LD, Sparrow D, Vokonas P, et al: Is the glass half empty or half full? A prospective study of optimism and coronary heart disease in the Normative Aging Study. Psychosom Med 63:910–916, 2001

Kubzansky LD, Wright RJ, Cohen S, et al: Breathing easy: a prospective study of optimism and pulmonary function in the Normative Aging Study. Ann Behav Med 24:345–353, 2002

Kubzansky LD, Martin L, Buka SL: Early manifestations of personality and adult emotional functioning. Emotion 4:364–377, 2004

Lader M, Marks I: Clinical Anxiety. London, Heinemann, 1973

Lazarus RS: Emotions and adaptation: conceptual and empirical relations, in Nebraska Symposium on Motivation. Lincoln, NE, University of Nebraska Press, 1968, pp 175–276

Lazarus RS: Emotion and Adaptation. New York, Oxford University Press, 1991a

Lazarus RS: Progress on a cognitive-motivational-relational theory of emotion. Am Psychol 46:819–834, 1991b

Lazarus RS: The stable and the unstable in emotion, in The Nature of Emotion. Edited by Ekman P, Davidson RJ. New York, Oxford University Press, 1994, pp 70–85

Leventhal H, Patrick-Miller L: Emotion and illness: the mind is in the body, in Handbook of Emotions. Edited by Lewis M, Haviland JM. New York, Guilford, 1993, pp 365–380

McEwen BS: Protective and damaging effects of stress mediators. N Engl J Med 338:171–179, 1998

Melnechuk T: Emotions, brain, immunity, and health: a review, in Emotions and Psychopathology. Edited by Clynes M, Panksepp J. New York, Plenum, 1988, pp 181–246

Murphy JM, Olivier DC, Monson RR, et al: Depression and anxiety in relation to social status. Arch Gen Psychiatry 48:223–229, 1991

Murphy JM, Horton NJ, Monson RR, et al: Cigarette smoking in relation to depression: historical trends from the Stirling County Study. Am J Psychiatry 160:1663–1669, 2003

Nolen-Hoeksema S, Larson J, Grayson C: Explaining the gender difference in depressive symptoms. J Pers Soc Psychol 77:1061–1072, 1999

Ohman A: Fear and anxiety as emotional phenomena: clinical phenomenology, evolutionary perspectives, and information-processing mechanisms, in Handbook of Emotions. Edited by Lewis M, Haviland JM. New York, Guilford, 1993, pp 511–536

Paykel ES, Weissman MM: Social adjustment and depression: a longitudinal study. Arch Gen Psychiatry 28:659–663, 1973

Pennebaker JW: Writing about emotional experiences as a therapeutic process. Psychol Sci 8:162–166, 1997

Pennebaker J, Beall SK: Confronting a traumatic event: toward and understanding of inhibition and disease. J Abnorm Psychol 95:274–281, 1986

Peterson C, Seligman MEP, Yurko KH, et al: Catastrophizing and untimely death. Psychol Sci 9:127–130, 1998

Rasmussen K, Ravnsbaek J, Funch-Jenson P, et al: Oesophageal spasm in patients with coronary artery spasm. Lancet 1:174–176, 1986

Relman AS: Integrative medicine: who needs it and why (letter). Arch Intern Med 160:1205, 2000

Ryff CD, Singer B: The contours of positive human health. Psychol Inq 9:1–28, 1998

Salovey P, Rothman AJ, Detweiler JB, et al: Emotional states and physical health. Am Psychol 55:110–121, 2000

Scherer KR: Emotion as a process: function, origin and regulation. Soc Sci Inf 21:555–570, 1982

Seligman MEP: Learned Optimism. New York, Knopf, 1991

Shedler J, Mayman M, Manis M: The illusion of mental health. Am Psychol 48:1117–1131, 1993

Siegler IC: Hostility and risk: demographic and lifestyle variables, in Anger, Hostility, and the Heart. Edited by Siegman AW, Smith TW. Hillsdale, NJ, Lawrence Erlbaum Associates, 1994, pp 199–214

Siegman AW: Cardiovascular consequences of expressing and repressing anger, in Anger, Hostility, and the Heart. Edited by Siegman AW, Smith TW. Hillsdale, NJ, Lawrence Erlbaum Associates, 1994, pp 173–197

Smith TW, Frohm KD: What's so unhealthy about hostility? Construct validity and psychosocial correlates of the Cook and Medley Ho scale. Health Psychol 4:503–520, 1985

Spielberger CD, Sarason JG: Stress and Anxiety. Washington, DC, Hemisphere, 1978

Williams RB, Schneiderman N, Relman AS, et al: Resolved: psychosocial interventions can improve clinical outcomes in organic disease. Rebuttals and closing arguments. Psychosom Med 64:564–567, 2002

Wright RJ, Rodriguez M, Cohen S: Review of psychosocial stress and asthma: an integrated biopsychosocial approach. Thorax 53:1066–1074, 1998

Zautra AJ: Emotions, Stress, and Health. New York, Oxford University Press, 2003

Something Old, Something New, Something Borrowed, Something Blue

The Story of "Gulf War Syndrome"

Simon Wessely, F.R.C.Psych.

Matthew Hotopf, Ph.D.

THE GULF WAR AND ITS AFTERMATH

The Gulf War

Iraq invaded Kuwait on August 2, 1990. Shortly after, coalition forces led by the United States began a military deployment known as Operation Desert Shield. On January 17, 1991, an active air campaign began against Iraq, Operation Desert Storm, and on February 24 a ground war began that lasted only 4 days. It was a resounding military success. Iraqi forces were beaten in the field and expelled from Kuwait. The main contributor to the coalition was the United States, with 697,000 personnel. Substantial contributions also came from the United Kingdom (53,000), Saudi Arabia, Egypt, Oman, France, Syria, Kuwait, Pakistan, Canada, Bahrain, Morocco and Qatar. Twenty-five other countries also contributed smaller numbers.

Not only was the campaign a military success, it was also a medical success. It is only during the modern era that deaths from battle have exceeded deaths from disease for most armies. Traditionally, fighting in hostile environments such as the desert has been associated with morbidity and mortality, often substantial, from causes not related to enemy action, such as heat stroke, dehydration, and infectious disease. Yet during the Gulf War there was no evidence for any deaths from those sources among American or British personnel (Hyams et al. 1995). Military medical authorities must have ended the campaign relieved not to have had to deal with large-scale casualties and delighted with the success of their preventive measures.

Gulf War Syndrome

Now, more than a decade later, all that sounds a little hollow. Military success was not reflected by regime change, which would require a second war. Few remember the genuine medical achievements of the campaign, and instead, when asked about the Gulf War and health, most people answer, "Ah yes, that's where Gulf War syndrome began."

Shortly after the cessation of hostilities reports started to emerge from the United States of clusters of unusual illnesses occurring among Gulf War veterans. Claims were made that previously fit veterans had developed unusual diseases, illnesses, and symptoms. Reports emerged also of children with birth defects being born to Gulf War veterans.

These reports were invariably anecdotal and impressionistic. Details remained obscure; when many of these clusters were formally investigated either there was no objective evidence of any new illness or it could not be shown that the illness represented anything more than normally occurring conditions. Meanwhile, formal epidemiological research was at last commissioned (discussed later), but by the time these studies began to report, Gulf War syndrome (GWS) had captured the public imagination.

Long before the machinery of scientific research had rolled into action, GWS had been the focus of a remarkable barrage of publicity and media attention. We found it impossible to document the number and range of this coverage, but there can be no doubt that by the mid-1990s GWS had become a media *cause celebre* on both sides of the Atlantic.

In this chapter we suggest a tentative explanation of Gulf War–related illnesses. We argue for the importance of three related factors. The first factor we propose is the events of the Gulf War itself. We suggest that the initial trigger for Gulf War–related illnesses were the peculiar physical and psychological hazards of modern warfare and the methods used to protect troops from such hazards. In particular we consider the threat of chemical and biological warfare and the methods used to reduce that threat. The second factor relates to events after the conflict and the interaction between the media, government, and military that served to foster a climate of suspicion and rumor. The third factor links the particular hazards of modern warfare to Western contemporary societal attitudes on environmental risks and concerns. Many of the hazards encountered during the Gulf campaign had resonance with a common, and often passionate, societal agenda that gave the narratives of the Gulf veterans a particular resonance and link to wider civilian concerns.

THE EVIDENCE SO FAR

Results of the Studies

Case Series

The first coordinated response to the problem was to invite any veteran with health problems to come forward for detailed medical evaluation. This began in the United States with health registries established by both the Veterans Administration and the Department of Defense to provide systematic clinical evaluations and was then repeated in the United Kingdom with the establishment of the Medical Assessment Programme.

There have now been several analyses of those attending these programs, who now number more than 3,000 in the United Kingdom and more than 100,000 in the United States. The results have not suggested any unusual pattern of illness; instead, the largest diagnostic category has been medically unexplained symptoms and syndromes (Coker et al. 1999; Joseph 1997; Lee et al. 2001; Roy et al. 1998). These programs have served a very important function, however, because attendance is not random and is associated with a wide variety of war-related exposures (Smith et al. 2002). The therapeutic effect of a sound assessment, information, and provision of services and/or reassurance should not be underestimated.

Scientifically, other than providing evidence of significant concerns in the veteran community, such programs can give only limited scientific information because of their nonrandom selection. However, one would expect that if service in the Gulf was associated with either disease new to medical science (as with the first appearance of AIDS at the beginning of the 1980s) or a dramatic elevation of a recognized but hitherto rare condition, then this would have been detected. Neither has happened (Gray et al. 2004).

Epidemiology

The most comprehensive analyses have been made of the mortality of both the United States and United Kingdom Gulf War cohorts. The results show that, contrary to media reports, there has been no increase in mortality in either cohort (Kang and Bullman 1996, 2001; MacFarlane et al. 2000) other than an increase in accidental death (U.S. and U.K.) or suicide (U.S. only) as observed in the aftermath of other conflicts.

The first large epidemiological study of Gulf War–related illness was a questionnaire-based study of a random sample of Gulf War veterans and appropriate military control subjects from the state of Iowa (Iowa Persian Gulf Study Group 1997). This showed increased rates of symptom reporting in the Gulf War cohort. Symptom-defined conditions including chronic fatigue syndrome, depression, posttraumatic stress disorder (PTSD), and others were all elevated.

In the King's United Kingdom study we compared a random sample of 4,246 U.K. Gulf War veterans drawn from all three Armed Services and including both those serving and those not serving, with similar numbers of nondeployed personnel and an active-duty control group, namely, members of the United Kingdom Armed Forces who had served in the difficult and dangerous environment of Bosnia from the start of the United Nations peacekeeping mission there (1992–1997; Unwin et al. 1999). The results were striking. U.K. Gulf War veterans were between two and three times more likely to report each and every one of the 50 symptoms inquired about. Whatever the symptom, the rate was at least twice as high in the Gulf War cohort than in either the nondeployed or the Bosnia cohorts. Health perception was decreased in the Gulf War cohort, but physical functioning was only very slightly different and still above expected nonmilitary norms. Hence the Gulf War veterans experienced more symptoms, endorsed more conditions, and felt worse, but were still physically functioning well as a group, than either the nondeployed cohort or those deployed to Bosnia (Unwin et al. 1999).

Figure 11–1 illustrates these findings (Unwin et al. 1999). Each data point represents an individual symptom. To the left are common symptoms, such as fatigue or headache, whereas to the right are unusual symptoms, such as lump in throat, night sweats, or passing urine more often. It is clear that there is no difference between those deployed to Bosnia and those in the military in general in 1991. It is equally clear that the Gulf War cohort are different; frankly, visual inspection alone leaves no doubt as to the substantial differences between the groups. Yet the shape of the curve between the Gulf War veterans and the two control groups does not differ.

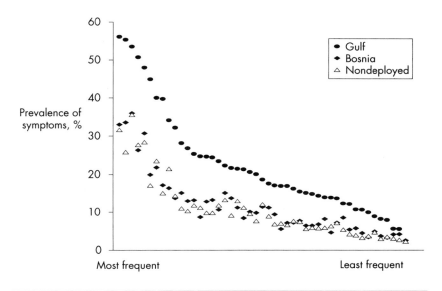

FIGURE 11–1. Self-reported symptoms in three military cohorts.

Likewise, we asked about 50 symptoms, but other symptoms were not inquired after, which prompted some commentators to suggest that we had some how "missed" the real symptoms of GWS. Yet this graph shows that to be unlikely—one can assume that any other symptom would appear in the Bosnia or nondeployed group at its expected frequency and in the Gulf War group at twice the rate. The position on the x axis for any given symptom is determined by its relative frequency in the control population. Further statistical analyses have merely confirmed what is visually clear (Everitt et al. 2002; Ismail et al. 1999). Other epidemiologically based samples from Hawaii and Pennsylvania (Stretch et al. 1995), Boston (Proctor et al. 1998), active service United States Army Air Force personnel (Fukuda et al. 1998), Kansas (Steele 2000), the SeaBees (Gray et al. 1999a) and the large Veterans Administration study (Kang et al. 2000) all show essentially the same findings.

In a recent review, Barrett et al. (2003) concluded that overall, Gulf War veterans report two to three times the rates of common symptoms as their nondeployed colleagues. Likewise, there is a consensus that health perception and quality of life are impaired among Gulf War–era deployed compared with nondeployed personnel (Kang et al. 2000; Proctor et al. 2001; Voelker et al. 2002). Significantly, all of these studies, including our own, are limited by the use of self-report measures. Self-reported symptoms are not a good guide to findings on clinical examination (McCauley et al. 1999). High rates of reported symptoms do not necessarily reflect high rates of physical disorder. Indeed, if that were the case it would contradict a considerable body of literature on the nature of somatic symptoms in the community. These symptoms are exceedingly common and often persistent. Yet fewer than one in five are found to have a discrete physical explanation (Kroenke and Mangelsdorff 1989), suggesting that simple assumptions linking symptom with disease are frequently misleading (Mayou et al. 1995).

What exactly is the size of observed increase in morbidity? Symptoms in the community are distributed dimensionally, but if one imposes certain arbitrary but not implausible cutoffs or case definitions, then the excess burden of "caseness," or ill health, seems to be 20%–30% (Cherry et al. 2001a; Fukuda et al. 1998; Gray et al. 2002; Steele 2000).

Is there evidence of something simpler, an increase in an already known and defined physical condition? In general, the answer is no. None of the case series give any hint of an increase in any particular physical condition; if such registries contained considerable numbers of any particular diagnostic condition, for example, lupus or an unusual cancer, then given that there is a fixed denominator (Gulf War service), even case registries would be sufficient to note an excess. However, this has not happened (Macfarlane et al. 2004; Smith et al. 2000).

There have been some exceptions. We have found an increase in seborrheic dermatitis (Higgins et al. 2002), although this has attracted little attention and no comment. What has understandably attracted attention is the possibility of an increase in a rare but usually fatal neurological disorder, amyotrophic lateral sclerosis (ALS), known as motor neuron disease (MND) in the United Kingdom. A large-scale study in the United States that used multiple methods of data collection, including newspaper articles and Web site appeals, reported 40 cases in among U.S. Gulf War veterans. This significant increase was sufficient for the U.S. government to declare the disease to be service related (Horner et al. 2003). However, it is worthy of note that there has been no increase in mortality due to neurological disease, which would be expected given that ALS is a fatal disease. Instead, it remains possible, as has been argued, that there has been an overascertainment of cases in the Gulf War veterans compared with the control subjects (Rose 2004). Regardless, although ALS is a devastating disease for those affected, it is still very rare in veteran populations and cannot account for anything more than a fraction of the observed increase in morbidity in Gulf War veterans, which is not accompanied by evidence of peripheral nervous system involvement.

Who Is at Risk?

If the Gulf War health effect were confined only to a particular subset of the entire deployment, this would provide valuable clues as to etiology. However, this has not happened. The predictors of ill health are not particularly surprising and tend to be nonspecific. Lower rank, for example, which is highly correlated with education, is firmly associated with ill health (Ford et al. 2001; Ismail et al. 2000; Wolfe et al. 1998).

Some studies have found differences between the services, with, for example, the Navy being less at risk (Steele 2000), but in the United Kingdom we have found no differences in the burden of ill health between the three services. Several U.S. studies have reported that reservists and women are at increased risk (Carney et al. 2003; Gray et al. 2002). We did not find this, but the U.K. Armed Forces used far fewer reservists and women during the conflict, which might explain these differences. An association with a particular time period of the conflict might provide clues to a discrete environmental exposure and has been reported by one study (Steele 2000) but not another (Spencer et al. 1998).

Is There a Gulf War Syndrome?

The term *Gulf War syndrome* has acquired remarkable media and popular salience, but is there any such thing? A syndrome implies a unique constellation of signs and/or symptoms. For there to be a *Gulf War syndrome*, not only must there be evidence of such a unique constellation but also it must be found in the context of the Gulf War conflict and not elsewhere (Wegman et al. 1998).

Robert Haley (Haley et al. 1997b), a Dallas-based epidemiologist, was the first to argue in favor of a unique Gulf War syndrome, using factor analysis. However, his data came from a much-studied single naval reserve construction battalion already known to have high rates of illness. The study had a 41% response rate and a sample size of 249 and did not have a control group, military or nonmilitary. As numerous commentators have pointed out, this makes it difficult to establish whether the proposed new syndrome is indeed linked to Gulf War service (Landrigan 1997). Undeterred, Haley has continued to pursue the trail of a unique Gulf War syndrome with tenacity and has claimed to have found specific evidence of damage to the basal ganglia and pons (Haley 2003). He has found the cause of this to be exposure to chemical weapons and/or pesticides and has stated that "there is substantial evidence and general acknowledgment that large numbers of military personnel were repetitively exposed to low environmental levels of the organophosphate chemical nerve agent sarin and pesticides" (Haley et al. 1999). According to Haley, exposures to chemical weapons and pesticides has led to specific central and peripheral nerve damage since the end of the conflict, and this risk will continue to increase over time, like a Sword of Damocles hanging over the heads of the veterans. However, a series of expert review committees and panels have failed to be convinced by the suggestion of widespread use of chemical weapons, and the suggestions of specific localized brain damage need to be replicated.

Beyond Haley's work, studies that use epidemiologically defined subjects and appropriate controls have generally not found evidence of a unique Gulf War syndrome. True, clusters of symptoms can be found. For example, there is general agreement that Gulf War veterans are affected more by a cluster of symptoms that can be collectively grouped as "cognitive/psychological," and most find a factor labeled by Haley as "arthromyoneuropathy" but that others prefer to call musculoskeletal. Yet the most important question is not whether such clusters exist, but are they unique to Gulf War veterans?

For example, in our study we did indeed find evidence to support a particular factor structure to symptoms in the Gulf War cohort, but this was no different from the factor structure in the Bosnia or nondeployed control subjects. The Gulf War group had more symptoms experienced at greater intensity, but there was no difference in the way these symptoms could be organized (Ismail et al. 1999). A series of controlled studies in the United States drew similar conclusions (Bourdette et al. 2001; Doebbeling et al. 2000; Fukuda et al. 1998; Knoke et al. 2000). Only Kang et al. (2002) found something different in a very large study of deployed and nondeployed veterans. Five of six factors were very similar between the groups, but there was one "Gulf" factor containing symptoms such as blurred vision, loss of balance, tremors/shaking, and speech difficulty. Those loading on this factor reported substantially more "Gulf" exposures such as depleted uranium, botulism vaccine (not used by U.K. forces), chemical agent–resistant coating (CARC) paint, contaminated food, and nerve gas. Once again, this raises the question of the direction of causality and/or recall bias.

There is evidence of an increase in other unexplained syndromes in Gulf War veterans, including such concepts as chronic fatigue syndrome, fibromyalgia, and multiple chemical sensitivities (Bourdette et al. 2001; Gray et al. 2002; Reid et al. 2001). Yet this is really only another way of reporting that the overall burden of symptoms is increased—explaining one symptom-defined condition (GWS) by another does not advance knowledge very far.

The balance of evidence is currently against there being a distinct Gulf War syndrome. In many ways, it is a side issue that has attracted more interest and polemic than it deserves. The key question is whether or not there is a Gulf War health effect, and this is established beyond reasonable doubt. Whether this amounts to a unique illness, identifiable only by complex statistical techniques, seems to be a secondary issue.

The argument among academics is academic, because regardless of the emerging professional consensus, GWS is established as a popular media and social reality. Investigating how and why this concept developed is important, but the answers will not come from social as much as the clinical sciences.

The Position Elsewhere

Thus far we have considered the position solely from a United States/ United Kingdom perspective. Yet many countries participated in the coalition forces, and we are now starting to hear from them as well.

The first non-U.S. country to publish a detailed examination of its Gulf War veterans was Canada (Goss Gilroy, Inc. 1998). The results were remarkably consistent with what had already been reported from the United States and would be reported from the United Kingdom, Denmark, and most recently Australia.

Each country's experience has also given examples of natural variations and experiments that will, in time, prove informative. For example, Canada sent three vessels to the Persian Gulf—two used pyridostigmine prophylaxis, and one did not. Yet rates of illness were identical among the three ships (Goss Gilroy, Inc. 1998). Likewise, Danish Gulf War veterans also have elevated rates of symptomatic ill health (Ishoy et al. 1999), yet nearly all were only involved in peacekeeping duties after the end of hostilities and neither used pyridostigmine prophylaxis nor received vaccinations against biological agents. Australian health concerns seemed to have surfaced considerably later than those in the United States or United Kingdom (McKenzie et al. 2004).

The French experience remains enigmatic. French authorities have consistently denied that any health problems have emerged in their Gulf War forces. Likewise, although one or two articles have appeared in the French press about GWS in other countries, there have been very few media reports of similar stories in France, which largely appeared in 2000 and then seem to have ceased, prompted by the death of a single French Gulf War veteran from neoplastic disease (Reuters 2000). If the French were not affected, this would be important epidemiological evidence, because the pattern of forces protection used by the French differed from that of both the Americans and the British, and in particular, anthrax vaccination was not used. One must, however, be cautious about the lack of evidence. First, no systematic study has yet been reported, although one is under way, and keep in mind the official denials of any problem in this country prior to the publication of systematic studies. Second, the cultural pattern of illnesses in French society differs from that in the English-speaking and Scandinavian regions. Illness entities such as chronic fatigue syndrome or multiple chemical sensitivity are hardly acknowledged or recognized (Girault 2002; Mouterde 2001).

Summary

The conclusion of these studies is, therefore, that *something* about Gulf War service has affected the symptomatic health of large numbers of those who took part in the campaign from most of the Coalition countries. At the same time, no compelling evidence has emerged to date of either distinct biomedical abnormalities or premature mortality.

THE POSITIONS
- -

We probably will never know the precise explanation for the increase in ill health seen in members of the armed forces of several coalition countries who took part in the Gulf War. It is almost certain there is no single explanation. Instead, we propose three different explanatory models, each of them a different approach and conceptualization of the problem.

The First Position: Gulf War Illness Is the Result of Biological Hazards in the Gulf

The most popular explanation for the Gulf War health effect among the media and, we suspect, the general public is that the cause of GWS lies in the particular hazards of that conflict. Most attention has been given to the measures taken to protect the combatants from the threat of chemical and biological warfare. These included immunizations against biological weapons such as plague and anthrax and pyridostigmine tablets to protect against exposure to anticholinesterase-based nerve agents such as sarin. Other hazards included exposure to depleted uranium or to the smoke from the oil fires ignited by the retreating Iraqi forces.

Evidence is conflicting. A small group of U.S. Gulf War veterans were definitely exposed to depleted uranium in the form of shrapnel fragments and are being intensively monitored. Some subtle changes were soon reported in neuropsychological and neuroendocrine function (McDiarmid et al. 2000). Ten years after exposure, urine uranium remains persistently elevated (McDiarmid et al. 2004), but renal function remains normal, which is a crucial observation because renal toxicity is the main long-term hazard of uranium exposure, contrary to the popular perception that it is only weakly radioactive. There is some evidence of a mutagenic effect in those with depleted uranium shrapnel fragments still in their bodies (McDiarmid et al. 2004), but immune competence was normal. More surprising was the finding that personnel who were involved in the same "friendly fire" incidents but who did not receive depleted uranium shrapnel wounds also had significant elevations of uranium levels in their urine, presumably via inhalation or contamination (Gwiazda et al. 2004).

Smoke from the burning oil wells received much publicity at the end of the land war, and perhaps for that reason it was closely monitored on the spot. A series of environmental monitoring studies concluded that in general most toxins were below accepted lower limits, but there was an increase in level of fine particulate, although even that was not unusual for a desert region (U.S. Army Environmental Hygiene Agency 1994). A recent paper reported that levels of polycyclic aromatic hydrocarbon biomarkers, which would be expected to be elevated, were actually lower in Gulf War veterans exposed to the oil fires than control subjects who had remained in Germany (Poirier et al. 1999), whereas no links were found between modeled exposures (as opposed to self-reported exposures) and respiratory health (Lange et al. 2002).

Pyridostigmine bromide, a reversible inhibitor of acetylcholinesterase, was used as a prophylaxis against exposure to nerve gas. Although side effects were frequently reported during its use in the Gulf War campaign, these were short lived. No acute toxicity was observed (Keeler et al. 1991). This is important, because long-term organophosphorus toxicity, which is certainly a hazard, has only been clearly documented in the aftermath of acute toxicity (Fulco et al. 2000). The Canadian experience also argued against a prominent role for pyridostigmine bromide, which has been used in civilian practice for the treatment of myasthenia gravis for many years, and in higher dosages than used by the armed forces, without apparent adverse effect. It has even been used as a treatment for the fatigue associated with postpolio syndrome (Trojan and Cashman 1995). The extensive cumulative experience with pyridostigmine bromide in civilian neurological practice argues against an important role for it in Gulf War–related illnesses (Albers and Berent 2000; Presidential Advisory Committee on Gulf War Veterans' Illnesses 1997).

Thus the evidence does not support an important role for pyridostigmine bromide administration, but with two caveats. An elegant mouse experiment has suggested that pyridostigmine bromide, which normally does not penetrate the blood–brain barrier, may do so under stressful conditions (Friedman et al. 1996), but this was not confirmed in guinea pigs (Grauer et al. 2000). Second, hazard may have resulted from interactions with other agents. A study of chickens confirmed the safety of pyridostigmine, permethrin (a pesticide), and *N*,*N*-diethyl-*m*-toluamide (DEET, an insect repellent) individually but reported neurotoxicity when given in combination, albeit in high dosage (Abou-Donia et al. 1996), and rats given similar combinations have slower locomotion rates (Hoy et al. 2000).

Perhaps host variation may explain differences in individual susceptibility. Haley claimed that polymorphisms in the enzyme detoxification pathways for organophosphate compounds are related to symptoms (Haley et al. 1999), which is theoretically plausible (Furlong 2000) but has not been confirmed in two studies from the United Kingdom (Hotopf et al. 2003; Mackness et al. 2000). Finally, animal experiments have failed to confirm any adverse delayed neurobehavioral effects from low-dose pyridostigmine alone or in combination with low-dose sarin but confirmed that pyridostigmine did convey some protection against sarin, the purpose for which it is administered (Scremin et al. 2003).

The role of pesticides, and in particular organophosphate pesticides, has also been much discussed. Large quantities of pesticides in various forms were used by all the combatants to reduce the risk of infectious disease. In general, providing these were used appropriately and by trained personnel, little hazard should have resulted (Parliamentary Office of Science and Technology 1997). However, whether this actually happened in practice is unclear. There have now been numerous expert committee reports on both sides of the Atlantic, but most particularly in the United Kingdom. There is no disputing the acute toxic effects of organophosphates on the human nervous system, but there remains considerable uncertainty and controversy about the effects of low-level chronic exposure (Committee on Toxicity of Chemicals in Food 1999; Presidential Advisory Committee on Gulf War Veterans' Illnesses 1997; Royal College of Physicians and Psychiatrists 1998; U.S. General Accounting Office 1997). Even when chronic low-dose exposure has been documented, this is not synonymous with evidence of damage to the nervous system (Albers et al. 2004). Information mismanagement has played a part in making this a controversial issue.

Detailed studies of the peripheral nervous system in both United States and our own epidemiologically derived samples have failed to find evidence of neuropathy (Bourdette et al. 2001), including normal findings on the sensitive single fiber electromyography paradigm, which is strong evidence against any chronic peripheral nerve damage (Amato et al. 1997; Sharief et al. 2002). The results of the massive Veterans Administration epidemiological survey of Gulf War veterans and their families recently have been published. More than 1,000 Gulf War veterans and an equal number of control subjects were studied for evidence of peripheral nerve damage. None was found (Davis et al. 2004). Again the main dissenting opinion has come from Robert Haley in Dallas, even though his own study of his highly selected small population did not reveal any clinically detectable neurological involvement (Haley et al. 1997a).

In the United States, but not in the United Kingdom, there was much attention given to the possibility that troops had been exposed to low levels of the nerve agents sarin and cyclosarin following the probable accidental destruction of an Iraqi arms dump at Khamisiyah. There was no contemporary evidence of chemical weapon detections or clinical evidence of exposure, and since then little evidence has been found that those possibly exposed to the plume thought to have resulted from the incident had any difference in postwar illness or neurological damage (Davis et al. 2004; Gray et al. 1999b; McCauley et al. 2002). Later studies using better exposure estimate models failed to find any suspicious pattern of hospitalization in those possibly exposed, with the exception of a small increase in hospital episodes for cardiac dysrhythmias (Smith et al. 2003), which provides a tantalizing link with the rich historical literature on cardiac dysfunction in service personnel, going back via effort syndrome as far as "soldier's heart" in the American Civil War. A recent animal study failed to show any adverse effects from low-dose sarin (Pearce et al. 1999), and we should not forget that, dissenting opinions aside, there is no reliable evidence to suggest deliberate use of chemical or biological weapons during the conflict.

There is also little evidence of central nervous system damage as indicated by objective evidence of neuropsychological deficits (David et al. 2002). Subjective symptoms of cognitive difficulties are of course very common; however, as in the literature of chronic fatigue syndrome, these do not relate very well to objective indices of neuropsychological difficulties but do relate to symptoms of PTSD or depression (David et al. 2002; Lindem et al. 2003). In conclusion, "it is unlikely that the tens of thousands of Gulf War veterans with unexplained health problems are suffering from the results of exposure to neurotoxic chemicals" (Spencer et al. 2001).

Some of the most suggestive evidence comes from studies of the possible effects of the vaccination program used to protect the armed forces against the threat from biological weapons, although this may partly reflect the fact that quantifying exposure to vaccines, although difficult, is not impossible, unlike some of the other postulated hazards.

The United States program involved immunization against anthrax and botulism, whereas the United Kingdom chose to protect its armed forces against plague and anthrax, with the additional use of pertussis vaccine as adjuvant to speed up the response to anthrax (Ministry of Defence 2000). We found a relationship between receiving both multiple vaccinations in general and those against chemical and biological agents in particular and the persistence of symptoms, despite controlling for obvious confounders. The finding that multiple vaccinations in other contexts, including deployment to Bosnia, were not associated with any increase experience of symptoms suggests some interaction between multiple vaccination and active service deployment to the Persian Gulf (Hotopf et al. 2000; Unwin et al. 1999). The Manchester group likewise found a relationship between reported receipt of multiple vaccinations and subsequent symptoms (Cherry et al. 2001b).

What does all this mean? Rook and Zumla (1997) argued from a theoretical perspective that the particular medical countermeasures used by the United Kingdom Armed Forces, namely the combination of anthrax, pertussis, and multiple immunizations, given sometimes under stressful conditions, could bias the immune system toward a Th2-cytokine pattern. An American study of help-seeking veterans failed to find compelling evidence of any immunological dysfunction (Everson et al. 2002), nor did a study of Dutch veterans who had served with the United Nations in Cambodia and experienced similar symptoms to Gulf War veterans (Soetekouw et al. 1999). We used a nested case–control design to study sick Gulf War veterans, well Gulf War veterans, and sick veterans from other deployments. We found evidence of ongoing Th1 activation associated with ill health in the Gulf War veterans detectable some 9 years after the conflict and a biased generation of memory cells secreting the suppressor cytokine interleukin 10. Although this is not in keeping with the original hypothesis, the demonstration of ongoing immune activation remains significant and requires explanation (Skowera et al. 2004).

There are also some general objections to the view that the cause of the ill health experienced by Gulf War veterans is only the physical and/or toxic hazards of the campaign (Presidential Advisory Committee on Gulf War Veterans' Illnesses 1997). Some studies have found that certain symptom patterns are related to certain self-reported exposures (Haley and Kurt 1997; Wolfe et al. 1998), but others have not (Gray et al. 1999a, 2002; Iowa Persian Gulf Study Group 1997; Kroenke et al. 1998; Unwin et al. 1999). In general it seems that most exposures are linked to most outcomes, if judged by retrospective self-recall. If one accepts recall as accurate, then the links would be via the aggregate stressors of war; alternatively, if one does not accept this, the links would be a product of recall bias and search after meaning influenced by current health. These are not mutually exclusive: we found, when asking veterans identical questions about Gulf War exposures over time, that recall varied according to current health perception. If this has improved, fewer exposures were recalled, whereas if subjective health had declined, the opposite was true (Wessely et al. 2003). If self-recall of hazard exposure is not stable (Spencer et al. 2001) and is influenced by state markers (Wessely et al. 2003), then this changes the interpretation of studies that find specific links between recall of hazards and specific symptoms, raising the possibility that the symptom came first. Finally, the time latency between the war and onset of symptoms is also unusual if symptoms were related to war exposure (Kroenke et al. 1998)

In summary, there is some evidence to suggest that some of the new hazards to which the armed forces were exposed during the Gulf War may be associated with unexpected side effects and perhaps later ill health. Some claims need replication, and others remain implausible. Position 1 thus has partial support.

The Second Position: Gulf War Illness Is a Modern Manifestation of Postconflict Ill Health

The first argument, that the cause of the Gulf War health effect lies in the unique nature of modern warfare, would be substantially weakened if it could be shown that similar clinical syndromes have arisen after other conflicts that did not involve the particular hazards of the Gulf War.

That similar syndromes have indeed been found after other conflicts has been most clearly argued by Craig Hyams and colleagues (1996) in a seminal paper. Interpretable medical records and accounts really only commence from the middle of the nineteenth century, but from then onward the literature does contain clinical descriptions of ex-servicemen (always men) with conditions that show considerable similarities to the Gulf War narratives. These condition have received many different labels; soldier's heart, later termed effort syndrome, owes its provenance to the Crimean and American Civil War. Shell shock and neurasthenia dominate the writings of the First World War, whereas Agent Orange Syndrome and PTSD emerge after Vietnam.

Hyams's argument rests entirely on a reading of secondary sources, but we have recently concluded a study based on primary sources as well. We began by locating clinical case histories from the Crimean War and Indian Mutiny (Jones and Wessely 1999) that begin the theme of chronic, unexplained symptoms. This was then continued in a systematic study of U.K. war pension files from the Boer War, through the First and Second World Wars, and ending with clinical files from the Gulf War Medical Assessment Programme (Jones et al. 2002).

The results showed that postconflict syndromes that show considerable similarities to Gulf War illness have been reported after all the major conflicts involving the British armed forces. The names have changed, of course, but there has also been some shift in the symptom patterns recorded, from the debility/weakness picture of Victorian neurasthenia to the more neuropsychiatric (including cognitive and depressive symptoms) of modern times. Of course, we cannot know if this represents a true cultural shift in symptoms or merely a shift in recognition and reporting.

The second position therefore states that sending young men (and increasingly women) to war invariably results in some casualties that cannot be explained on a solely physical injury basis and that the symptoms experienced are similar to those experienced by Gulf War veterans.

The implication is that this reflects the psychological cost of warfare on the combatants. Yet the Gulf War was not a particularly "stressful" conflict in the traditional sense. The active ground war only last a few days. Casualties among the coalition forces were exceptionally light. It would be historically wrong to extrapolate from the prolonged privation, fear, and danger of, for example, the trenches to the Gulf War. In support of that is our evidence that the actual rate of the quintessential psychiatric injury of war, PTSD, is indeed elevated in U.K. Gulf War veterans but not to the extent that could explain the overall increase in ill health (Ismail et al. 2002). The relative risk was very similar to that in an overall meta-analysis of nine studies of psychiatric disorder in Gulf War veterans that reported an odds ratio of 3.2 for the risk of PTSD (Stimpson et al. 2003), but the attributable risk was low; in other words, most symptomatic Gulf War veterans did not have PTSD.

Some may be surprised at this latter observation, because there does exist a number of studies that report considerable posttraumatic symptomatology in Gulf War veterans. However, it is worth pointing out a number of caveats. First of all, these studies are based on questionnaires rather than standardized psychiatric interviews, and it is well known that pencil and paper tests always overestimate the extent of psychiatric morbidity. Second, symptoms do not equate with disorder—for that, one needs not just symptoms, which are common, but disability, which is less so. Third, there is a tendency to assume that all psychiatric disorders in veterans of war are PTSD, but in fact our data and those of others suggests that depression and substance abuse are more common.

Yet it would be equally wrong to claim that Gulf War veterans were not exposed to stress or fear of any sort. There is a firm consensus that physical symptomatology is related to stressful exposures in all sorts of circumstances, and of course going to war is no exception (Ford et al. 2001; Storzbach et al. 2000). Most particularly, the real threat posed by chemical and biological exposures cannot be underestimated (Betts 1998; Stokes and Banderet 1997). Such weapons "engender fear out of all proportion to their threat" (O'Brien and Payne 1993)—they are as much, if not more, weapons of psychological as physical warfare (Holloway et al. 1997). Even in training, up to 20% of those who took part in exercises using simulated exposure to irritant gases showed moderate to severe psychological anxiety (Fullerton and Ursano 1990).

Ignoring the current controversy over weapons of mass destruction, there was no doubting back in 1991 that Iraq possessed such weapons and had used them extensively during the Iran–Iraq war and against Kurdish civilians. It was anticipated that they would be used in the forthcoming campaign. Countermeasures were untested and probably insufficient. Effective measures, such as wearing the full nuclear-biological-chemical suits, were uncomfortable and induced a state of partial sensory deprivation. Surveys of U.S. forces during Desert Shield confirmed that the threat of chemical and biological warfare was the most common expressed fear of the coming conflict. The ground war may have only taken a few days, but the deployment itself lasted over many months. During Desert Storm there were several thousand documented chemical alarm alerts. Subsequently the consensus of opinion is that none were true positives and that Iraq did not use its chemical and biological arsenal. However, at the time, each alert had to be assumed to be genuine. Thus even if traditional military stressors were not a prominent feature of the active campaign, a well-founded and realistic anxiety about the threat of dread weapons could still be important. It does not take much imagination to accept the very potent psychological effects of operating in an environment where one could be subject to chemical attack or of believing, even erroneously, that one has been the victim of such an attack (Fullerton and Ursano 1990; Riddle et al. 2003).

Indeed, believing oneself to be exposed to such weapons has been frequently found to be associated with the development of symptoms (Nisenbaum et al. 2000; Unwin et al. 1999), sometimes very strongly (Haley et al. 1997b; Proctor et al. 1998; Stuart et al. 2003). The psychological impact generated by the knowledge that such weapons existed, even if they were not used, is substantial.

The Third Position: Gulf War Syndrome Can Be Found in People Who Have Never Been to the Gulf or Served in the Armed Forces

We have argued that either some hazard of Gulf War service alone (position 1) or war service in general (position 2) is linked to subsequent ill health.

But may the features of Gulf War illness actually have nothing to do with warfare at all?

This seems a surprising proposition. However, patients with multiple unexplained symptoms, all of them reported in the narratives of Gulf War veterans, are also encountered in civilian medical practice and literature. In the popular literature, first-person accounts and patient-oriented literature (in the media and the Internet) exist with considerable similarities to those of some Gulf War veterans. One finds such material under diverse headings such as "ME" (myalgic encephalomyelitis), total allergy syndrome, electrical hypersensitivity, dental amalgam disease, silicone breast implant disease, hypoglycemia, chronic Lyme disease, sick building syndrome, and many more.

Turning to the professional literature, studies are now reporting that the rates of various symptom-defined conditions originally described in the civilian population are also elevated in the Gulf War cohorts. Chief among these are chronic fatigue syndrome (Kang et al. 2003; Kipen et al. 1999) and/or multiple chemical sensitivity (Black et al. 2000; Reid et al. 2001). These syndromes, which also include fibromyalgia, irritable bowel syndrome, and others, overlap not only with each other (Wessely et al. 1999) but also with Gulf War illness.

That symptom-based conditions overlap with Gulf War illness is not surprising given that all the epidemiological studies confirm that Gulf War veterans experience an increased reporting of each and every one of the symptoms that make up the case definitions of all these syndromes found in civilian practice. This does not mean, however, that these conditions and the others are all the same, or that Gulf War illness is the same. It does mean that they all overlap, that discrete boundaries cannot be drawn between them (or if they can, we currently have no idea where these boundaries are). It also means that any explanation of GWS must explain how similar conditions can be found either in nondeployed military personnel or in civilians as well.

ATTRIBUTIONS AND EXPLANATIONS

The Military: From Effort Syndrome to Gulf War Syndrome

It is a truism to state that people, whether civilians or soldiers, need to explain their distress. Indeed, an intriguing body of research confirms that in the clinical setting patients prefer a firm, albeit inaccurate, label for their symptoms as opposed to an honest expression of uncertainty (Thomas 1978). We have already discussed the various labels given in the past to postconflict syndromes and suggested that there is considerable overlap between the different names given at different times. Yet where did those labels come from, and can one read any significance into the choice of label? The answer seems to be yes. Some of the labels applied to unexplained illnesses in the armed services clearly are related to the particular nature of the recent conflict. Soldier's heart arose because of the contemporary concern that the straps securing the heavy back pack sworn by the Union soldiers in the American Civil War was compressing the muscles, arteries, and nerves in the region of the heart. The epidemic of "rheumatic" conditions that occurred after the Boer War was a response to the presumed health dangers of sleeping out in wet conditions on the High Veldt. Shell shock took its name from the presumed effects of concussion caused by the passage of the shell, let alone its actual detonation. Again, one must remember that the exploding shell remains the predominant image of the First World War and epitomized both then and now the particular trauma and anxiety of that conflict—for the first time, the main cause of death was the unseen enemy.

Another popular term was neurasthenia. As originally described in civilian life, neurasthenia was a condition affecting successful people, usually males, and was a response to the stresses and strains of contemporary life. Overwork, exhaustion, long hours, the new demands of capitalism, and so on were the kind of explanations that dominated the early (but not late) literature—it was an illness of successful men, "captains of industry." Hence when it emerged that army captains on the Western front were developing similar unexplained conditions associated with extreme exhaustion, it was not difficult to translate the civilian neurasthenia concept into the military context. Sir Frederick Mott (1919), one of the most influential medical figures of the period, wrote that "neurasthenia...was more likely to be acquired in *officers of a sound mental constitution than men of the ranks*, because in the former the prolonged stress of responsibility which, in the officer worn out by the prolonged stress of war and want of sleep, causes anxiety lest he should fail in his critical duties."

After Vietnam came two new syndromes, one ostensibly psychological, the other somatic. PTSD was socially created to deal with the guilt and trauma of an unpopular lost campaign (Scott 1990; Young 1995). The other, Agent Orange Syndrome (Hall 1989), can be seen as the forerunner of GWS. Thus the labels given to previous postconflict syndromes can be seen to derive from both the specifics of that particular campaign and the general health beliefs of the time. We have already listed the main health concerns of the Gulf War—depleted uranium, vaccinations, pollution, chemical warfare, and so on. How do these map onto wider civilian health concerns?

The Civilian Perspective

People who feel ill need an explanation for their malaise. Sometimes doctors can provide such an explanation, but often they cannot (Kroenke and Mangelsdorff 1989), and in those circumstances, when medicine fails to provide clear answers, people most often turn to their environment to provide those explanations. The choice they make is culturally determined, because it must depend on contemporary and accepted views of health and disease.

In a previous time ill health and misfortune were commonly interpreted in terms of demonic possession, spirits, and satanic influence. Such explanations have now lost their cultural resonance in the developed world. To a large extent these have been replaced by explanations based on environmental hazards and threats.

It is evident that the range and scope of symptoms, illnesses, and conditions blamed on the environment has increased since the 1980s. There are many social, historical, and cultural reasons why this should be—reflecting increasing global concern about the effects of chemicals, radiation, and infectious diseases and the collective memories of recent health disasters. The generation that fought the Gulf War was born in a world already sensitized by "Silent Spring" and the thalidomide tragedy and came to maturity in a background of the AIDS epidemic, mad cow disease, and numerous well-publicized environmental tragedies such as Chernobyl, Seveso, and Bhopal. It is a moot point indeed if our environment really is more threatening than it was—the food, water, and air of any given post–Industrial Revolution city of the nineteenth century does not bear comparison with their modern counterparts (Dalrymple 1998; Shorter 1997)—but we are certainly more aware of these dangers than our predecessors.

It is the role of environmental attribution that provides a link between the otherwise varied new illnesses and health hazards that figure so prominently in the media, such as dental amalgam disease, electromagnetic radiation, myalgic encephalomyelitis, organophosphate toxicity, candida, sick building syndrome, multiple chemical sensitivity, and so on. Although the postulated pathophysiological mechanisms are many and varied, all are associated with the presence of multiple unexplained symptoms, and all are in one way or another blamed on some unwelcome external environmental hazard such as chemicals, pollution, viruses, and radiation or on an internal toxic substance introduced from outside, such as silicone breast implants or dental amalgam. Thus in civilian life what unites these disparate conditions is not only the clinical evidence of multiple unexplained symptoms but also the cognitive schema linking them with ideas of environmental hazard and toxicity. Petrie and Wessely (2002) suggested that all these new syndromes can be collectively considered as "illnesses of modernity" or to use a phrase that was very much in vogue in the latter half of the nineteenth century, "diseases of modern life."

One result of this heightened environmental awareness has been a gradual transformation of popular models of illness and disease. In place of the demons and spirits comes the belief that we as a society are oppressed by mystery gases, viruses and toxins, all of which are invisible and some of which are as elusive as the demons of old. One can see this in the changing pattern of attributions given by patients with unexplained symptoms (Stewart 1990). Guy's Poisons Unit, for example, reported that only since the 1980s have they started to see patients with multiple symptoms attributed to environmental poisoning (Hutchesson and Volans 1989).

Many scientists now profess themselves baffled by the public anxieties expressed over the possible adverse effects of pesticides, not to mention genetically modified foods and cell phones (Burke 1999), but these make sense in the light of the last paragraph. At the turn of the nineteenth century, science and technology held great hopes for the future—the introduction of chemicals into food was to be welcomed because it promised greater, and not lesser, food safety, and *chemical* was not the term of abuse it has now become. Those days have passed. Science is certainly not a force for evil, nor have we become a nation of Luddites, but both science and technology are clearly seen in more ambiguous terms than previously. Few can deny the heightened anxiety by the public and mass media over the safety of the environment and the suspicions about the food we eat, the water we drink, and the air we breathe. As Barsky (1988b) pointed out, "the world seems generally filled with peril, jammed with other health hazards in addition to disease...nothing in our environment can be trusted, no matter how comfortable or familiar."

Likewise, few can doubt the growing strength of the environmental movement. We are far more aware of the risks of our environment than ever before. Activism to combat environmental pollution and toxic waste has been described as a new social movement (Matterson-Allen and Brown 1990), one that has gradually shifted its focus from its origins in the birth of the ecology movement after "Silent Spring," which was very much about the challenge to biodiversity posed by pollution, to a new focus on risks to human health. The word *risk* is itself a quintessentially modern word, and there is even an epidemic of the word risk in the scientific, and most particularly epidemiological, journals (Skolbekken 1995).

There is a complex relationship between environmental concerns and symptoms. There is no doubt that being exposed to environmental hazard, such as chemicals, leads to increased fears and concerns (Bowler et al. 1994).

This increase occurs whether the exposure is real or perceived. These fears in turn lead to increased symptom reporting, perhaps via activation of the stress response. The strength of a subject's opinions on environmental matters was associated with symptom reporting in those exposed to a hazardous waste site but also in those who were not (Lipscomb et al. 1992; Roht et al. 1985). Those who described themselves as "very worried" about local environmental conditions were 10 times more likely to complain of headaches than those not so concerned (Shusterman et al. 1991). Finally, people who experience more symptoms, for whatever reason, may have an increased level of concern about their environment as they look for explanations for their ill health. The consequence is a vicious circle linking exposure (whether real or perceived), beliefs, and symptoms.

It is therefore possible that as the general level of concern increases, so might the overall burden of symptoms. This is perhaps one explanation for the oft observed "paradox of health"—that we live longer, healthier lives than at any time in human history but experience more symptoms and feel worse (Barsky 1988a).

Concerns About Reproduction

At the same time as fears over health surfaced, so did fears about reproductive health. Numerous emotional media stories emerged of veterans fathering children with severe birth defects. It was impossible not to be moved by these individual tragedies and impossible not to understand and sympathize why the parents of children so afflicted should search for explanations and generally find these in the father's military service. These fears remain prominent—a common response we have encountered among the veterans who have completed our qualitative survey is the intention to delay having children until these issues are resolved, which may of course create the very outcome they are striving to avoid.

The evidence for an association with "hard outcomes" such as congenital malformations is mixed. No increase was found comparing 34,000 live births to Gulf War veterans with 41,000 births to nondeployed military personnel (Cowan et al. 1997). Araneta et al. (2003) reported an increased rate of certain cardiac abnormalities and renal agenesis. Doyle et al. (2004) carried out the only United Kingdom study of reproductive health in which it was attempted to obtain data from the entire Gulf War cohort and Gulf War–era controls, albeit only partially successfully. They found no evidence for a link between fathers' Gulf War service and the risk of stillbirth, most structural abnormalities, chromosomal malformations, or syndromes. Malformations of the urinary system and nonspecific musculoskeletal malformations were elevated, but the risk was reduced when the analysis was restricted to medically verified outcomes only. There was also an increased risk of early (but not late) miscarriage or stillbirths in pregnancies fathered by male (but not female) Gulf War veterans. However, the authors speculated that this may relate to the lower-than-expected rate in the nondeployed control subjects (Doyle et al. 2004).

Reproductive fears are one area in which there is a lack of historical continuity. These fears are largely absent from the voluminous records and narratives of the First World War. The first example we can find is an isolated report that Australian veterans returning from the Pacific War expressed these fears, which they blamed on the malaria prophylaxis they had taken, but fears about hazard to the next generation is not a common Second World War belief either. It first surfaces as a major issue in veterans' health during the Vietnam era as part of the Agent Orange controversy. One may speculate whether the cumulative and widespread knowledge of the medical effects of radiation after Hiroshima and the thalidomide tragedy are the triggers for this change. Now such fears seem to be an integral part of most environmental accidents and exposures. Following the Chernobyl radiation disaster there was a decrease in the birth rate across Western Europe and an increase in induced abortions (Bertollini et al. 1990; Knudson 1991)—the International Atomic Energy Agency estimated that some where between 100,000 and 200,000 pregnancies were therapeutically aborted in Western Europe for this reason (Ketchem 1987). There was also a major increase in therapeutic abortions after the Seveso incident (Pocchiari et al. 1979). Spontaneous abortions and delayed pregnancy became an issue in the Balkans during aerial bombing of chemical plants (Fineman 1999).

The Soldier Becomes a Civilian Again

The situation of the soldier returning from war, especially if accompanied by rapid separation from service, is a complex one. On joining up individuals join military society and become part of a group where their loss of autonomy is offset by a feeling of belonging and a clearly defined role within the organization. Deployment to war is a unique experience of shared adversity when the reality of military service cannot be avoided and where individual fears are shared and managed by group membership. War provides an exaggerated, perhaps extreme, version of the entire range of human experiences—excitement, love, friendship, and achievement as well as fear, hate, and guilt (Bourke 1999).

After combat everything is changed. Readjustment to routine soldering occurs and the process of assimilation and accommodation of the experience of war continues. Some may experience guilt or shame at acts of commission or omission. Pride and a feeling of achievement may be felt, whereas others may become angry and accusatory at those whom they see as letting them down in time of threat. The search for meaning may continue for years.

Leaving the service may be desired for many reasons. These include the simple end of their engagement as well as being unable to equal the combat experience or desiring never to have to repeat it. Once "separated," modern servicemen and women return to a risk-aversive society in which individual rights, not duties or obligations, count—the obverse of military society. A realistic knowledge of military experience by civilian society has become less with the end of national conflicts or national service; fewer and fewer civilians have any contact with the military. Contemporary understanding of military service is more likely to be driven by Hollywood's depictions than personal experience. Films that portray the veteran as victim are common, a situation abhorrent to most servicemen and women. A few, however, do construe their experience in this way encouraged by the media.

Military and veteran culture also reflects the general changing relationship between individual and society. One sign of this is the loss of Crown Indemnity by the Ministry of Defence and the subsequent avalanche of litigation against the military authorities. However, it is simplistic, and probably erroneous, to assume that the rise in symptoms among Gulf War veterans is related to the rise in litigation, as some skeptics have suggested. Instead, it is more likely that litigation arises as a consequence, rather than a cause, of these concerns. Furthermore, there is little difference in the health complaints and concerns of United States versus United Kingdom veterans (Kang et al. 2000), but whereas United Kingdom veterans can and are litigating against the military, their American counterparts are statute barred from any similar activity.

We do not subscribe to simplistic notions of war, stress, and posttraumatic stress, but neither do we see war as of no psychological or social significance. We suggest that nearly everyone is changed by exposure to combat, either for better or worse. In the words of one World War II veteran, "everything since [war] has just been a footnote."

The Gulf War and Modernity

Turning to the hazards of the Gulf War, we can also see that these have particular resonance to general societal issues and concerns. There is, for example, a powerful antivaccination lobby that receives frequent media coverage, as exemplified by the controversy over whooping cough vaccination and, more recently MMR vaccination (Jefferson 2000). Likewise, the intense concerns around the use of depleted uranium munitions seem less related to its toxic properties (those of a heavy metal) and more to the powerful emotional impact of its assumed link with radioactivity (actually weak), engendered by the term *uranium.*

All commentators agree that the Gulf War was the most "high tech" military conflict up to that time, the first time the so-called Revolution in Military Affairs had been seen in action, and the first demonstration of the overwhelming superiority of American military technology. All of this might be expected to reduce traditional military stressors from more direct, low-tech combat. However, the introduction of new technologies is not without risks of its own—the introduction of new technologies into civilian industries is often accompanied by a rise in nonspecific complaints and is also blamed by many for particular syndromes such as repetitive strain injury (Smith and Carayon 1996). Scandinavian researchers have coined the term "Techno Stress" to describe this phenomenon (Arnetz and Wiholm 1997; Berg et al. 1992).

One reason why technological/chemical incidents and disasters have a stronger association with long-term subjective health effects than natural disasters may relate to the differing time courses of the threats (Havenaar et al. 2002). Technological threats or disasters give rise not only to more health-related fears but also to genuine uncertainty about the long-term risks from such exposures (Havenaar et al. 2002). Hence it is difficult for experts to confirm or deny such fears, particularly those related to possible outcomes that occur endemically in affected communities anyway, such as cancer, miscarriage, or reproductive abnormalities. The lack of certainty of long-term health risks, such as seen in the Three Mile Island episode (Prince-Embury and Rooney 1988), can be applied to many of the nontraditional military hazards of the Gulf War, providing a further link between civilian and military health (Bowler and Schwarzer 1991).

Distrust, Conspiracy, and Confidence

The importance of public confidence and political (mis-)judgment in shaping health concerns may be illustrated by one United States/United Kingdom comparison. In the United States there was been considerable concern and outcry over the role of the probably accidental discharge of sarin gas at the Khamisiyah arms dump, but this has not been a major issue in the United Kingdom. What has been a major issue is the role of exposure to organophosphate pesticides. One reason may be that both issues were accompanied by misinformation. In Great Britain it was originally denied that any organophosphate pesticides had been used—a clear misjudgment.

This was corrected, but the result was to focus attention on this particular risk and fuel the cries of "cover up." Something similar transpired with regard to Khamisiyah in the United States.

Indeed, one can go further and say that the initial actions of the United Kingdom authorities could hardly have been worse in terms of maintaining the confidence and trust of the armed forces and the populace. First, records that now would give crucial information, such as vaccination records, were destroyed. We do not generally subscribe to the conspiracy theorists and instead see this as a low-level decision to get rid of unnecessary paperwork that was no longer of interest. Armies fight wars, they do not plan epidemiological surveys. Yet it handed a weapon to Internet conspiracy buffs who have flocked to the Gulf War issues in droves.

Second, when concerns first began to surface in the United Kingdom, there was an attitude, expressed in Parliament by a senior Minister, that this was a "storm in a teacup." There were also coded hints that rotten apples could be found in every basket, that those complaining really should be able to "pull themselves together," and that this would not happen to troops who were properly led and trained. This sentiment was not expressed in so many words, but the meaning was clear. This is not a new view—similar sentiments were expressed to and by the Shell Shock Commission of 1922 (Bogacz 1989)—but the modern change in the balance between the duties and rights of individuals, and media scrutiny on a previously unknown scale, means such views are now less acceptable.

Third, there was a delay in commissioning research that might allay fears. In the United Kingdom, control of the research agenda was given to the scientists in the form of the Medical Research Council. One can understand the logic of this decision, but the result was that the opportunity to use research as part of the risk management (and essentially political) process was lost. Clemenceau's famous dictum was that war is too important to be left to the generals. Nowadays one might add that research is too important to be left to the scientists.

The results of all these events was a serious lack of trust of governmental and military authorities. This was partly a response to the specific errors related to Gulf War illness and partly a result of other known misjudgments or denials usually from the Cold War era, including such events as involuntary experiments carried out on some service personnel during that period. Given that risk communication and management are critically dependent upon a trust between the community that feels exposed and those responsible for managing that risk (Slovic 1999), these misjudgments may have been integral to the further development and shaping of GWS after the conflict.

Most commentators also ascribe a role to the media. Certainly, attendances at the assessment program for Gulf War veterans tends to peak after media stories on the topic, but this proves little. It would be naïve to blame, as some do, the media for GWS. Public concern and media coverage go hand in hand; GWS was a "good story" precisely because it touched on so many contemporary issues of general public concern. Public concerns and media coverage are consistent with each other, even if neither necessarily reflect an "objective" appraisal or reality (Funkhouser 1973). It is, however, true that the news media are more likely to report negative, trust-destroying stories than ones that enhance trust (Slovic 1999).

CONCLUSION

Remaining Questions

Many important research questions remain unanswered. A few will be addressed in the next few years. Many clinical studies will report, some of them based on epidemiologically based samples, others not. The interpretation of these results will be far easier in the former than in the latter. Animal studies will also add pieces to the jigsaw. Having said this, we must also face reality. It is now more than a decade since the end of the first Gulf War. Possibilities of further direct etiological research diminish with each year. The chances of finding new evidence on exposures during the conflict are now remote.

The Lessons

It might be argued that each military deployment is unique in its historical and military context, and so it is. Yet the story of GWS can only make sense when seen in the wider context. The origins of GWS can be traced to factors outside the 1991 conflict, and these same factors continue to operate today, perhaps even heightened by the Gulf War experience both in reality and mythology. Will the future hold more "Gulf War syndromes"?

   In the decade after the first Gulf War, newspaper reports have appeared concerning, for example, the "horrendous range of symptoms" now experienced by Canadian United Nations peacekeepers in Croatia (Gilmour 1999) and Dutch peacekeepers in Cambodia (De Vries et al. 2000; Soetekouw et al. 1999). Similar reports have emerged in the German and Belgian presses concerning their soldiers in Kosovo. Concerns include exposure to depleted uranium munitions, contaminated sandbags (Kondro 1999), or pollutants released from the destruction of factories during the North Atlantic Treaty Organization (NATO) bombing campaign against Serbia.

The outcome of the 1992 El Al crash in Amsterdam reproduced many of the features of GWS (Yzermans 2002). There has likewise been an epidemic of papers in the medical journals concerning preparations to deal with a chemical or biological terrorism incident, all of which have been concerned with the acute emergency response. We have argued elsewhere that the insidious but perhaps ultimately more damaging long-term effects have been ignored (Hyams et al. 2002).

The current uncertainty over the chronic health effects of low-level exposure to chemical and nuclear materials will continue and will further increase public anxiety. Because health officials cannot provide blanket assurances that harm will not result from acute, non–symptom-producing exposure, distrust of medical experts and government officials can result (Prince-Embury and Rooney 1988). The potential effects of low-level chemical and radiation exposure is a long-standing controversy (Birchard 1999). It is unlikely that these complex scientific and political issues will be resolved in the near future, nor is it likely that research studies conducted after well-publicized disasters will convincingly answer basic scientific questions because of the difficulties eliminating research biases in highly charged circumstances (David and Wessely 1995; Neutra 1985; Roht et al. 1985). As a result, numerous unconfirmed and controversial hypotheses about the effects of low-level exposures will flourish, just as they did after the Gulf War. We can expect more contested diagnoses in the future (Shriver et al. 2002). As we write this, American and British forces are engaged in Iraq, and there have been a handful of reports starting to emerge that describe many of the same concerns that began to appear soon after the end of the first Gulf War, but it is too early to speculate on the size, scale, and nature of the problem.

Gulf War Syndrome: The Postmodern Illness

In a characteristically provocative article, Gray (1999) described the features of what he calls "postmodern medicine": a distrust of science, a readiness to resort to litigation, a greater attention to risk, and better access to information (of whatever quality). He also pointed out, as indeed have many others, how consumer and patient values have already replaced paternalistic and professional values: where doctors used to lead, they now follow. The monolithic role of the doctor has been challenged by "lay experts" whose ability to influence public debate and policy increases just as that of the doctor or scientist diminishes. The "lay expert" may be the survivor of a disaster or the sufferer from a disease (Bury 1998). The Gulf War veteran may fulfill both roles.

GWS is therefore a paradigmatic postmodern illness. It is perhaps the first major health condition that was constructed almost entirely without the assistance of medicine in any shape or form. This is postmodern. Previous syndromes in the military have arisen for many reasons—shell shock was not invented by Myers in his seminal 1915 paper, but without his contribution it is improbable that the term would have gained widespread acceptance. In modern civilian practice, the success of chronic fatigue syndrome depended in part on the rise in patient consumerism and the reaction against medical paternalism, but key triggers were the paper describing the original Royal Free epidemic that gave rise to the term "myalgic encephalomyelitis" in the United Kingdom or the National Institutes of Health papers on "chronic Epstein-Barr" virus infection in the United States (Wessely et al. 1998). Without them, chronic fatigue syndrome would have taken a different course, if it had emerged at all. Sick building syndrome, like GWS, arose out of confusion, but a key part in its success was the persistent and vocal activities of a handful of doctors and scientists who, in the words of one commentator, "unequivocally diagnosed as a pathological state something that had not been scientifically demonstrated" (Bardana 1997).

Yet for GWS the shape of the syndrome seems to have been determined in the popular and political imaginations long before scientists or doctors had anything to say on the matter. GWS, we argue, developed without the assistance of science or medicine. Certainly populist and occasionally maverick scientists have emerged into the limelight of GWS and have played roles in subsequent events, but GWS may be the first truly postmodern illness because it developed from the congruence of veterans' narratives, veterans' disquiet and distrust, and a powerful media agenda (Zavestoski et al. 2004). Medical professionals and scientists generally have reacted to events and not shaped them.

The story of GWS may well reflect the shape of things to come. Classic conventional warfare between states is becoming increasingly hard to imagine—no state can match the firepower of an advanced military technology such as the United States. Modern professional militaries could no longer sustain the type of large-scale conventional casualties that were a feature of the two world wars, and we should be thankful for that. Yet as some perceptive commentators have pointed out, reducing the numbers of direct casualties as far as our modern professional armies are concerned, as has happened in the NATO nations, does not appear to have reduced the cost of war, direct or indirect. Harvey Sapolsky (2003) perceptively used the example of GWS to make the case that war is becoming too expensive, and with over one-third of the United States personnel committed to the Gulf now receiving service-related disability payments, he may well have a point. Likewise, the example of GWS also serves as a reminder that the pattern of risks and threats faced by modern militaries has changed and that these new, hard to understand, hard to measure, and hard to manage risks such as pollution, chemicals, and depleted uranium present a more potent challenge to the efficiency of a modern military than the conventional risks of direct trauma (Wessely 2005).

Final Words

So what did happen after the first Gulf War? The story began with the experiences of veterans' reporting symptoms. These may have been triggered as an unexpected reaction to measures taken to protect the armed forces against modern warfare—the "something new" of our title. These must be added to the unchanging psychological toll of warfare and the legacy of previous postconflict syndromes—"something old." All have been taken up by a powerful media and shaped into a particular syndrome under the influence of popular nonmilitary views of health, disease, and illness— "something borrowed"—with further impetus from the actions, or inactions, of government. Finally, although direct traumatic psychological injury is not prominent, mood disorder also plays a role—"something blue."

REFERENCES

Abou-Donia M, Wilmarth K, Jensen K, et al: Neurotoxicity resulting from coexposure to pyridostigmine bromide, DEET, and permethrin: implications of Gulf War chemical exposures. J Toxicol Environ Health 48:35–56, 1996

Albers J, Berent S: Controversies in neurotoxicology. Neurol Clin 18:741–763, 2000

Albers J, Berent S, Garabrant D, et al: The effects of occupational exposure to chlorpyrifos on the neurologic examination of the central nervous system: a prospective cohort study. J Occup Environ Med 46:367–378, 2004

Amato A, McVey A, Cha C, et al: Evaluation of neuromuscular symptoms in veterans of the Persian Gulf War. Neurology 48:4–12, 1997

Araneta MS, Edmonds L, Destiche D, et al: Prevalence of birth defects among infants of Gulf War veterans in Arkansas, Arizona, California, Georgia, Hawaii and Iowa 1989–1993. Birth Defects Res 67:246–260, 2003

Arnetz B, Wiholm C: Technological stress: psychophysiological symptoms in modern offices. J Psychosom Res 43:35–42, 1997

Bardana E: Sick building syndrome: a wolf in sheep's clothing. Ann Allergy Asthma Immunol 79:283–293, 1997

Barrett DG, Doebbeling BN, Clauw DJ, et al: Prevalence of symptoms and symptom-based conditions among Gulf War veterans: current status of research findings. Epidemiol Rev 24:218–227, 2003

Barsky A: The paradox of health. N Engl J Med 318:414–418, 1988a

Barsky A: Worried Sick: Our Troubled Quest for Wellness. Toronto, Ontario, Canada, Little, Brown and Co, 1988b

Berg M, Arnetz B, Liden S, et al: Techo-stress: a psychophysiology study of employees with VDU-associated skin complaints. J Occup Med 34:698–700, 1992

Bertollini R, Di Lallo D, Mastrolacovo P, et al: Reduction in births in Italy after the Chernobyl accident. Scand J Work Environ Health 16:96–101, 1990

Betts R: The new threat of mass destruction. Foreign Aff 77:26–41, 1998

Birchard K: Experts still arguing over radiation doses. Lancet 354:400, 1999

Black D, Doebbeling B, Voelker M, et al: Multiple chemical sensitivity syndrome: symptom prevalence and risk factors in a military population. Arch Intern Med 160:1169–1176, 2000

Bogacz T: War neurosis and cultural change in England 1914–1922: work of the War Office Committee of Enquiry into Shellshock. J Contemp Hist 24:227–256, 1989

Bourdette D, McCauley L, Barkhuizen A, et al: Symptom factor analysis, clinical findings, and functional status in a population-based case-control study of Gulf War unexplained illness. J Occup Environ Med 43:1026–1040, 2001

Bourke J: An Intimate History of Killing. London, England, Granta, 1999

Bowler R, Schwarzer R: Environmental anxiety: assessing emotional distress and concerns after toxin exposure. Anxiety Res 4:167–180, 1991

Bowler R, Mergler D, Huel G, et al: Psychological psychosocial and psychophysiological sequelae to a community affected by a railroad disaster. J Trauma Stress 7:601–624, 1994

Burke D: The recent excitement over genetically modified food, in Risk Communication and Public Health. Edited by Bennett P, Calman K. Oxford, England, Oxford Medical Publications, 1999, pp 140–151

Bury M: Postmodernity and health, in Modernity and Health. Edited by Scambler G, Higgs P. London, England, Routledge, 1998, pp 1–28

Carney CS, Voelker M, Woolson R, et al: Women in the Gulf War: combat experience, exposures, and subsequent health care use. Mil Med 168:654–651, 2003

Cherry N, Creed F, Silman A, et al: Health and exposures of United Kingdom Gulf War veterans, part 1: the pattern and extent of ill health. Occup Environ Med 58:291–298, 2001a

Cherry N, Creed F, Silman A, et al: Health and exposures of United Kingdom Gulf War veterans, part II: the relationship of health to exposure. Occup Environ Med 58:299–306, 2001b

Coker W, Bhatt B, Blatchley N, et al: Clinical findings for the first 1000 Gulf war veterans in the Ministry of Defence's medical assessment programme. BMJ 318:290–294, 1999

Committee on Toxicity of Chemicals in Food: Organophosphates. London, England, Department of Health, 1999

Cowan D, Gray G, DeFraites R: Birth defects among children of Persian Gulf War veterans. N Engl J Med 337:1175–1176, 1997

Dalrymple T: Mass Listeria: The Meaning of Health Scares. London, England, Andre Deutsch, 1998

David A, Wessely S: The legend of Camelford: medical consequences of a water pollution accident. J Psychosom Res 39:1–10, 1995

David A, Hull L, Unwin C, et al: Cognitive functioning and disturbances of mood in UK veterans of the Persian Gulf War: a comparative study. Psychol Med 32:1357–1360, 2002

Davis L, Murphy F, Alpern R, et al: Clinical and laboratory assessment of distal peripheral nerves in Gulf War veterans and spouses. Neurology 63:1070–1077, 2004

De Vries M, Soetekouw PM, Bleijenberg G, et al: Fatigue in Cambodia veterans. Q J Med 93:283–289, 2000

Doebbeling B, Clarke W, Watson D, et al: Is there a Persian Gulf War syndrome? Evidence from a large population-based survey of veterans and nondeployed controls. Am J Med 108:695–704, 2000

Doyle PM, Davies G, Maconochie I, et al: Miscarriage, stillbirth and congenital malformation in the offspring of UK veterans of the first Gulf war. Int J Epidemiol 33:74–86, 2004

Everitt B, Ismail K, David A, et al: Searching for a Gulf War syndrome using cluster analysis. Psychol Med 32:1371–1378, 2002

Everson M, Shi K, Alreidge P, et al: Immunological responses are not abnormal in symptomatic Gulf War veterans. Ann N Y Acad Sci 966:327–343, 2002

Fineman M: Yugoslav city battling toxic enemies. Los Angeles Times, July 6, 1999

Ford J, Campbell K, Storzbach D, et al: Posttraumatic stress symptomatology is associated with unexplained illness attributed to Persian Gulf War military service. Psychosom Med 63:842–849, 2001

Friedman A, Kaufer D, Shemer J, et al: Pyridostigmine brain penetration under stress enhances neuronal excitability and induces early immediate transcriptional response. Nat Med 2:1382–1385, 1996

Fukuda K, Nisenbaum R, Stewart G, et al: Chronic multisymptom illness affecting air force veterans of the gulf war. JAMA 280:981–988, 1998

Fulco C, Liverman C, Sox H (eds): Gulf War and Health, Vol 1: Depleted Uranium, Sarin, Pyridostigmine Bromide, Vaccines. Washington, DC, Institute of Medicine, 2000

Fullerton C, Ursano R: Behavioral and psychological responses to chemical and biological warfare. Mil Med 155:54–59, 1990

Funkhouser G: The issues of the sixties: an exploratory study in the dynamics of pubic opinion. Public Opin Q 37:62–75, 1973

Furlong C: PON1 status and neurologic symptom complexes in gulf war veterans. Genome Res 10:153–155, 2000

Gilmour B: Hazardous duty. Edmonton Journal, September 9, 1999

Girault V: Chronic fatigue, an underrated syndrome. Presse Med 31:531, 2002

Goss Gilroy, Inc: Health Study of Canadian Forces Personnel Involved in the 1991 Conflict in the Persian Gulf. Ottawa, Canada, Goss Gilroy, Inc, 1998

Grauer E, Alkalia D, Kapon J, et al: Stress does not enable pyridostigmine bromide to inhibit brain cholinesterase after parenteral administration. Toxicol Appl Pharmacol 164:301–304, 2000

Gray G, Kaiser KS, Hawksworth AW, et al: Increased postwar symptoms and psychological morbidity among U.S. Navy Gulf War veterans. Am J Trop Med Hyg 60:758–766, 1999a

Gray G, Smith T, Knoke J, et al: The postwar hospitalization experience of Gulf War veterans possibly exposed to chemical munitions destruction at Khamisiyah, Iraq. Am J Epidemiol 150:532–540, 1999b

Gray G, Reed R, Kaiser K, et al: Self reported symptoms and medical conditions among 11,868 Gulf War-era veterans: the SeaBee Health Study. Am J Epidemiol 155:1033–1044, 2002

Gray G, Kang H, Graham J, et al: After more than 10 years of Gulf War veteran medical examinations, what have we learned? Am J Prev Med 26:443–452, 2004

Gray JA: Postmodern medicine. Lancet 354:1550–1553, 1999

Gwiazda RH, McDiarmid M, Smith D: Detection of depleted uranium in urine of veterans from the 1991 Gulf War. Health Phys 86:12–18, 2004

Haley R: Gulf war syndrome: narrowing the possibilities. Lancet 2:272–273, 2003

Haley R, Kurt T: Self-reported exposure to neurotoxic chemical combinations in the Gulf War: a cross-sectional epidemiologic survey. JAMA 277:231–237, 1997

Haley R, Hom J, Roland P, et al: Evaluation of neurologic function in Gulf War veterans: a blinded case-control study. JAMA 277:223–230, 1997a

Haley R, Kurt T, Hom J: Is there a Gulf War syndrome? Searching for syndromes by factor analysis of symptoms. JAMA 277:215–222, 1997b

Haley R, Billecke S, La Du B: Association of low PON1 Type Q (type A) arylesterase activity with neurologic symptom complexes in Gulf War veterans. Toxicol Appl Pharmacol 157:227–233, 1999

Hall W: The logic of a controversy: the case of Agent Orange in Australia. Soc Sci Med 29:537–544, 1989

Havenaar J, Cwikel J, Bromet J (eds): Toxic Turmoil: Psychological and Societal Consequences of Ecological Disasters. New York, Plenum, 2002

Higgins E, Kant K, Harman K, et al: Skin disease in Gulf War veterans. Q J Med 95:671–676, 2002

Holloway H, Norwood A, Fullerton C, et al: The threat of biological weapons: prophylaxis and mitigation of psychological and social consequences. JAMA 278:425–427, 1997

Horner R, Kamins K, Feussner J, et al: Occurrence of amyotrophic lateral sclerosis among Gulf War veterans. Neurology 61:742–749, 2003

Hotopf M, David A, Hull L, et al: The role of vaccinations as risk factors for ill-health in veterans of the Persian Gulf War. BMJ 320:1363–1367, 2000

Hotopf M, Nikolaou V, Collier D, et al: Paraoxonase in Persian Gulf War veterans. J Occup Environ Med 45:668–675, 2003

Hoy J, Cornell J, Karlix J, et al: Repeated coadministrations of pyridostigmine bromide, DEET, and permethrin alter locomotor behavior of rats. Vet Hum Toxicol 42:72–76, 2000

Hutchesson E, Volans G: Unsubstantiated complaints of being poisoned: psychopathology of patients referred to the National Poisons unit. Br J Psychiatry 154: 34–40, 1989

Hyams K, Hanson K, Wignall F, et al: The impact of infectious diseases on the health of US troops deployed to the Persian Gulf during Operations Desert Shield and Desert Storm. Clin Infect Dis 20:1497–1504, 1995

Hyams K, Wignall F, Roswell R: War syndromes and their evaluation: from the US Civil War to the Persian Gulf War. Ann Intern Med 125:398–405, 1996

Hyams K, Murphy F, Wessely S: Combating terrorism: recommendations for dealing with the long term health consequences of a chemical, biological or nuclear attack. J Health Polit Policy Law 27:273–291, 2002

Iowa Persian Gulf Study Group: Self-reported illness and health status among Persian Gulf War veterans: a population-based study. JAMA 277:238–245, 1997

Ishoy T, Suadicani P, Guldager B, et al: State of health after deployment in the Persian Gulf: The Danish Gulf War Study. Dan Med Bull 46:416–419, 1999

Ismail K, Everitt B, Blatchley N, et al: Is there a Gulf war syndrome? Lancet 353:179–182, 1999

Ismail K, Hotopf M, Hull L, et al: Occupational risk factors for ill health in UK Gulf war veterans. J Epidemiol Community Health 54:834–838, 2000

Ismail K, Kent K, Brugha T, et al: The mental health of UK Gulf war veterans: phase 2 of a two-phase cohort study. BMJ 325:576–579, 2002

Jefferson T: Real or perceived adverse effects of vaccines and the media-a tale of our times. J Epidemiol Community Health 54:402–403, 2000

Jones E, Wessely S: Chronic fatigue syndrome after the Crimean War and the Indian Mutiny. BMJ 319:1645–1647, 1999

Jones E, McCartney H, Everitt B, et al: Post-combat syndromes from the Boer War to the Gulf: a cluster analysis of their nature and attribution. BMJ 324:324–327, 2002

Joseph S: A comprehensive clinical evaluation of 20,000 Persian Gulf War veterans. Mil Med 162:149–156, 1997

Kang H, Bullman T: Mortality among U.S. veterans of the Persian Gulf War. N Engl J Med 335:1498–1504, 1996

Kang H, Bullman T: Mortality among U.S. veterans of the Persian Gulf War. Am J Epidemiol 154:399–405, 2001

Kang HK, Mahan CM, Murphy FM: Illnesses among United States veterans of the Gulf War: a population-based survey of 30,000 veterans. J Occup Environ Med 42:491–501, 2000

Kang HM, Lee K, Murphy F, et al: Evidence for a deployment-related Gulf War syndrome by factor analysis. Arch Environ Health 57:61–68, 2002

Kang HK, Natelson B, Mahan C, et al: Post-traumatic stress disorder and chronic fatigue syndrome-like illness among Gulf War veterans: a population-based survey of 30,000 veterans. Am J Epidemiol 157:141–148, 2003

Keeler J, Hurst C, Dunn M: Pyridostigmine used as a nerve agent pretreatment under wartime conditions. JAMA 266:693–695, 1991

Ketchem L: Lessons of Chernobyl: SNM members dry to decontaminate world threatened by fallout. J Nucl Med 6:933–942, 1987

Kipen HM, Hallman W, Natelson BH: Prevalence of chronic fatigue and chemical sensitivities in Gulf Registry veterans. Arch Environ Health 54:313, 1999

Knoke J, Smith TC, Gray G, et al: Factor analysis of self reported symptoms: does it identify a Gulf War syndrome? Am J Epidemiol 152:379–388, 2000

Knudson L: Legally induced abortions in Denmark after Chernobyl. Biomed Pharmacother 45:229–232, 1991

Kondro W: Soldiers claim ill health after contact with contaminated soil in Croatia. Lancet 354:494, 1999

Kroenke K, Mangelsdorff A: Common symptoms in ambulatory care: incidence, evaluation, therapy and outcome. Am J Med 86:262–266, 1989

Kroenke K, Koslowe P, Roy M: Symptoms in 18,495 Persian Gulf War veterans. J Occup Environ Med 40:520–528, 1998

Landrigan P: Illness in Gulf War veterans: causes and consequences. JAMA 277:259–261, 1997

Lange JL, Doebbeling BN, Heller JM, et al: Exposures to the Kuwait oil fires and their association with asthma and bronchitis among gulf war veterans. Environ Health Perspect 110:1141–1146, 2002

Lee H, Gabriel R, Bale A, et al: Clinical findings of the second 1000 UK Gulf War veterans who attended the Ministry of Defence's Medical Assessment Programme. Journal of the Royal Army Medical Corps, 147:153–160, 2001

Lindem KH, White RF, Proctor SP, et al: Neuropsychological performance in Gulf War–era veterans: traumatic stress symptomatology and exposure to chemical-biological warfare agents. J Psychopathol Behav Assess 25:105–119, 2003

Lipscomb JA, Satin KP, Neutra RR: Reported symptom prevalence rates from comparison populations in community-based environmental studies. Arch Environ Health 47:263–269, 1992

MacFarlane G, Thomas E, Cherry N: Mortality amongst United Kingdom Gulf War veterans. Lancet 356:17–21, 2000

Macfarlane G, Maconochie N, Hotopf M, et al: Incidence of cancer among UK Gulf War veterans: cohort study. BMJ 327:1373–1375, 2004

Mackness B, Durrington P, Mackness M: Low paraoxonase in Persian Gulf War veterans self reporting Gulf War Syndrome. Biochem Biophys Res Commun 276:729–733, 2000

Matterson-Allen S, Brown P: Public reaction to toxic waste contamination: analysis of a social movement. Int J Health Serv 20:484–500, 1990

Mayou R, Bass C, Sharpe M: Overview of epidemiology, classification and aetiology, in Treatment of Functional Somatic Symptoms. Edited by Mayou R, Bass C, Sharpe M. Oxford, England, Oxford University Press, 1995, pp 42–65

McCauley L, Joos S, Lasarev M, et al: Gulf war unexplained illnesses: persistence and unexplained nature of self-reported symptoms. Environ Res 81:215–223, 1999

McCauley L, Lasarev M, Sticker D, et al: Illness experience of Gulf War veterans possibly exposed to chemical warfare agents. Am J Prev Med 23:200–206, 2002

McDiarmid M, Keogh J, Hooper F, et al: Health effects of depleted uranium on exposed gulf war veterans. Environ Res 82:168–180, 2000

McDiarmid MA, Engelhardt S, Oliver M, et al: Health effects of depleted uranium on exposed Gulf War veterans: a 10-year follow-up. J Toxicol Environ Health A 67:277–296, 2004

McKenzie D, Ikin J, McFarlane A, et al: Psychological health of Australian veterans of the 1991 Gulf War: an assessment using the SF-12, GHQ-12 and PCL-S. Psychol Med 34:1419–1430, 2004

Ministry of Defence: British Chemical Warfare Defence During the Gulf Conflict (1990–1991). London, England, Ministry of Defence, 2000

Mott F: War Neuroses and Shell Shock. London, England, Hodder & Stoughton, 1919

Mouterde O: Myalgic encephalomyelitis in children. Lancet 357:562, 2001

Neutra R: Epidemiology for and with a distrustful community. Environ Health Perspect 62:393–397, 1985

Nisenbaum R, Barrett DH, Reyes M, et al: Deployment stressors and a chronic multisymptom illness among Gulf War veterans. J Nerv Ment Dis 188:259–266, 2000

O'Brien L, Payne RG: Prevention and management of panic in personnel facing a chemical threat: lessons from the Gulf. J R Army Med Corps 139:41–45, 1993

Parliamentary Office of Science and Technology: Gulf War Illnesses: Dealing With the Uncertainties. London, England, Parliamentary Office of Science and Technology, 1997

Pearce P, Crofts H, Muggleton N, et al: The effects of acutely administered low dose sarin on cognitive behaviour and the electroencephalogram in the common marmoset. J Psychopharmacol 13:128–135, 1999

Petrie K, Wessely S: Modern worries and medicine. BMJ 324:690–691, 2002

Pocchiari F, Silano V, Zampieri A: Human health effects from accidental release of tetrachlorodibenzo-p-dioxin (TCDD) at Seveso, Italy. Ann N Y Acad Sci 320:311–320, 1979

Poirier M, Weston A, Schoket B, et al: Polycyclic aromatic hydrocarbon biomarkers of internal exposure in US Army soldiers serving in Kuwait in 1991. Polycyclic Aromatic Compounds 17:197–208, 1999

Presidential Advisory Committee on Gulf War Veterans' Illnesses: Final Report. Washington, DC, U.S. Government Printing Office, 1997

Prince-Embury S, Rooney J: Psychological symptoms of residents in the aftermath of the Three-Mile Island nuclear accident in the aftermath of technological disaster. J Soc Psychol 128:779–790, 1988

Proctor S, Heeren T, White R, et al: Health status of Persian Gulf War veterans: self-reported symptoms, environmental exposures, and the effect of stress. Int J Epidemiol 27:1000–1010, 1998

Proctor S, Harley R, Wolfe J, et al: Health-related quality of life in Gulf War veterans. Mil Med 166:510–519, 2001

Reid S, Hotopf M, Hull L, et al: Multiple chemical sensitivity and chronic fatigue syndrome in UK Gulf War veterans. Am J Epidemiol 153:604–609, 2001

Riddle JB, Smith T, Ritchie EC, et al: Chemical warfare and the Gulf War: a review of the impact on Gulf veterans' health. Mil Med 168:600–605, 2003

Reuters: French army wary of first Gulf War syndrome charge. Paris, France, May 29, 2000

Roht L, Vernon S, Weir F, et al: Community exposure to hazardous waste disposal sites: assessing reporting bias. Am J Epidemiol 122:418–433, 1985

Rook G, Zumla A: Gulf war syndrome: is it due to a systemic shift in cytokine balance towards a Th2 profile? Lancet 349:1831–1833, 1997

Rose M: Gulf war service an uncertain trigger for ALS. Neurology 61:730–731, 2004

Roy M, Koslowe P, Kroenke K, et al: Signs, symptoms and ill-defined conditions in Persian Gulf War veterans: findings from the Comprehensive Clinical Evaluation Program. Psychosom Med 60:663–668, 1998

Royal College Of Physicians and Psychiatrists: Organophosphate sheep dip: clinical aspects of long-term low-dose exposure. Salisbury, Wiltshire, Royal College of Physicians, 1998

Sapolsky H: War needs a warning label. Breakthroughs 12:3–8, 2003

Scott W: PTSD in DSM-III: a case in the politics of diagnosis and disease. Soc Probl 37:294–310, 1990

Scremin O, Shih T, Huynh L, et al: Delayed neurologic and behavioral effects of subtoxic does of cholinesterase inhibitors. J Pharmacol Exp Ther 304:1111–1119, 2003

Sharief M, Delamont R, Rose M, et al: Neurophysiologic evaluation of neuromuscular symptoms in UK Gulf War veterans: a controlled study. Neurology 59:1518–1525, 2002

Shorter E: Multiple chemical sensitivity: pseudodisease in historical perspective. Scand J Work Environ Health 23:35–42, 1997

Shriver TE, Webb GR, Adams B: Environmental exposures, contested illness, and collective action: the controversy over Gulf War illness. Humboldt Journal of Social Relations 27:73–105, 2002

Shusterman D, Lipscomb J, Neutra R, et al: Symptom prevalence and odor-worry interaction near hazardous waste sites. Environ Health Perspect 94:25–30, 1991

Skolbekken J: The risk epidemic in medical journals. Soc Sci Med 40:291–305, 1995

Skowera A, Sawicka E, Varela-Calvino R, et al: Cellular immune activation in Gulf War veterans. J Clin Immunol 24:66–73, 2004

Slovic P: Trust, emotion, sex, politics, and science: surveying the risk assessment battlefield. Risk Anal 19:689–702, 1999

Smith M, Carayon P: Work organization, stress and cumulative trauma disorders, in Beyond Biomechanics: Psychosocial Aspects of Musculoskeletal Disorders in Office Work. Edited by Moon S, Sauter S. London, England, Taylor & Francis, 1996, pp 23–44

Smith T, Gray G, Knoke J: Is systemic lupus erythematosus, amyotrophic lateral sclerosis, or fibromyalgia associated with Persian Gulf War Service: an examination of Department of Defence hospitalization data. Am J Epidemiol 151:1053–1059, 2000

Smith T, Ryan MAK, Gray GC, et al: Ten years and 100,000 participants later: occupational and other factors influencing participation in U.S. Gulf War health registries. J Occup Environ Med 44:758–768, 2002

Smith T, Weir JC, Heller JM, et al: Gulf War veterans and Iraqi nerve agents at Khamisiyah: postwar hospitalization data revisited. Am J Epidemiol 158:457–467, 2003

Soetekouw P, De Vries M, Preijers F, et al: Persistent symptoms in former UNTAC soldiers are not associated with shifted cytokine balance. Eur J Clin Invest 29:960–963, 1999

Spencer P, McCauley LA, Barkhuizen A, et al: Gulf War veterans: service periods in theatre, differential exposures, and persistent unexplained illness. Toxicol Lett 102–103:515–521, 1998

Spencer P, McCauley L, Lapidus J, et al: Self-reported exposures and their association with unexplained illness in a population based case-control study of Gulf War veterans. J Occup Environ Med 43:1041–1056, 2001

Steele L: Prevalence and patterns of gulf war illness in Kansas veterans: association of symptoms with characteristics of person, place and time of military service. Am J Epidemiol 152:992–1002, 2000

Stewart D: The changing faces of somatization. Psychosomatics 31:153–158, 1990

Stimpson NT, Weightman AL, Dunstan F, et al: Psychiatric disorders in veterans of the Persian Gulf War of 1991: systematic review. Br J Psychiatry 182:391–403, 2003

Stokes J, Banderet L: Psychological aspects of chemical defense and warfare. Mil Psychol 9:395–415, 1997

Storzbach D, Binder LM, McCauley L, et al: Psychological differences between veterans with and without Gulf War unexplained symptoms. Psychosom Med 62:726–735, 2000

Stretch R, Bliese P, Marlowe D, et al: Physical health symptomatology of Gulf War–era service personnel from the states of Pennsylvania and Hawaii. Mil Med 160:131–136, 1995

Stuart J, Ursano R, Fullerton C, et al: Belief in exposure to terrorist agents: reported exposure to nerve or mustard gas by Gulf War veterans. J Nerv Ment Dis 191:431–436, 2003

Thomas K: The consultation and the therapeutic illusion. BMJ i:1327–1328, 1978

Trojan D, Cashman N: An open trial of pyridostigmine in post poliomyelitis syndrome. Can J Neurol Sci 22:223–227, 1995

U.S. Army Environmental Hygiene Agency: Biological Surveillance Initiative: Appendix F of Final Report Kuwait Oil Fire Health Risk Assessment, 5 May–3 December 1991. Aberdeen Proving Ground, MD, U.S. Army Environmental Hygiene Agency, 1994

U.S. General Accounting Office: Gulf War Illnesses: Improved Monitoring of Clinical Progress and Reexamination of Research Emphasis Are Needed. Washington, DC, U.S. General Accounting Office, 1997

Unwin C, Blatchley N, Coker W, et al: The health of United Kingdom servicemen who served in the Persian Gulf War. Lancet 353:169–178, 1999

Voelker M, Saag K, Schwartz D, et al: Health-related quality of life in Gulf War–era military personnel. Am J Epidemiol 155:899–907, 2002

Wegman D, Woods N, Bailar J: Invited commentary: how would we know a Gulf War syndrome if we saw one? Am J Epidemiol 146:704–711, 1998

Wessely S: Risk, psychiatry and the military. Br J Psychiatry 186:459–466, 2005

Wessely S, Hotopf M, Sharpe M: Chronic Fatigue and Its Syndromes. Oxford, England, Oxford University Press, 1998

Wessely S, Nimnuan C, Sharpe M: Functional somatic syndromes: one or many? Lancet 354:936–939, 1999

Wessely S, Unwin C, Hotopf M, et al: Is recall of military hazards stable over time? Evidence from the Gulf War. Br J Psychiatry 183:314–322, 2003

Wolfe J, Proctor S, Duncan Davis J, et al: Health symptoms reported by Persian Gulf War veterans two years after return. Am J Ind Med 33:104–113, 1998

Young A: The Harmony of Illusions: Inventing Post-Traumatic Stress Disorder. Princeton, NJ, Princeton University Press, 1995

Yzermans J: The chaotic aftermath of an airplane crash in Amsterdam: a second disaster, in Toxic Turmoil: Psychological and Societal Consequences of Ecological Disasters. Edited by Havenaar CJ, Bromet EJ. New York, Plenum, 2002, pp 85–99

Zavestoski SB, McCormick S, Mayer B, et al: Patient activism and the struggle for diagnosis: Gulf War illness and other medically unexplained physical symptoms in the U.S. Soc Sci Med 58:161–175, 2004

Schizophrenia

Use of National Medical Databases to Study Medical Illness and Mortality in Schizophrenia

Preben Bo Mortensen, M.D., Dr.Med.Sci.

STUDIES OF MORTALITY and physical illness in relation to schizophrenia and other mental disorders have a long history. The increased mortality in asylums was described in the 1840s (Simpson 1988). During the first half of the twentieth century, the high mortality and morbidity from tuberculosis was a major health problem among schizophrenia patients, giving rise to changes in both services and research (see e.g., Alström 1942). Unexpected disease associations have also had a long history. For example, low rates of cancer among schizophrenia patients were suspected in the 1920s (Büel 1925; Mortensen 1994), and speculations about an inverse relationship between schizophrenia and epilepsy was one of the factors leading to the development of convulsive treatment and electroconvulsive therapy.

A number of facts have emerged from this long history of research. We know that mortality in schizophrenia is increased not only from suicide and other unnatural causes but also from cardiovascular diseases, respiratory diseases, and most other natural causes (Allebeck and Wistedt 1986; Harris and Barraclough 1998; Hiroeh et al. 2001; Mortensen 2002; Mortensen and

Juel 1993). Cancer seems to be the exception among causes of death because mortality generally has not been found to be increased.

The consistent findings of an elevated mortality from natural causes in schizophrenia contrasts with the relatively limited number of studies addressing the causes of this increased risk. Apart from being linked to the disease process of schizophrenia itself, a number of likely explanations for this finding exist. Lifestyle factors such as increased frequency of tobacco smoking, poor dietary habits, or even low socioeconomic status in patients with schizophrenia could account for some of this elevated mortality (Bennedsen 1998). However, to date no mortality studies of schizophrenia have been conducted in which these factors have been taken into account. Poor diagnoses and treatment of comorbid physical disorders could be another likely explanation. Indeed, difficulties and shortcomings in the diagnosing of physical disorders in mentally ill patients have been noted by a number of authors, but again, the impact of mortality has not been studied directly. Finally, psychopharmacological treatment might be suspected to influence mortality. Few studies relate neuroleptic treatment to cardiovascular death (e.g., Enger et al. 2004), but generally there has been very limited confounder control including risk factors for cardiovascular diseases, tobacco smoking, or a comorbid disease such as diabetes. Studies have often been small, and so far there is not conclusive evidence regarding the potential role of neuroleptics in relation to cardiovascular death. The findings regarding breast cancer and neuroleptics are described in further detail later, but overall there is very limited knowledge about long-term effects upon the physical health of users of neuroleptics.

MEDICAL COMORBIDITY

Generally, morbidity has been studied much less than mortality. This has been pointed out by several authors (Adler and Griffith 1991; Jeste et al. 1996) as well as the difficulty in diagnosing comorbid medical illnesses, the possible links to psychopharmacological treatment, and the supposedly increased rates of morbidity. However, this has not led to much further research, and there would still be several good reasons to study medical comorbidity. First, the elevated mortality would make it likely that a number of diseases occur more frequently among patients with schizophrenia. Second, both from the perspective of preventing the excess mortality as well as from the general clinical perspective, it would be highly relevant to elucidate the frequency and causes of medical comorbidity in schizophrenia patients. Finally, both elevated and reduced rates of specific disorders in groups of patients with another disease than schizophrenia may provide clues in the search for the etiology of other disorders. Perhaps surprisingly, this has probably been the most frequent reason for studying medical comorbidity in schizophrenia patients.

However, the relative lack of comorbidity studies is not only due to any lack of interest in the topic but can be due to the difficulties inherent in the study of one, perhaps uncommon, disorder in a group of patients with another relatively uncommon disorder. First, an important problem is statistical power. Generally, studies of comorbidity may require several thousands of patients to be followed for long periods of time, perhaps decades, and this would obviously be very difficult to do in most settings. Another problem is comparable background data—that is, precise estimates of the expected number of cases of the disorder in the study in the same population. In practice, this means that it may be very difficult to perform these studies without access to systematically collected morbidity data in the format of medical databases or registers. Because many of the examples of studies of comorbidity described in this chapter are based on Danish registers, a brief introduction is provided here.

DANISH REGISTERS AS A RESEARCH RESOURCE

Denmark has a population of approximately 5.3 million people. One feature of importance to register-based research is the health care system. There is no significant private hospital sector and generally no fee for service. All secondary health care has been recorded systematically on an individual basis for several years, typically since the 1960s or 1970s. Other individual data have been collected, such as income, education, and occupation. Through Danish registers, it is possible to link a relatively large proportion of the population to their first-degree relatives. The key feature of the Danish registration system is that every resident in Denmark since 1968 has been assigned a unique person identifier, the CPR number. This identifier consists of 10 digits of which the first 6 are the date of birth and the last 4 indicate gender, century of birth, and other information. A crucial feature about the identifier is that it can be logically checked for errors, making it very difficult to fabricate a nonexisting CPR number. Also, the identifier is used across all public registrations system in Denmark, making it possible to link across registers and also across long time spans. Individuals are protected from violation against their privacy through legislation (http://www.datatilsynet.dk/eng/index.html), and data cannot be accessed by employers, insurance companies, or anyone else without the consent of the registered individual. However, the legislation also opens the possibility for researchers to access linked anonymous information. So far, these safeguards have been successful in that there has been no breach of confidentiality in relation to use of data for research since the identification number was introduced in 1968. Of particular importance for these studies is the Danish Psychiatric Case Register, which has been described in detail by Munk-Jørgensen and Mortensen (1997). It covers all psychiatric hospitals and, since 1995, all hospital-based outpatient facilities and community psychiatry services. Other important data sources consist of the National Patients Register (Andersen et al. 1999), which covers all general hospital admissions and outpatient contacts; the Medical Birth Register (Knudsen and Olsen 1998); the Register of Causes of Death (Juel and Helweg-Larsen 1999); a number of specialized disease registers such as the Cancer Registry (Storm et al. 1997); and recently also a national prescription registry containing all prescribed drugs on an individual basis.

Although it is, of course, a huge advantage to have these data sources, there are also some shortcomings. First, variables are only collected for administrative purposes, meaning that some of the variables one would like to have access to are not available, including lifestyle factors such as tobacco smoking. Another problem is that diagnoses are only clinical diagnoses made by the treating consultant. Third, the diagnoses-specific data are generally only available at the secondary health care level, meaning that diseases mostly treated by general practitioners are not registered.

WHAT IS KNOWN ABOUT COMORBIDITY?

Generally, studies are often case reports or are based on small selected samples. In the more epidemiologically oriented studies, one must often consider possible ascertainment bias as confounders and treatment effects. However, there would be consensus regarding some findings.

Cardiovascular Diseases

Cardiovascular diseases are probably increased among patients with schizophrenia. It has not been studied directly in many studies, but the increased cardiovascular mortality would certainly suggest this. Also, this could plausibly be linked to increased rates of smoking and other risk factors (McCreadie 2003). There also would be good theoretical reasons to believe that neuroleptic treatment could influence cardiovascular morbidity both through inducing short-term electrocardiographic changes (Buckley and

Sanders 2000) as well as long-term effects on weight gain (Sussman 2003). However, only a few studies have actually linked an elevated risk to the use of typical neuroleptics (Enger et al. 2004), and none of them have had good confounder control. So at present there is no definite evidence linking cardiovascular disease to the use of neuroleptic treatment. Although risk factors such as tobacco smoking have an increased occurrence, and dietary practices may not follow the general recommendations, no preventive trials exist at present trying to reduce exposure to general risk factors for cardiovascular diseases among schizophrenia patients.

Cancer

Some literature suggests that there might be a reduced occurrence of cancer in schizophrenic patients. Studies in the postneuroleptic era have suggested that the incidence of cancer may indeed be reduced (Mortensen 1995). One Finnish study, however, found increased rates of cancer, especially lung cancer (Lichtermann et al. 2001), whereas some Danish studies have found reduced rates of cancer in male patients, with lower rates of smoking-related cancer as well as cancer of the prostate, testes, and malignant melanoma (Mortensen 1989, 1995). The reasons for these findings are not clear, but neuroleptic treatment may have reduced cancer risk (Mortensen 1987, 1992). There are only very few small direct studies, but a number of experimental studies based on laboratory animals and cell cultures, a number of case reports describing unexpected regression of tumors in relation to neuroleptic treatment, and very few epidemiological studies may suggest that even low doses of phenothiazines may have antitumor effects (Jones 1985). In contrast, neuroleptics have been implied as a potential risk factor for breast cancer (Halbreich et al. 1996; Schyve et al. 1978). This has been suggested both for theoretical reasons due to the effect of neuroleptics in elevating prolactin levels and in some epidemiological studies finding elevated rates among psychotic patients. However, a recent Danish study (Oksbjerg et al. 2003) showed that elevated rates of breast cancer among women with schizophrenia could be explained by reproductive factors, meaning that the low parity of schizophrenic women alone would be enough to explain elevated rates in the magnitude that has been reported in the literature. Therefore, currently there is no empirical basis to issue warnings regarding associations between breast cancer risk and neuroleptics, whereas the possible tumor-inhibiting effect of neuroleptics also needs to be examined further. Another question is whether the reduced cancer rate in schizophrenic males might be an etiological clue. It has been suggested that there may be a genetically based inverse relationship between cancer and schizophrenia. Lichtermann et al. (2001) found reduced cancer rates in relatives of schizophrenic patients. However, in a recent large, population-based Danish study (Dalton et al. 2004a, 2004b) no change in cancer risk was found among parents of schizophrenic patients, with the exception of a slightly increased rate of lung cancer among mothers of patients. Their results also suggested that the findings could be due to selection bias, because they compared the rates among relatives, primarily parents, of the schizophrenia patients with general population rates for cancer, and as people who become parents may well be positively selected also in relation to a number of lifestyle factors, this may explain the findings (Dalton et al. 2004b). In summary, some forms of cancer may be reduced, especially among schizophrenic males, and this may in part be due to the effect of treatment. However, there is less evidence that there is genetically determined antagonism between schizophrenia and cancer.

Epilepsy

Another recurring theme in the study of physical comorbidity in schizophrenia has been epilepsy. Several studies have reported an association between epilepsy, especially temporal lobe epilepsy, and an increased risk of developing schizophrenia or schizophrenialike psychoses. This has been reported in several studies, including Bredkjær et al. (1998). In a study that was recently submitted (Qin et al. 2005) in a population-based cohort study of 2.1 million persons with information about parents and siblings, this was also confirmed. Interestingly, they also found that a family history of epilepsy also slightly increased the risk of developing schizophrenia, although the individuals themselves had not been diagnosed with epilepsy. This effect, however, was confined to individuals without a family history of severe mental disorders. This could possibly indicate some genetic overlap between psychoses and epilepsy, but at present, this is speculative.

Autoimmune Disorders

Several studies have reported reduced rates of rheumatoid arthritis (Eaton et al. 1992). Although part of this negative association could be due to reduced sensitivity to pain or more sedentary lifestyle, it may also reflect a true reduction in rheumatoid arthritis rates (Mors et al. 1999). Another autoimmune disorder is type 1 diabetes. Although a positive association between schizophrenia and diabetes has been reported both in patients themselves and among first-degree relatives (Gilvarry et al. 1996; Marinow 1971), studies are generally small, and whether there indeed is an association must yet be considered undetermined. The relationship between neuroleptic treatment and glucose metabolism is described in more detail elsewhere in this volume (Chapter 14).

Another group of diseases with an autoimmune component is intestinal diseases. Celiac disease or gluten intolerance was suggested by Dohan (1973) to have links to schizophrenia; he suggested that an inherited defect interacted as an environmental trigger of gluten and precipitated schizophrenia in some individuals. This finding is interesting from an etiological point of view because genes of importance for celiac disease and schizophrenia have been suggested in loci relatively close to each other (Eaton et al. 2004), if gluten indeed is involved in the etiology of even a small percentage of schizophrenia cases, this would be of both theoretical and preventive importance. However, the finding should be considered suggestive but inconclusive because the number of cases with the combination of celiac disease and schizophrenia is very small in this study.

CONCLUSION

Studies of medical comorbidity in schizophrenia have a long history. However, although the elevated mortality is well established and although prevention of some of this excess mortality will probably have higher impact on the longevity of patients with schizophrenia than even suicide prevention, very little is known about the causes of the excess mortality, and no preventive trials have been conducted. Also, the general study of medical comorbidity could have many clinically relevant aspects, and the relative absence of knowledge about long-term health effects of neuroleptic treatment would suggest that there is a great need for pharmaco-epidemiological studies in this area. Finally, disease associations may serve as clues in the search for etiology. In this context, the combination of registers or other similar systems and biobanks may provide new ways of exploring the associations between diseases, taking the step from describing associations to understanding the biological mechanisms.

REFERENCES

Adler LE, Griffith JM: Concurrent medical illness in the schizophrenic patient: epidemiology, diagnosis, and management. Schizophr Res 4:91–107, 1991

Allebeck P, Wistedt B: Mortality in schizophrenia: a ten-year follow-up based on the Stockholm County inpatient register. Arch Gen Psychiatry 43:650–653, 1986

Alström CH: Mortality in mental hospitals with especial regard to tuberculosis. Acta Psychiatr Neurol Suppl XXIV:1–422, 1942

Andersen TF, Madsen M, Jorgensen J, et al: The Danish National Hospital Register: a valuable source of data for modern health sciences. Dan Med Bull 46:263–268, 1999

Bennedsen BE: Adverse pregnancy outcome in schizophrenic women: occurrence and risk factors. Schizophr Res 33:1–26, 1998

Bredkjær SR, Mortensen PB, Parnas J: Epilepsy and non-organic non-affective psychosis: national epidemiologic study. Br J Psychiatry 172:235–238, 1998

Buckley NA, Sanders P: Cardiovascular adverse effects of antipsychotic drugs. Drug Saf 23:215–228, 2000

Büel E: Maligne tumoren bei geisteskrankenheiten. Allg Z Psychiatry 80:314–321, 1925

Dalton SO, Laursen TM, Mortensen PB, et al: Major life event: diagnosis of schizophrenia in offspring and risk for cancer. Br J Cancer 90:1364–1366, 2004a

Dalton SO, Laursen TM, Mellemkjær L, et al: Risk for cancer in parents of patients with schizophrenia. Am J Psychiatry 161:903–908, 2004b

Dohan FC: Coeliac disease and schizophrenia. BMJ 3:51–52, 1973

Eaton W, Hayward C, Ram R: Schizophrenia and rheumatoid arthritis: a review. Schizophr Res 6:181–192, 1992

Eaton W, Mortensen PB, Agerbo E, et al: Coeliac disease and schizophrenia: population based case control study with linkage of Danish national registers. BMJ 328:438–439, 2004

Enger C, Weatherby L, Reynolds RF, et al: Serious cardiovascular events and mortality among patients with schizophrenia. J Nerv Ment Dis 192:19–27, 2004

Gilvarry CM, Sham PC, Jones PB, et al: Family history of autoimmune diseases in psychosis. Schizophr Res 19:33–40, 1996

Halbreich U, Shen J, Panaro V: Are chronic psychiatric patients at increased risk for developing breast cancer? Am J Psychiatry 153:559–560, 1996

Harris EC, Barraclough B: Excess mortality of mental disorder. Br J Psychiatry 173:11–53:11–53, 1998

Hiroeh U, Appleby L, Mortensen PB, et al: Death by homicide, suicide, and other unnatural causes in people with mental illness: a population-based study. Lancet 358:2110–2112, 2001

Jeste DV, Gladsjo A, Lindamer LA, et al: Medical comorbidity in schizophrenia. Schizophr Bull 22:413–430, 1996

Jones GR: Cancer therapy: phenothiazines in an unexpected role. Tumori 71:563–569, 1985

Juel K, Helweg-Larsen K: The Danish registers of causes of death. Dan Med Bull 46:354–357, 1999

Knudsen LB, Olsen J: The Danish Medical Birth Registry. Dan Med Bull 45:320–323, 1998

Lichtermann D, Ekelund J, Pukkala E, et al: Incidence of cancer among persons with schizophrenia and their relatives. Arch Gen Psychiatry 58:573–578, 2001

Marinow A: Diabetes in chronic schizophrenia. Dis Nerv Syst 32:777–778, 1971

McCreadie RG: Diet, smoking and cardiovascular risk in people with schizophrenia: descriptive study. Br J Psychiatry 183:534–539, 2003

Mors O, Mortensen PB, Ewald H: A population-based register study of the association between schizophrenia and rheumatoid arthritis. Schizophr Res 40:67–74, 1999

Mortensen PB: Neuroleptic treatment and other factors modifying cancer risk in schizophrenic patients. Acta Psychiatr Scand 75:585–590, 1987

Mortensen PB: The incidence of cancer in schizophrenic patients. J Epidemiol Community Health 43:43–47, 1989

Mortensen PB: Neuroleptic medication and reduced risk of prostate cancer in schizophrenic patients. Acta Psychiatr Scand 85:390–393, 1992

Mortensen PB: The occurrence of cancer in first admitted schizophrenic patients. Schizophr Res 12:185–194, 1994

Mortensen PB: The epidemiology of cancer in schizophrenic patients (thesis). Denmark, Aarhus University, 1995

Mortensen PB: Mortality and physical illness in schizophrenia. in The Epidemiology of Schizophrenia. Edited by Murray RM, Jones PB, Susser E, et al. New York, Cambridge University Press, 2002, pp 275–287

Mortensen PB, Juel K: Mortality and causes of death in first admitted schizophrenic patients. Br J Psychiatry 163:183–189, 1993

Munk-Jørgensen P, Mortensen PB: The Danish Psychiatric Central Register. Dan Med Bull 44:82–84, 1997

Oksbjerg DS, Munk LT, Mellemkjaer L, et al: Schizophrenia and the risk for breast cancer. Schizophr Res 62:89–92, 2003

Qin P, Huilan X, Laursen TM, et al: Risk for schizophrenia and schizophrenialike psychosis among patients with epilepsy: a population-based cohort study. BMJ 331:23, 2005

Schyve PM, Smithline F, Meltzer HY: Neuroleptic-induced prolactin level elevation and breast cancer: an emerging clinical issue. Arch Gen Psychiatry 35:1291–1301, 1978

Simpson JC: Mortality studies in schizophrenia, in Handbook of Schizophrenia: Nosology, Epidemiology and Genetics of Schizophrenia. Edited by Tsuang MT, Simpson JC. New York, Elsevier, 1988, pp 245–274

Storm HH, Michelsen EV, Clemmensen IH, et al: The Danish Cancer Registry: history, content, quality and use. Dan Med Bull 44:535–539, 1997

Sussman N: The implications of weight changes with antipsychotic treatment. J Clin Psychopharmacol 23:S21–S26, 2003

COX-2 Inhibition in Schizophrenia

Focus on Clinical Effects of Celecoxib Therapy and the Role of TNF-α

Norbert Müller, M.D., Ph.D.

Markus J. Schwarz, M.D.

Michael Riedel, M.D.

PSYCHIATRIC SYMPTOMS, especially schizophreniform and depressive symptoms, have been described both during inflammation and during different types of autoimmune disorders involving the central nervous system (CNS). These observations led to the suggestion that inflammation may be an important pathogenetic mechanism underlying schizophrenia. Our own investigations showed an inflammatory process in at least a subgroup of schizophrenic patients: signs of inflammation have been found in the cerebrospinal fluid as well as in postmortem CNS tissue of schizophrenic patients (Körschenhausen et al. 1996).

This study was supported by the Theodore and Vada Stanley Medical Research Institute.

TABLE 13–1. Influence of typhus infection on mental illness

Author	Patients	Unchanged	Healthy	Improved
Gaye	62	58 (94%)		4 (6%)
Nasse	21	6 (29%)	10 (48%)	5 (24%)
Campbell	22	16 (72%)	3 (14%)	3 (14%)
Rath	22	7 (32%)	5 (23%)	10 (45%)
Forel	12	8 (67%)	1 (8%)	3 (25%)
Jolly	12	—	3 (25%)	9 (75%)
		48%	20%	32%

Source.   Wagner von Jauregg 1887.

VACCINATION TREATMENT IN PSYCHOSIS

One of the pioneers of psychoneuroimmunology was Ritter Julius Wagner von Jauregg, the Nobel Prize–winning laureate for medicine in 1927. He developed the malaria therapy for syphilis. The immunological mechanism of this therapy is the activation of the immune system by attenuated antigens from strains of malaria in order to recognize and eliminate foreign antigens as non-self of the organism. Long before the development of the malaria therapy of syphilis, Wagner von Jauregg studied the effects of fever therapy in psychosis. The development of the fever therapy was based on observations of the effects of typhus infections—which recurred as epidemics during the nineteenth century—on mental illness. In 1887 Wagner von Jauregg published a type of meta-analysis in which he compared the observations of other psychiatrists from various countries during typhus epidemics (Table 13–1). These authors published the interesting observation that during typhus epidemics, the mentally ill (psychiatric patients) developed a much lower rate of infections than the "guards"—nurses during earlier times—did. On average, only 17% of the mentally ill subjects showed signs of an infection, whereas signs of an infection were observed in 39% of the guards (Wagner von Jauregg 1887). That means the guards developed a rate of infection that was twice as high as observed in psychiatric patients.

An even more interesting observation of several authors was that after recovering from the typhus infection, some of the patients also improved with respect to their mental illness. Up to 75% improved and up to 48% became mentally healthy after the infection. On average, 48% of the patients were unchanged after infection, whereas 32% were improved and 20% recovered from the mental illness. This observation of Wagner von

Jauregg and other authors led to the suggestion that certain infections might help in respect to mental illness. Consequently, this became the starting point for the further development of fever therapy. Wagner von Jauregg followed the subject of fever therapy and immune-mediated therapeutic mechanisms in psychosis during his further scientific life and published a paper in 1926 suggesting vaccination therapy in psychosis (Wagner von Jauregg 1926). For fever therapy, attenuated strains of *Salmonella typhii*, *Plasmodium malariae*, and *Mycobacterium tuberculosis* were used. However, due to the clinical side effects of vaccination with typhus, malaria, or tuberculosis (in particular to the often incalculable course of the infection and fever) and later to the introduction of therapy with neuroleptics, the focus of therapeutic and basic research changed from vaccination and immune system to dopaminergic neurotransmission and neuroleptic drugs. Nevertheless, the common immunological mechanisms of these therapies are of particular interest, because these three infectious agents induce the activation of the type 1 immune response, as we know today (Flesch et al. 1995; Mastroeni et al. 1992; Ramarathinam et al. 1993; Winkler et al. 1998).

Recent immunological studies point to an imbalance between the type-1 and type-2 immune response in schizophrenia, with an overactivation of the type-2 response and a lack of type-1 response. In conclusion, the distinct activation of the type-1 response without causing an infectious disorder would be expected to show advantageous effects in schizophrenia.

One class of modern drugs is well known to induce a shift from the type 1–like to a type 2–dominated immune response: the selective cyclo-oxygenase-2 (COX-2) inhibitors. Several studies have demonstrated the type-2 inducing effect of prostaglandin E_2 (PGE_2)—the major product of COX-2—whereas inhibition of COX-2 is accompanied by inhibition of type-2 cytokines and induction of type-1 cytokines (Pyeon et al. 2000; Stolina et al. 2000).

CYCLO-OXYGENASE-2 INHIBITION IN SCHIZOPHRENIA

Therefore, it seemed meaningful to study the effects of COX-2 inhibition using an add-on design together with a well-proven neuroleptic medication in schizophrenic patients (Müller et al. 2002). Celecoxib is a selective COX-2 inhibitor that accesses the CNS easily and has few adverse side effects. Risperidone was selected because it is an atypical neuroleptic with high efficacy in the therapy for both positive and negative symptoms of schizophrenia. In addition, a wealth of experience with risperidone treatment has been collected to date (Marder and Maibach 1994; Möller et al. 1998).

This study was performed as a prospective single-center, double-blind, placebo-controlled, randomized, add-on, parallel group evaluation of risperidone and celecoxib versus risperidone and placebo. Fifty schizophrenic patients were included in the study. Twenty-five (11 females and 14 males) were randomly assigned to the risperidone and celecoxib treatment group, and 25 (14 females and 11 males) to the risperidone and placebo group. All patients were hospitalized inpatients due to an acute exacerbation of their schizophrenic psychoses. Sixteen of the patients had been hospitalized for the first time, eight in the celecoxib group and eight in the placebo group.

CLINICAL OUTCOME OF CELECOXIB ADD-ON THERAPY IN SCHIZOPHRENIA

The celecoxib add-on therapy had a significant effect on the mean improvement in total Positive and Negative Symptom Scale (PANSS) score (between subjects factor *celecoxib* $F=3.8$, $df=1;47$, $P=0.05$). The difference between the two treatment groups was not homogeneous across time (multivariate *celecoxib* by *time* interaction $F=3.91$, $df=4;44$, $P=0.008$). The main effects of celecoxib were seen in the middle of the treatment period (quadratic interaction component $F=12.5$, $df=1;47$, $P=0.001$). In simple post hoc t tests, the difference between the two treatments groups is significant from week 2 ($t=2.06$, $df=48$, $P=0.05$) to week 4 (week 3 $t=2.64$, $df=48$, $P=0.01$; week 4 $t=2.54$, $df=48$, $P=0.01$). Regarding the mean improvement, none of the subscales showed a significant effect (positive symptoms: *celecoxib* $F=1.74$, $df=1;47$, $P=0.19$; negative symptoms: *celecoxib* $F=2.82$, $df=1;47$, $P=0.10$, global subscale: *celecoxib* $F=3.19$, $df=1;47$, $P=0.08$). The quadratic trend in the *celecoxib-time* interaction, however, was present in all subscales (positive symptoms: $F=4.77$, $df=1;47$, $P=0.03$; negative symptoms: $F=8.86$, $df=1;47$, $P=0.005$; global subscale: $F=6.16$, $df=1;47$, $P=0.02$). The celecoxib add-on treatment resulted in an earlier improvement in all subscales.

As predicted by our hypothesis, the celecoxib add-on therapy group had a significant better effect on the PANSS total scores. The largest improvements were seen between weeks 2 and 4. In practice this means an earlier treatment response under the add-on therapy. The acceleration of the treatment response was seen in a similar way in all subscales. These results show that the additional treatment with celecoxib has significant positive effects on the psychopathology of schizophrenia. Therapy with 400 mg celecoxib was well tolerated, and no clinically important side effects were observed.

EFFECTS OF CELECOXIB ADD-ON THERAPY TO TUMOR NECROSIS FACTOR-α

In order to evaluate the effects of the celecoxib therapy to the immune system in schizophrenia, markers of the peripheral immune system were measured in the blood of schizophrenic patients before the start of the therapy, weekly during therapy, and at the end of the study. The results of these examinations are mentioned elsewhere (Müller et al. 2004a). Here, we focus on the role of soluble tumor necrosis factor-alpha (TNF-α) receptor-1 levels.

The serum levels of the soluble TNF-α receptor-1 (sTNF-R1) in the blood of both groups of patients, the celecoxib group and the placebo group, were measured. After centrifugation, serum samples were frozen (–80°C) and stored until analysis. Levels of sTNF-R1 were estimated using a commercially available double-sandwich enzyme-linked immunosorbent assay according to the manufacturer's instructions. Each concentration was measured in duplicate.

For the analysis of sTNF-R1 we did not use the method according to the criterion "last observation carried forward" but values that were actually measured. Missing values were recorded as missing.

SOLUBLE TUMOR NECROSIS FACTOR RECEPTOR-1 LEVELS DURING THERAPY

The levels of the sTNF-R1 did not change significantly during the course of therapy. Before the start of the therapy the sTNF-R1 levels were 1,325±324 pg/mL in the celecoxib group and 1,280±375 pg/mL in the placebo-group. At the endpoint the sTNF-R1 levels were 1,224±303 pg/mL in the celecoxib group and 1,230±309 pg/mL in the placebo group. No statistically significant changes were observed in either group. Accordingly, no significant differences were found between the two therapy groups.

Interestingly, when we divided the patients into responders to therapy and nonresponders to therapy according to the criterion of at least 30% improvement on the PANSS total scale, we found a statistically significant difference only in the celecoxib group (Figure 13–1). In the group of nonresponders, sTNF-R1 levels were 1,414±338 pg/mL before the start of the therapy, whereas they were 1,135±193 pg/mL in the responders. This difference was significant using the two-tailed t test ($P<0.04$). The responders to celecoxib had significantly lower sTNF-R1 levels before the start of the therapy.

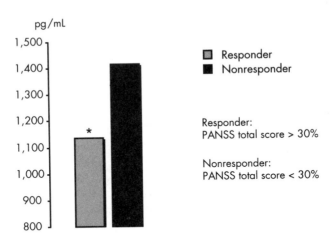

FIGURE 13–1.   Soluble TNF-α receptor-1 (p55) and response to COX-2 inhibition.

Note.   Low levels of TNF-α receptor-1 (p55) predict a better therapeutic response to celecoxib (*P<0.05).

DISCUSSION

The effects of celecoxib in the CNS have not yet been fully elucidated. There is no doubt that activation of COX-2 mediates inflammation and that COX-2 is expressed in brain tissue. COX-2 can be activated by cytokines like interleukin (IL)-2, IL-6, and IL-10, and cytokine-activated COX-2 expression mediates further inflammation. It is reported that IL-2 and soluble IL-2R (Licinio et al. 1993; McAllister et al. 1995), soluble IL-6 receptors as a functional part of the IL-6 system (Müller et al. 1997), and IL-10 (van Kammen et al. 1997) are increased in the cerebrospinal fluid of schizophrenic patients. The increase of cytokines in the CNS compartment may be accompanied by increased COX-2 expression. We suppose that celecoxib downregulates the cytokine-induced COX-2 activation in the CNS. Moreover, COX-2 inhibition seems to regulate the adhesion molecule expression (Bishop-Bailey et al. 1998). Adhesion molecule regulation is impaired in schizophrenia, possibly leading to an imbalance and a lack of communication between the peripheral and the CNS immune systems (Müller et al. 1999; Schwarz et al. 1998, 2000).

There might be a special subgroup of patients that benefits from cele-coxib more than others, because even an onset of psychotic symptoms during celecoxib therapy has been described (Lantz and Giambanco 2000). On the other hand, malaria is known to induce schizophrenia-like symptoms, whereas an attenuated malaria infection was used as antipsychotic therapy by Wagner von Jauregg.

Several factors that may play a role in the effect of celecoxib in schizophrenia could not be considered because of an existing lack of studies and experience. Those factors include the dosage of celecoxib, the degree of CNS penetration, the duration of therapy, the combination with other psychotropic drugs, and the duration until the onset of CNS effects of celecoxib. Thus, the ultimate therapeutic benefit of adjunctive celecoxib may require much more optimization of dosage, duration of treatment, and so on.

From a scientific viewpoint, the therapeutic effects of celecoxib without an additional neuroleptic drug would be more interesting. However, because neuroleptics are effective in antipsychotic treatment, ethics committees would not approve a study with a COX-2 inhibitor as the sole drug in acute schizophrenic patients before showing greater evidence for a therapeutic effect.

This study was planned according to the psychoneuroimmunological hypothesis that a lipophilic anti-inflammatory substance may lead to therapeutic benefits in schizophrenia. The result reveals one more indication that immune dysfunction in schizophrenia may be related to the pathomechanism of schizophrenia and is not just an epiphenomenon. The effects of the celecoxib therapy to the peripheral immune system, however, are weak. Nevertheless, an increase of soluble IL-2R levels (Müller et al. 2004a) is in accordance with our hypothesis that the COX-2 inhibition activates the type-1 immune response and downregulates the type-2 immune response, given that soluble IL-2R levels represent the type-1 response of the cellular immune system and B-cells and activated B-cells represent the type-2 response (Müller et al. 2004a).

TNF-α is derived from various cellular sources of the immune system, including activated macrophages and T-cells, and has several different functions. TNF-α is called an "early response cytokine" because it coordinates pro-inflammatory signals of the early immune response in the innate cellular immune system. Due to this function, TNF-α is assigned to the type-1 cytokines. TNF-receptor-1 (TNF-R1) is the primary signaling receptor for TNF-α (Mitzgerd et al. 2001), mediating the immunological and molecular effects of TNF-α (Alaaeddine et al. 1997). The levels of sTNF-R1—induced by shedding from the cell surface—are associated with the blood levels of TNF-α (Alaaeddine et al. 1997). In a large study including 361 patients it was shown that sTNF-R1 levels of schizophrenic patients were slightly decreased compared with healthy control subjects even after taking into account the confounding factors such as age, smoking, gender, infection, and medication (Haack et al. 1999). This finding of decreased sTNF-R1 serum levels in schizophrenia is in accordance with various findings pointing to a decreased type-1 immune response in schizophrenia. Several studies have demonstrated the type-2 immune response–inducing effect of PGE_2—the major product of COX-2—while inhibition of COX-2 is accompanied by inhibition of type-2 cytokines and induction of type-1 cytokines (Pyeon et al. 2000; Stolina et al. 2000). The COX-2 inhibition seems to balance the type-1/type-2 immune response by inhibition of PGE_2 and by stimulating the type-1 immune response (Litherland et al. 1999). It can be speculated that low levels of sTNF-R1 reflect a low degree of type-1 immune activation, and COX-2 inhibition has a high potency for the rebalancing of the type-1/type-2 immune response in patients with low levels of sTNF-R1. Whether this mechanism explains the predictive value of sTNF-R1 for the therapeutic effect of celecoxib in schizophrenia has to be elucidated in further studies.

In animal experiments it has been shown that the effects of TNF-α can be trophic or toxic (Yang et al. 2002), possibly depending on the type of target cells. In hippocampal neurons of rats (Barger et al. 1995; Cheng et al. 1994), TNF-α has been shown to be trophic, whereas it is toxic on cortical neurons (Yang et al. 2002). It can be speculated that low TNF-α levels in schizophrenias may be associated with hippocampal damage.

TUMOR NECROSIS FACTOR RECEPTOR-1 AS DEATH RECEPTOR

TNF-R1 has been shown to act as a death receptor: it contains an intracellular "death domain" and contributes to cell death when activated (Chen and Goeddel 2002; Tartaglia et al. 1993). Regarding the function of TNF-R1 as a death receptor, another function of low sTNF-R1 levels has to be taken into account. Schizophrenia is a neurodegenerative disorder, showing a loss in the brain volume during the course of the disease. The mechanism of this loss is still unknown. An increase of the schizophrenic deficit syndrome is found related to increasing duration of the disease, and the outcome of therapy is related to the duration of disease before the start of the treatment (duration of untreated psychosis) (Bottlender and Möller 2003). Regarding the brain volume, a meta-analysis showed that a loss of volume of total brain is observed (Wright et al. 2000)—in particular, in critical regions such as the hippocampus (Meisenzahl et al. 2002; Wright et al. 2000). An increase in the cerebrospinal fluid spaces of schizophrenic patients—indicating the loss of brain volume—have been described related to the duration of illness (Meisenzahl et al., unpublished data, 2005), although a reduction of CNS volume can be observed already in first-episode schizophrenic patients (Chua et al. 2003). There are also hints that the outcome in the therapy of schizophrenic patients is related to the brain volume—that is, that patients with large ventricular volume show poorer outcome of therapy (Lieberman et al. 2001).

Given the function of sTNF-R1 as a death receptor mediating apoptosis of cells, low levels of sTNF-R1 may reflect a small degree of apoptosis in patients with schizophrenia and a better outcome to therapy. Data from another study (our unpublished results) point to a strong relationship between the duration of the disease and therapy outcome of celecoxib, showing that celecoxib has favorable effects in particular in patients with a short duration of the disease. This is in accordance with the view that better therapeutic outcome is associated with low progression of the disease and low progression of cell loss. The relationship between low sTNF-R1 and better outcome was not found in the patients who only received risperidone. This result points out that sTNF-R1 might be a marker for the effects of anti-inflammatory therapy, not of neuroleptic therapy. The relationship between poor therapeutic outcome and loss of brain volume, however, was described for therapy with neuroleptics (Lieberman et al. 2001). The response to anti-inflammatory treatment might be more sensitive to the progression of the disorder. Selective COX-2 inhibitors seem to influence the levels of TNF-α and of sTNF-R1 (Casolini et al. 2002). On the other hand it has to be taken into account that the levels of sTNF-R1 are not increased in schizophrenic patients compared with control subjects, what would be expected if sTNF-R1 is a marker of neurodegeneration in the peripheral blood. The levels of sTNF-R1 in the peripheral blood, however, are influenced by various parameters that, under certain conditions, may mask neurodegeneration, in particular peripheral immunological or inflammatory processes.

The therapeutic effects of COX-2 inhibition are also discussed in other neuropsychiatric disorders such as Alzheimer's disease and affective disorders (Müller et al. 2004b). The possible specific action in schizophrenia has to be explored in further studies. It has to be taken into account that the therapeutic effect of celecoxib is not only mediated by immune mechanisms but by glutamatergic mechanisms as well. Regardless of the mechanism(s) involved, acute add-on treatment with celecoxib appears to have a beneficial effect on schizophrenic psychopathology, although this finding of a clinical effect of celecoxib needs to be replicated. Further investigations are needed in order to understand the antipsychotic mechanism of COX-2 inhibition and the role of TNF-α and TNF-receptors.

REFERENCES

Alaaeddine N, DiBattista JA, Pelletier JP, et al: Osteoarthritic synovial fibroblasts posses an increased level of tumor necrosis factor-receptor 55 (TNF-R55) that mediates biological activation by TNF-α. J Rheumatol 24:1985–1994, 1997

Barger SW, Horster D, Furukawa K, et al: Tumor necrosis factors alpha and beta protect neurons against amyloid beta-peptide toxicity: evidence for involvement of a kappa B-binding factor and attenuation of peroxide and Ca2+ accumulation. Proc Natl Acad Sci U S A 92:9328–9332, 1995

Bishop-Bailey D, Burke-Gaffney A, Hellewell PG, et al: Cyclooxygenase-2 regulates inducible ICAM-1 and VCAM-1 expression in human vascular smooth muscle cells. Biochem Biophys Res Commun 249:44–47, 1998

Bottlender R, Möller HJ: The impact of the duration of untreated psychosis (DUP) on the short- and long-term outcome in schizophrenia. Curr Opin Psychiatry Suppl 2:39–43, 2003

Casolini P, Catalani A, Zuena A, et al: Inhibition of COX-2 reduces the age-dependent increase of hippocampal inflammatory markers, corticosterone secretion and behavioral impairment in the rat. J Neurosci Res 68: 337–343, 2002

Chen G, Goeddel DV: TNF-R1 signaling: a beautiful pathway. Science 296:1634–1635, 2002

Cheng B, Christakos S, Mattson MP: Tumor necrosis factors protect neurons against metabolic-excitotoxic insults and promote maintenance of calcium homeostasis. Neuron 12:139–153, 1994

Chua SE, Lam IW, Tai KS, et al: Brain morphological abnormality in schizophrenia is independent of country of origin. Acta Psychiatr Scand 108:269–275, 2003

Flesch IE, Hess JH, Huang S, et al: Early interleukin 12 production by macrophages in response to mycobacterial infection depends on interferon gamma and tumor necrosis factor alpha. J Exp Med 181:1615–1621, 1995

Haack M, Hinze-Selch D, Fenzel T, et al: Plasma levels of cytokines and soluble cytokine receptors in psychiatric patients upon hospital admission: effects of confounding factors and diagnosis. J Psychiatry Res 33:407–418, 1999

Körschenhausen D, Hampel H, Ackenheil M, et al: Fibrin degradation products in postmortem brain tissue of schizophrenics: a possible marker for underlying inflammatory processes. Schizophr Res 19:103–109, 1996

Lantz MS, Giambanco V: Acute onset of auditory hallucinations after initiation of celecoxib therapy. Am J Psychiatry 157:1022–1023, 2000

Licinio J, Seibyl, JP, Altemus M, et al: Elevated levels of Interleukin-2 in neuroleptic-free schizophrenics. Am J Psychiatry 150:1408–1410, 1993

Lieberman J, Chakos M, Wu H, et al: Longitudinal study of brain morphology in first episode schizophrenia. Biol Psychiatry 49:487–499, 2001

Litherland SA, Xie XT, Hutson AD, et al: Aberrant prostaglandin synthase 2 expression defines an antigen-presenting cell defect for insulin-dependent diabetes mellitus. J Clin Invest 104:515–523, 1999

Marder SR, Meibach RC: Risperidone in the treatment of schizophrenia. Am J Psychiatry 151:825–831, 1994

Mastroeni P, Villarreal-Ramos B, Hormaeche CE: Role of T cells, TNF alpha and IFN gamma in recall of immunity to oral challenge with virulent salmonellae in mice vaccinated with live attenuated aro-Salmonella vaccines. Microb Pathog 13:477–491, 1992

McAllister CG, van Kammen DP, Rehn TJ, et al: Increases in CSF levels of interleukin-2 in schizophrenia: effects of recurrence of psychosis and medication status. Am J Psychiatry 152:1291–1297, 1995

Meisenzahl EM, Frodl T, Zetzsche T, et al: Investigation of a possible diencephalic pathology in schizophrenia. Psychiatry Res 115:127–35, 2002

Mitzgerd JP, Spieker MR, Doerschunk CM: Early response cytokines and innate immunity: essential roles for TNF receptor 1 and type I IL-1 receptor during *Escherichia coli* pneumonia in mice. J Immunol 166:4042–4048, 2001

Möller HJ, Gagiano DA, Addington CE, et al: Long-term treatment of schizophrenia with risperidone: an open-label, multicenter study of 386 patients. Int Clin Psychopharmacol 13:99–106, 1998

Müller N, Dobmeier P, Empel M, et al: Soluble IL-6 receptors in the serum and cerebrospinal fluid of paranoid schizophrenic patients. Eur Psychiatry 12:294–299, 1997

Müller N, Hadjamu M, Riedel M, et al: The adhesion-molecule receptor expression on T helper cells increases during treatment with neuroleptics and is related to the blood–brain barrier permeability in schizophrenia. Am J Psychiatry 156:634–636, 1999

Müller N, Riedel M, Scheppach C, et al: Beneficial anti-psychotic effects of celecoxib add-on therapy compared to risperidone alone in schizophrenia. Am J Psychiatry 159:1029–1034, 2002

Müller N, Ulmschneider M, Scheppach C, et al: COX-2 inhibition as a treatment approach in schizophrenia: immunological considerations and clinical effects of celecoxib add-on therapy. Eur Arch Psychiatry Clin Neurosci 254:14–22, 2004a

Müller N, Riedel M, Schwarz MJ: Psychotropic effects of COX-2 inhibitors: a possible new approach for the treatment of psychiatric disorders. Pharmacopsychiatry 37:1–4, 2004b

Pyeon D, Diaz FJ, Splitter GA: Prostaglandin E(2) increases bovine leukemia virus tax and pol mRNA levels via cyclooxygenase 2: regulation by interleukin-2, interleukin-10, and bovine leukemia virus. J Virol 74:5740–5745, 2000

Ramarathinam L, Niesel DW, Klimpel GR: *Salmonella typhimurium* induces IFN-gamma production in murine splenocytes: role of natural killer cells and macrophages. J Immunol 150:3973–3981, 1993

Schwarz MJ, Ackenheil M, Riedel M, et al: Blood-CSF-barrier impairment as indicator for an immune process in schizophrenia. Neurosci Lett 253:201–203, 1998

Schwarz MJ, Riedel M, Ackenheil M, et al: Decreased levels of soluble intercellular adhesion molecule-1 (sICAM-1) in unmedicated and medicated schizophrenic patients. Biol Psychiatry 47:29–33, 2000

Stolina M, Sharma S, Lin Y, et al: Specific inhibition of cyclooxygenase 2 restores antitumor reactivity by altering the balance of IL-10 and IL-12 synthesis. J Immunol 164:361–370, 2000

Tartaglia LA, Merill A, Wong GW, et al: A novel domain within the 55 kDa TNF receptor signals cell death. Cell 74:845–854, 1993

van Kammen DP, McAllister-Sistilli CG, et al: Relationship between immune and behavioral measures in schizophrenia, in Current Update in Psychoimmunology. Edited by Wieselmann G. New York, Springer Verlag, 1997, pp 51–55

Wagner von Jauregg J: Über die Einwirkung fieberhafter Erkrankungen auf Psychosen. Jahrbücher für Psychiatrie 7:94–131, 1887

Wagner von Jauregg J: Fieberbehandlung bei Psychosen. Wien Med Wochenschr 76:79–82, 1926

Winkler S, Willheim M, Baier K, et al: Reciprocal regulation of Th1- and Th2-cytokine-producing T cells during clearance of parasitemia in Plasmodium falciparum malaria. Infect Immun 66:6040–6044, 1998

Wright IC, Rabe-Hesketh S, Woodruff PW, et al: Meta-analysis of regional brain volumes in schizophrenia. Am J Psychiatry 157:16–25, 2000

Yang L, Lindholm K, Konishi Y, et al: Target depletion of distinct tumor necrosis factor receptor subtypes reveals hippocampal neuron death and survival through different signal transduction pathways. J Neurosci 22:3025–3032, 2002

Schizophrenia, Metabolic Disturbance, and Cardiovascular Risk

John W. Newcomer, M.D.

Dan W. Haupt, M.D.

ATYPICAL ANTIPSYCHOTIC DRUGS offer important benefits for many patients with disorders such as schizophrenia, including a reduced risk of the extrapyramidal side effects associated with older, conventional antipsychotics. However, certain atypical antipsychotics, like a few other drugs in medical practice (e.g., protease inhibitors, glucocorticoids), can produce substantial weight gain and increased adiposity in vulnerable individuals, and these agents have also been associated with an increased risk of dyslipidemia and type 2 diabetes. Although other adverse events during treatment can impact factors such as patient satisfaction and adherence to treatment, adverse events like weight gain, dyslipidemia, and hyperglycemia have the potential to substantially impact long-term medical comorbidity and medical mortality.

Elevated rates of medical comorbidity and mortality occur in patients with mental illness, including increased rates of type 2 diabetes mellitus (T2DM) and cardiovascular disease (Casey et al. 2004). Elevated plasma glucose is one of the five key modifiable risk factors for cardiovascular disease that emerged from the Framingham Heart Study and other large epidemiological studies of health risk factors, along with increased body weight, smoking, dyslipidemia, and hypertension (Wilson et al. 1998). Each factor alone confers an approximate twofold increase in relative risk of cardiovascular disease, with additive or greater effects observed for combinations of two or more risk factors, amplifying the potential for adverse outcomes. Primary and secondary prevention targeting these risk factors may be especially important in psychiatric populations. In a study of 88,000 patients aged 65 years and older who were hospitalized for myocardial infarction, the presence of any comorbid mental disorder was associated with a 20% increase in mortality (Druss et al. 2001).

A key risk factor for cardiovascular disease is excess adiposity, which can be indirectly estimated using the weight and height function of body mass index (BMI; kg/m^2). Increasing BMI beyond a threshold level of 25 kg/m^2 in adult populations is associated with increasing mortality (Gray 1989). The underlying health risks associated with increased adiposity include osteoarthritis; certain cancers including breast, prostate, and colon cancers; type 2 diabetes; and cardiovascular disease (Expert Committee on the Diagnosis and Classification of Diabetes Mellitus 2003; Resnick et al. 1998). The relative risk of a variety of medical diseases increases with adiposity (Calle et al. 1999). Importantly, not all body fat is associated with equal risk. Increases in abdominal adiposity, and particularly visceral abdominal fat, is strongly associated with decreases in insulin sensitivity (Banerji et al. 1997). Decreases in insulin sensitivity, sometimes referred to as *insulin resistance*, are associated with physiological changes including impaired glucose control, an atherogenic dyslipidemia that includes increases in plasma triglyceride and more dense LDL particles, increased blood pressure, increased risk of blood clotting, and increases in markers of inflammation, all of which are associated with an increased risk of cardiovascular disease (Reaven 1999). A patient with any three of the following would be considered to have metabolic syndrome based on Adult Treatment Panel guidelines from the National Cholesterol Education Program: obesity (measured as waist circumference ≥ 40 inches in males or 35 inches in females), low high-density lipoprotein cholesterol (<40 mg/dL in males or 50 mg/dL in females), high triglyceride levels (≥150 mg/dl), elevated blood pressure (≥130 mm Hg systolic or 85 diastolic), or increased fasting blood glucose (≥110 mg/dL; National Cholesterol Education Program 2001).

The long-term risks of hyperglycemia include microvascular (retinopathy, nephropathy, and neuropathies) and macrovascular disease, with the latter encompassing atherosclerosis-related cardiovascular disease (i.e., coronary heart disease, cerebrovascular disease, and peripheral vascular disease). Diabetes mellitus is additionally associated with a risk of short-term complications, including diabetic ketoacidosis and nonketotic hyperosmolar states, which although relatively uncommon, can be severe (American Diabetes Association 2003; Garg and Grundy 1990; Haffner et al. 1998; Harris 2000; Reaven 1999; Wilson et al. 1985). Mortality risk with diabetic ketoacidosis is approximately 2% in the most optimal clinical settings, rising as high as 20% in elderly samples, with mortality risk increasing in general with age, intercurrent illness, and delays in the initiation of insulin therapy.

Although insulin resistance and hyperglycemia below diabetic levels, as observed for example in the metabolic syndrome, are now recognized as important risk factors for cardiovascular disease, diabetes mellitus is now considered a "risk equivalent" for cardiovascular disease. This is based on well-replicated observations that the presence of diabetes is associated with an approximately 20% risk of myocardial infarction—the same risk as that observed in a patient who has already had a prior myocardial infarction (American Diabetes Association 2003). In operational terms, a patient with diabetes should be treated as though they have had their first heart attack; plasma glucose, lipids, and blood pressure must all be treated to target levels, with exercise and smoking cessation recommended.

The American Diabetes Association recently held a Consensus Position Conference concerning atypical antipsychotic agents and obesity and diabetes mellitus. The resulting position statement, co-sponsored by the American Psychiatric Association, the American Association of Clinical Endocrinologists, and the North American Association for the Study of Obesity, noted that clozapine and olanzapine treatment were associated with the greatest potential weight gain and consistent evidence for an increased risk of diabetes mellitus and dyslipidemia (American Diabetes Association 2004). This report emphasized that physicians should consider multiple factors when evaluating the risks and benefits of prescribing specific antipsychotic agents, including medical and psychiatric conditions, and the report emphasized that the potential benefits of drugs with metabolic liabilities might under certain circumstances outweigh the potential risks (e.g., clozapine therapy in treatment-resistant schizophrenia; American Diabetes Association 2004). The development of obesity, dyslipidemia, the metabolic syndrome, or T2DM within an individual patient can depend on the contributions of drug effects (e.g., known effects on weight gain) as well as the contributions of individual host factors (e.g., family history, disease, or lifestyle), with host factors often difficult to modify in psychiatric populations. The effect of increasing adiposity on metabolic risk (e.g., insulin resistance) within populations is well known, and obesity remains a key target of primary and secondary prevention efforts by public health agencies. Emerging data may address some unanswered questions, but additional studies are clearly needed in key areas such as whether and how antipsychotic medications might alter insulin sensitivity or secretion independent of the effects of increasing adiposity in vulnerable individuals. In the meantime, current knowledge provides valuable insights that can be used by clinicians to guide treatment and monitoring decisions and provide patients with the highest standard of care.

OBESITY, DIABETES, AND ANTIPSYCHOTICS

Certain antipsychotic medications can cause significant weight gain, which is a growing concern given the propensity for obesity and related conditions in general in industrialized countries (Mokdad et al. 2003), the increased prevalence of obesity and diabetes in the schizophrenic population (Allison and Casey 2001; Allison et al. 1999b), and the known health consequences of these conditions. Illustrating the increased risk faced by psychiatric populations even prior to the introduction of atypical antipsychotics, Allison et al. (1999b) analyzed data from the National Health and Nutrition Examination Survey III and reported that schizophrenia patients, particularly women, are more likely to be overweight or obese as compared to the general population. This conclusion is supported by smaller surveys; for example, a study of 226 patients being treated with depot formulations of conventional antipsychotics indicated that the prevalence of clinically relevant obesity was four times that of the general population (Silverstone et al. 1988).

Investigators have estimated that obesity accounts for 60%–90% of T2DM in the general population (Anderson et al. 2003). A recent study found that the prevalence of diabetes in 2001 was almost 8% in the general population of the United States, a 61% increase from 1990, and risk was significantly associated with overweight and obesity (Mokdad et al. 2003). The most obese patients (BMI ≥ 40 kg/m^2) were seven to eight times more likely to have diabetes, and even patients who were simply overweight (BMI 25 kg/m^2–29.9 kg/m^2) had approximately a 59% greater chance of having diabetes as compared with individuals with normal BMI. In addition, the risk of hypertension, hyperlipidemia, asthma, and arthritis were significantly increased in individuals who were overweight or obese (Mokdad et al. 2003).

The consequences of obesity are well studied and a source of major concern for public health agencies. An analysis of subjects from five different cohort studies found that almost 300,000 deaths in the United States in 1991 could be attributed to obesity-related mortality, and that more than 80% of those deaths occurred in subjects whose BMI was 30 kg/m² or greater (Allison et al. 1999a). Another study found that all-cause mortality associated with BMI occurred in roughly a U-shaped pattern and that the highest incidence of mortality was associated with the highest degrees of obesity (Calle et al. 1999). Again, even moderate overweight was associated with increased mortality, with all-cause risk for mortality in male nonsmokers with a BMI 26.5 kg/m² or greater significantly increased over those of normal weight. In summary, obesity and weight gain are major risk factors for insulin resistance and diabetes (Pi-Sunyer 1993), leading to concerns about the weight gain induced by some psychotropic treatment regimens, particularly certain antipsychotic medications.

The hypothesis that weight gain is only a risk factor in the general population but not related to the risk of diabetes during antipsychotic treatment (Boehm et al. 2004) would seem to depend on unknown protective factors to block the adverse effects of adiposity that have been well established in a variety of species and human populations. Given the evidence for higher, rather than lower, prevalence of diabetes in psychiatric populations in almost all of the datasets examined to date, it seems unlikely that such protective factors are operating in individuals with psychiatric illness. Therefore, it would seem prudent to assume that antipsychotic-induced weight gain, just like any other increase in total fat mass, may be associated with a variety of adverse physiological effects.

Antipsychotic medications can *cause* weight gain in humans, rather than weight gain and treatment being merely associated. Causality is established by large placebo-controlled randomized clinical trials, the gold standard of evidence-based medicine. Comparing drug effects relative to placebo, absolute weight gain observed in various trials and head-to-head comparisons all indicate that the relative incidence and magnitude of weight gain is not equal among the different specific antipsychotic medications. A meta-analysis of both conventional (e.g., thioridazine, chlorpromazine) and newer antipsychotics (e.g., clozapine, olanzapine) revealed substantial differences in the degree of weight gain after 10 weeks of treatment (Allison et al. 1999a). The estimated mean weight changes at 10 weeks for selected study drugs ranged from a maximal gain of 4 kg or more with olanzapine and clozapine to approximately 2 kg for risperidone and less than 0.25 kg with ziprasidone. A pooled analysis of 932 patients treated with aripiprazole for 4–6 weeks found weight changes of less than 0.75 kg (Marder et al. 2003). Another meta-analysis of 10-week weight gain extended findings to amisulpride, which demonstrated approximately 0.8 kg mean weight increase over this time frame (Leucht et al. 2004). A large retrospective study of 636 schizophrenic outpatients receiving a single antipsychotic (risperidone, olanzapine, quetiapine, or haloperidol) for at least 4 weeks found that the proportion of patients with clinically relevant weight gain (≥7%) was higher with olanzapine (45.7%) than with risperidone (30.6%) or haloperidol (22.4%). Olanzapine and risperidone were associated with greater risk for weight gain than haloperidol (Bobes et al. 2003).

Studies of the long-term effects of antipsychotic drugs on weight, in contrast to short-term effects, are more relevant to clinical practice, where long-term treatment is the routine. Pooled doses of aripiprazole and ziprasidone have been associated with mean weight gain of approximately 1 kg per year; amisulpride with approximately 1.5 kg per year (Leucht et al. 2004); quetiapine and risperidone with 2–3 kg per year; and olanzapine with more than 6 kg per year (AstraZeneca 2004; Janssen Pharmaceutica 2003; Kinon 1998; Nemeroff 1997; Otsuka America Pharmaceutical and Bristol-Myers Squibb 2004; Pfizer 2004). Mean weight gain of more than 10 kg was observed in patients treated with olanzapine at dosages between 12.5 mg and 17.5 mg, the highest dosages tested in large-scale pivotal trials (Nemeroff 1997).

INSULIN RESISTANCE, DIABETES MELLITUS, AND ANTIPSYCHOTIC TREATMENT

A range of evidence suggests that treatment with certain antipsychotic medications, in comparison with no treatment or treatment with alternative antipsychotics, is associated with increased risk of insulin resistance, hyperglycemia, and T2DM (Casey et al. 2004). Interpretation of this literature has been complicated by reports that patients with major mental disorders such as schizophrenia have an increased prevalence of abnormalities in glucose regulation (e.g., insulin resistance) prior to the introduction of antipsychotics (Kasanin 1926). Waitzkin (1966a, 1966b) found that approximately 12% of 359 untreated schizophrenia patients younger than 50 years, and 15% of 213 untreated schizophrenia patients older than 50 years, had diabetes, compared with a U.S. population prevalence of about 6% in 2000 (American Diabetes Association 2000). These early studies did not control for age, weight, adiposity, ethnicity, or diet, with most experts hypothesizing that differences between patients and control subjects on key factors such as diet and activity level can contribute to at least some of the abnormalities observed.

A recent cross-sectional study in 26 hospitalized first-episode antipsychotic-naïve schizophrenic patients found that 15% of these patients had impaired fasting glucose (Ryan et al. 2003). Compared with control subjects matched for lifestyle and anthropometric measures, the schizophrenic patients exhibited higher mean fasting glucose concentrations (95.8 mg/dL vs. 88.2 mg/dL), insulin levels (9.8 µU/mL vs. 7.7 µU/mL), and cortisol levels (499.4 nmol/L vs. 303.2 nmol/L) (Ryan et al. 2003). The elevated plasma cortisol levels observed in this sample probably contributed to some of the increase in insulin resistance and plasma glucose. However, hyper-cortisolemia is not typically observed in treated patients with schizophrenia (Newcomer et al. 2002), so this study may have overestimated the degree of insulin resistance and hyperglycemia that might be expected to persist past the acute psychotic and/or agitated condition that led to hospitalization. In any case, this study complements earlier reports in support of the view that patients with schizophrenia and perhaps other major mental disorders may have increased risk for insulin resistance and T2DM, independent of exposure to antipsychotic medications. Increased vulnerability to insulin resistance and T2DM prior to drug exposure could alternatively be viewed as 1) a reason to doubt subsequent drugs effects on these endpoints, or 2) a reason to increase clinical attention to drug effects on adiposity or other factors that could further enhance risk.

ANTIPSYCHOTIC MEDICATIONS AND ADVERSE METABOLIC EVENTS

Evidence spanning case reports and case series, prospective observational studies, retrospective database analyses, and controlled experimental studies including randomized clinical trials have identified an association between certain antipsychotic medications and adverse metabolic events that include hyperglycemia, dyslipidemia, insulin resistance, exacerbation of existing type 1 diabetes mellitus (T1DM) and T2DM, new-onset T2DM, and diabetic ketoacidosis (Casey et al. 2004). Adverse effects on glucose and lipid metabolism (e.g., diabetes and dyslipidemia) have more frequently and consistently been associated with treatment using clozapine and olanzapine. Relatively fewer reports have described similar events in association with quetiapine or risperidone treatment. Current evidence detailing limited short- and long-term weight gain is consistent with little or no evidence for adverse effects on metabolic outcomes for ziprasidone, amisulpride, and the most recently launched drug, aripiprazole (Casey et al. 2004; Haupt and Newcomer 2001; Yang and McNeely 2002).

Although the relative risk of diabetes during treatment appears to match the rank order of weight gain liability with the different agents, weight gain may not explain all observed metabolic adverse events. Newcomer et al. (2002) measured effects of conventional and atypical antipsychotics on glucose regulation in chronically treated nondiabetic patients with schizophrenia compared with untreated healthy control subjects, with all patient and control groups matched for adiposity and age. Using a modified oral glucose tolerance test, patients receiving olanzapine and clozapine demonstrated significantly higher fasting and postload plasma glucose values compared with patients receiving conventional antipsychotics or untreated healthy control subjects. The risperidone-treated group did not differ from the conventional antipsychotic group but had higher postload glucose levels than the control group. Both olanzapine- and clozapine-treated patients had higher calculated insulin resistance in comparison with those treated with conventional agents, whereas risperidone-treated patients and typical antipsychotic-treated patients did not differ from the control patients. Henderson et al. (2000) conducted a 5-year naturalistic study of 82 outpatients with schizophrenia who were treated with clozapine. Thirty of the 82 patients (36.6%) were diagnosed with diabetes during follow-up, and although many experienced significant weight gain, others became diabetic in the absence of significant weight gain. Retrospective analyses of clozapine-, olanzapine-, and risperidone-associated cases of new-onset diabetes in the U.S. Food and Drug Administration's MedWatch database have suggested that although the majority of new-onset T2DM cases were associated with substantial weight gain or obesity, approximately 25% were not (Koller and Doraiswamy 2002; Koller et al. 2001, 2003a).

There are three levels of evidence that detail the association between certain antipsychotic medications and adverse metabolic events: 1) case reports, case series, and uncontrolled observational studies, typically useful for hypothesis generation; 2) retrospective database analyses, some using population-based datasets, often useful for hypothesis testing (discussed later, methodological issues can limit interpretability); and 3) controlled experimental studies, including randomized clinical trials, generally recognized as hypothesis testing.

Analyses of case reports to the MedWatch database concerning clozapine, olanzapine, and risperidone have suggested that most new-onset T2DM cases occur within the first 6 months of treatment initiation, are typically associated with substantial weight gain or obesity (i.e., 75%), and affect individuals without a family history of diabetes in as many as half of cases, with some cases having a close temporal relationship between treatment initiation and discontinuation and the development and/or resolution of the adverse event (Koller and Doraiswamy 2002; Koller et al. 2001, 2003a). Koller and colleagues, utilizing the MedWatch surveillance database and published reports, reported on hyperglycemia associated with treatment with clozapine (Koller et al. 2001), olanzapine (Koller and Doraiswamy 2002), and risperidone (Koller et al. 2003b). Two hundred forty-two cases of new-onset T2DM were reported in patients taking clozapine, 80 cases of metabolic acidosis or ketosis, and 25 deaths during hyperglycemic episodes. Koller and Doraiswamy (2002) identified 237 cases of diabetes or hyperglycemia associated with olanzapine treatment; 188 cases were new-onset diabetes. Eighty patients had metabolic acidosis or ketosis, and 15 patients died. Improved glycemic control was established in some patients subsequent to drug withdrawal or dose reduction. One hundred thirty-one reports of risperidone-associated hyperglycemia or diabetes were identified, 78 with newly diagnosed diabetes, 26 with acidosis or ketosis, and 4 deaths.

Doraiswamy and colleagues reported on the incidence of pancreatitis associated with clozapine, olanzapine, risperidone, or haloperidol treatment (Koller et al. 2003b), noting that most cases of pancreatitis associated with these antipsychotics occurred within the first 6 months of therapy. Reports of pancreatitis occurred at higher rates in patients treated with clozapine (40%) and olanzapine (33%) in contrast to risperidone (16%) and haloperidol (12%). Wirshing et al. (2002) conducted a chart review of 215 patients taking antipsychotics including clozapine, olanzapine, risperidone, quetiapine, haloperidol, and fluphenazine to assess the effects that these medications have on metabolic parameters such as serum glucose or lipid concentrations. The authors found that clozapine, olanzapine, and haloperidol were associated with statistically significant increases in fasting glucose concentrations, whereas clozapine and olanzapine were associated with significant increases in serum triglyceride concentrations. Each antipsychotic assessed was associated with an increase in fasting serum glucose concentration, ranging from 21% with olanzapine to 3% with risperidone.

Several studies have noted an association between the use of selected atypical antipsychotics and increased insulin secretion consistent with increased insulin resistance. Melkersson et al. (1999) reported elevated insulin levels in 46% of patients receiving clozapine therapy compared with 21% of patients receiving typical antipsychotics. A study of olanzapine found that 71% of a limited number of patients ($n = 14$) exhibited elevated serum insulin levels. Additionally, the median serum concentration of insulin was significantly higher than the reference normal value. An in vitro study on pancreatic beta-cells found that clozapine, but not several other antipsychotics, increased basal insulin release (Melkersson et al. 2001). Similarly, increases in mean insulin and glucose levels were observed in six patients with schizophrenia treated with clozapine (Yazici et al. 1998).

There are currently more than 20 reported retrospective analyses that aim to test the strength of the association between treatment with specific medications and the presence of diabetes mellitus using large administrative or health plan databases. These analyses are funded primarily by pharmaceutical companies, and a limited number have been published in indexed journals to date. The common underlying approach has been to measure the association within an existing database between use of specific antipsychotic medications and the presence of one or more surrogate indicators of diabetes mellitus (e.g., prescription of hypoglycemic agent or relevant ICD-9 codes). The majority of these studies suggest that those drugs associated with more weight gain (e.g., olanzapine) are also associated with increased risk of diabetes in comparison with no treatment, conventional treatment, or a drug producing less weight gain (e.g., risperidone). Although explicit tests of the relationship of diabetes risk to weight gain are not possible with these studies, no study indicates that a drug with high weight-gain potential (e.g., olanzapine) has a lower risk of diabetes in comparison to any alternative treatment condition. A minority of studies detect no difference between groups or a nonspecific increase in the association for all treated groups versus untreated control subjects.

Limitations on the interpretation and generalizability of these retrospective database analyses include variable methodology, use of insurance or health plan versus population-based datasets in many but not all cases, uncontrolled cohort effects without access to relevant clinical parameters that might allow statistical controls (e.g., baseline and treatment-related weights, diet, family history, prior treatment history, and laboratory values), variable numbers of subjects exposed to comparison drugs for different periods of time leading to unequal sample sizes, limited comparability or exclusion of certain drugs, and importantly a limited history of prior antipsychotic and other drug exposures that makes it difficult to control for critical prior treatment effects (e.g., a 20-kg weight gain on prior treatment can impact current risk of T2DM).

The most important problem with retrospective database analyses involves the use of insensitive, unreliable, surrogate diagnostic indicators for diabetes (e.g., prescription of hypoglycemic drug, ICD-9 codes). Based on American Diabetes Association estimates that approximately 33% of individuals in the general population with T2DM are undiagnosed, many individuals with psychiatric disorders will have no associated hypoglycemic prescription or diabetes-related ICD-9 code to be detected in this type of analysis. Given that antipsychotic-related differences in diabetes prevalence are probably less than 33%, this suggests that measurement error may complicate detection of potential relevant target signals. The significant problem with signal-to-noise ratio in studies of this type suggests that variable results, including potential failure to detect the target signal, can be expected.

The third level of evidence for an association between antipsychotics and metabolic outcomes concerns controlled experimental studies and randomized clinical trials. Although several of the latter are currently in progress, a small number have been completed and are available for review. Growing evidence supports the key observation that treatments producing the largest increases in weight and adiposity are also associated with the most consistent and clinically significant adverse effects on insulin sensitivity, blood glucose, and blood lipids. Five studies have reported significant increases in plasma insulin, suggesting decreased insulin sensitivity (i.e., insulin resistance) during olanzapine treatment in comparison with various control conditions (Ebenbichler et al. 2003; Glick et al. 2001; Melkersson and Hulting 2001; Newcomer et al. 2002; Simpson et al. 2002), and some of these report a significant increase in insulin resistance during olanzapine therapy compared with baseline levels (Ebenbichler et al. 2003; Glick et al. 2001). Two studies report elevated insulin levels in 31%–71% of patients receiving olanzapine treatment (Melkersson and Dahl 2003; Melkersson et al. 2000), while significant improvements in insulin resistance and beta-cell function were also observed in a study of 40 patients with schizophrenia following the switch from olanzapine to risperidone therapy (Berry and Mahmoud 2002). These studies are consistent with the evidence from general population samples that conditions that increase adiposity will tend to be associated with increases in insulin resistance, potentially leading to compensatory insulin secretion in those persons with pancreatic beta-cell reserve and hyperglycemia in those individuals with relative beta-cell failure.

One randomized, double-blind trial was conducted in 157 schizophrenic patients, consisting of an 8-week fixed-dose period and a 6-week variable-dose period of clozapine, olanzapine, risperidone, or haloperidol (Lindenmayer et al. 2003). Patients were assessed for fasting plasma glucose and cholesterol concentrations at the end of both the 8-week and 6-week periods to determine the effect of these antipsychotics on these metabolic parameters. There were significant increases in glucose levels at the end of the 6-week variable-dose period for patients treated with olanzapine and at the end of the 8-week fixed-dose period for patients given clozapine or haloperidol. Cholesterol levels were increased at the end of the 6-week variable-dose period for patients given olanzapine and at the end of the 8-week fixed-dose period for the patients given clozapine or olanzapine. This study was complicated by baseline and related endpoint weights in some groups that are not characteristic of those usually seen in clinical practice or other trials, underscoring the need to control for previous treatments and baseline status in future trials. A pooled analysis of safety data from short-term (4–6 week) controlled trials of aripiprazole in schizophrenia found that changes in fasting serum glucose concentrations were similar between patients treated with aripiprazole and placebo (Marder et al. 2003). A 26-week controlled study of aripiprazole for relapse prevention in 310 patients with schizophrenia found no clinically significant change from baseline in fasting glucose concentration (Pigott et al. 2003).

The limited amount of controlled experimental data evaluating the metabolic effects of quetiapine therapy limit definitive assessment of the metabolic risks associated with its use. Findings to date suggest that quetiapine therapy is not associated with a consistent increase in the risk of developing diabetes or dyslipidemia. However, a possible increase in metabolic risk would be predicted to occur in association with any treatment course that produces increases in weight and adiposity, with quetiapine typically producing modest weight gain. A 6-week randomized study of atypical antipsychotics in 56 patients with schizophrenia (Atmaca et al. 2003) showed significant changes in triglyceride levels from baseline with quetiapine therapy. Quetiapine-treated patients ($n=14$) showed an increase in triglyceride levels from baseline at week 6 (11.64 mg/dL, $P<0.05$), although the mean increase was approximately three times less than that observed with clozapine (36.28 mg/dL) or olanzapine (31.23 mg/dL) therapy. In this particular dataset, body weight also showed a significant mean increase from baseline that was approximately twice that observed routinely in larger datasets, suggesting that effects on lipids in this dataset might be larger than that observed routinely in larger, more representative, datasets.

Fasting glucose, insulin, and lipid parameters have been assessed in a randomized, double-blind, 6-week study comparing olanzapine and ziprasidone therapy in 269 inpatients with an acute exacerbation of schizophrenia or schizoaffective disorder (Glick et al. 2001). Significant increases from baseline in median fasting plasma insulin levels ($P<0.0001$) and Homeostasis Model Assessment calculated insulin resistance ($P<0.0001$) were observed during olanzapine but not ziprasidone treatment. Median body weight increased by 7.2 lb (3.3 kg) from baseline with olanzapine treatment compared with 1.2 lb (0.5 kg) with ziprasidone—median body weight was significantly higher in the olanzapine group than the ziprasidone group at endpoint ($P<0.0001$). In this relatively young sample, with a significant compensatory hyperinsulinemic response, fasting plasma glucose did not change significantly in either olanzapine- or ziprasidone-treated subjects. Significant increases from baseline in median fasting total cholesterol (20 mg/dL, $P<0.0001$), low-density lipoprotein cholesterol

(13 mg/dL, *P*<0.0001), and triglyceride (26 mg/dL, *P*=0.0003) levels were observed with olanzapine therapy. In contrast, minimal changes were observed with ziprasidone therapy, and median total and low-density lipoprotein cholesterol, and triglyceride levels were significantly higher in the olanzapine group at endpoint (*P*<0.003).

The metabolic syndrome, as defined by the National Cholesterol Education Program Adult Treatment Panel III and other sources, is an important risk factor for the development of diabetes and coronary heart disease (Lorenzo et al. 2003; Sattar et al. 2003). In the first published example of a prospective randomized evaluation of drug effects on the incidence of the metabolic syndrome, pooled data were used from two 26-week double-blind, randomized controlled trials (McQuade et al. 2003; Pigott et al. 2003) evaluating the effects of aripiprazole. One trial compared aripiprazole with placebo in stable, chronic schizophrenic patients (*n*=310) and the second trial compared aripiprazole with olanzapine in patients in acute relapse of schizophrenia (*n*=314). In a pooled analysis of the two trials (L'Italien 2003), the cumulative incidence of metabolic syndrome (±SE) varied across the different treatment conditions, with an incidence of 19.2%±4.0% during olanzapine treatment, 12.8%±4.5% on placebo treatment, and 7.6%±2.3% on treatment with aripiprazole. A log-rank test indicated significant differences among the three incidence rates (*P*=0.003; aripiprazole vs. olanzapine, 69% relative risk reduction) (Casey et al. 2003; L'Italien 2003)

CONCLUSION

A variety of data concerning the use of atypical antipsychotics indicate that some drugs in this class are associated with a significant risk of weight gain and disordered glucose and lipid metabolism. It is not clear that weight gain is a prerequisite for the development of insulin resistance, impaired glucose tolerance, dyslipidemia, or diabetes. Additional research needs to be done to examine the pharmacological factors that contribute to these adverse events in vulnerable individuals.

Prudent clinicians can monitor patients taking atypical antipsychotics for weight increase and related metabolic changes, particularly within the first several months of treatment. The American Psychiatric Association recommends that fasting plasma glucose, lipid levels, and blood pressure be assessed within 3 months after initiation of antipsychotic drug therapy. Subsequent assessments of plasma glucose should be scheduled at least annually, and more often for patients with other risk factors for diabetes. If patients exhibit clinical signs and symptoms of hyperglycemia (e.g., poly-uria or polydipsia), clinicians should quickly assess plasma glucose concentrations and begin the process of treating and correcting any abnormalities. This would include medical or endocrine consultation, with any needed acute modification of the treatment regimen (e.g., hypoglycemia agents); the active education of patients and families about advisable lifestyle changes; and consideration of the risks and benefits of switching antipsychotic medication if necessary to one that carries less relative risk of precipitating weight gain or diabetes. Clinicians should also recognize that some medication combinations may further exacerbate weight gain (e.g., an atypical antipsychotic and a mood stabilizer like valproate). For patients who exhibit increased risk of diabetes prior to treatment (e.g., overweight or obese individuals), education should be initiated immediately, and selection of a medication regimen should take the patient's comorbid condition into account. With careful monitoring and individualized treatment, patients can enjoy maximum benefit from atypical antipsychotics, and physicians can continue to deliver the highest level of care.

REFERENCES

Allison DB, Casey DE: Antipsychotic-induced weight gain: a review of the literature. J Clin Psychiatry 62 (suppl):22–31, 2001

Allison DB, Mentore JL, Heo M, et al: Antipsychotic-induced weight gain: a comprehensive research synthesis. Am J Psychiatry 156:1686–1696, 1999a

Allison DB, Fontaine KR, Heo M, et al: The distribution of body mass index among individuals with and without schizophrenia. J Clin Psychiatry 60:215–220, 1999b

American Diabetes Association: Diabetes Facts and Figures. Alexandria, VA, American Diabetes Association, 2000

American Diabetes Association: Standards of medical care for patients with diabetes mellitus. Diabetes Care 26 (suppl):S33–S50, 2003

American Diabetes Association: Consensus development conference on antipsychotic drugs and obesity and diabetes. Diabetes Care 27:596–601, 2004

Anderson JW, Kendall CW, Jenkins DJ: Importance of weight management in type 2 diabetes: review with meta-analysis of clinical studies. J Am Coll Nutr 22:331–339, 2003

AstraZeneca: Seroquel (Quetiapine) Package Insert. New York, AstraZeneca, 2004

Atmaca M, Kuloglu M, Tezcan E, et al: Serum leptin and triglyceride levels in patients on treatment with atypical antipsychotics. J Clin Psychiatry 64:598–604, 2003

Banerji MA, Lebowitz J, Chaiken RL, et al: Relationship of visceral adipose tissue and glucose disposal is independent of sex in black NIDDM subjects. Am J Physiol 273:E425–E432, 1997

Berry S, Mahmoud R: Improvement of insulin indices after switch from olanzapine to risperidone. Eur Neuropsychopharmacol 12 (suppl):S316, 2002

Bobes J, Rejas J, Garcia-Garcia M, et al: Weight gain in patients with schizophrenia treated with risperidone, olanzapine, quetiapine or haloperidol: results of the EIRE study. Schizophr Res 62:77–88, 2003

Boehm G, Racoosin JA, Laughren TP, et al: Consensus development conference on antipsychotic drugs and obesity and diabetes: response to consensus statement. Diabetes Care 27:2088–2090, 2004

Calle EE, Thun MJ, Petrelli JM, et al: Body-mass index and mortality in a prospective cohort of U.S. adults. N Engl J Med 341:1097–1105, 1999

Casey DE, L'Italien GJ, Waldeck R, et al: Metabolic syndrome comparison between olanzapine, aripiprazole, and placebo. Poster Presented at the annual meeting of the American Psychiatric Association, San Francisco, CA, May 2003

Casey DE, Haupt DW, Newcomer JW, et al: Antipsychotic-induced weight gain and metabolic abnormalities: implications for increased mortality in patients with schizophrenia. J Clin Psychiatry 65 (suppl):4–18, 2004

Druss BG, Bradford WD, Rosenheck RA, et al: Quality of medical care and excess mortality in older patients with mental disorders. Arch Gen Psychiatry 58:565–572, 2001

Ebenbichler CF, Laimer M, Eder U, et al: Olanzapine induces insulin resistance: results from a prospective study. J Clin Psychiatry 64:1436–1439, 2003

Expert Committee on the Diagnosis and Classification of Diabetes Mellitus: Report of the Expert Committee on the Diagnosis and Classification of Diabetes Mellitus. Diabetes Care 26 (suppl):S5–S20, 2003

Garg A, Grundy SM: Management of dyslipidemia in NIDDM. Diabetes Care 13:153–169, 1990

Glick ID, Fryburg D, O'Sullivan RL, et al: Ziprasidone's benefits versus olanzapine on weight gain and insulin resistance. Presented at the 154th annual meeting of the American Psychiatric Association, New Orleans, LA, May 2001

Gray DS: Diagnosis and prevalence of obesity. Med Clin North Am 73:1–13, 1989

Haffner SM, Lehto S, Ronnemaa T, et al: Mortality from coronary heart disease in subjects with type 2 diabetes and in nondiabetic subjects with and without prior myocardial infarction. N Engl J Med 339:229–234, 1998

Harris MI: Health care and health status and outcomes for patients with type 2 diabetes. Diabetes Care 23:754–758, 2000

Haupt DW, Newcomer JW: Hyperglycemia and antipsychotic medications. J Clin Psychiatry 62 (suppl):15–26, 2001

Henderson DC, Cagliero E, Gray C, et al: Clozapine, diabetes mellitus, weight gain, and lipid abnormalities: a five-year naturalistic study. Am J Psychiatry 157:975–981, 2000

Janssen Pharmaceutica: Risperdal (Risperidone) Package Insert. Titusville, NJ, Janssen Pharmaceutica, 2003

Kasanin J: The blood sugar curve in mental disease. Arch Neurol Psychiatry 16:414–419, 1926

Kinon BJ: The routine use of atypical antipsychotic agents: maintenance treatment. J Clin Psychiatry 59 (suppl):18–22, 1998

Koller EA, Doraiswamy PM: Olanzapine-associated diabetes mellitus. Pharmacotherapy 22:841–852, 2002

Koller E, Schneider B, Bennett K, et al: Clozapine-associated diabetes. Am J Med 111:716–723, 2001

Koller EA, Cross JT, Doraiswamy PM, et al: Pancreatitis associated with atypical antipsychotics: from the Food and Drug Administration's MedWatch surveillance system and published reports. Pharmacotherapy 23:1123–1130, 2003a

Koller EA, Cross JT, Doraiswamy PM, et al: Risperidone-associated diabetes mellitus: a pharmacovigilance study. Pharmacotherapy 23:735–744, 2003b

L'Italien GJ: Pharmacoeconomic impact of antipsychotic-induced metabolic events. Am J Manag Care 3:S38–S42, 2003

Leucht S, Wagenpfeil S, Hamann J, et al: Amisulpride is an "atypical" antipsychotic associated with low weight gain. Psychopharmacology (Berl) 173:112–115, 2004

Lindenmayer JP, Czobor P, Volavka J, et al: Changes in glucose and cholesterol levels in patients with schizophrenia treated with typical or atypical antipsychotics. Am J Psychiatry 160:290–296, 2003

Lorenzo C, Okoloise M, Williams K, et al: The metabolic syndrome as predictor of type 2 diabetes: the San Antonio heart study. Diabetes Care 26:3153–3159, 2003

Marder SR, McQuade RD, Stock E, et al: Aripiprazole in the treatment of schizophrenia: safety and tolerability in short-term, placebo-controlled trials. Schizophr Res 61:123–136, 2003

McQuade RD, Jody D, Kujuwa M, et al: Long-term weight effects of aripiprazole versus olanzapine. Poster presented at the annual meeting of the American Psychiatric Association, San Francisco, CA, May 2003

Melkersson KI, Dahl ML: Relationship between levels of insulin or triglycerides and serum concentrations of the atypical antipsychotics clozapine and olanzapine in patients on treatment with therapeutic doses. Psychopharmacology (Berl) 170:157–166, 2003

Melkersson KI, Hulting AL: Insulin and leptin levels in patients with schizophrenia or related psychoses: a comparison between different antipsychotic agents. Psychopharmacology (Berl) 154:205–212, 2001

Melkersson KI, Hulting AL, Brismar KE: Different influences of classical antipsychotics and clozapine on glucose-insulin homeostasis in patients with schizophrenia or related psychoses. J Clin Psychiatry 60:783–791, 1999

Melkersson KI, Hulting AL, Brismar KE: Elevated levels of insulin, leptin, and blood lipids in olanzapine-treated patients with schizophrenia or related psychoses. J Clin Psychiatry 61:742–749, 2000

Melkersson K, Khan A, Hilding A, et al: Different effects of antipsychotic drugs on insulin release in vitro. Eur Neuropsychopharmacol 11:327–332, 2001

Mokdad AH, Ford ES, Bowman BA, et al: Prevalence of obesity, diabetes, and obesity-related health risk factors, 2001. JAMA 289:76–79, 2003

National Cholesterol Education Program: Executive summary of the Third Report of The National Cholesterol Education Program (NCEP) Expert Panel on Detection, Evaluation, and Treatment of High Blood Cholesterol In Adults (Adult Treatment Panel III). JAMA 285:2486–2497, 2001

Nemeroff CB: Dosing the antipsychotic medication olanzapine. J Clin Psychiatry 58 (suppl):45–49, 1997

Newcomer JW, Haupt DW, Fucetola R, et al: Abnormalities in glucose regulation during antipsychotic treatment of schizophrenia. Arch Gen Psychiatry 59:337–345, 2002

Otsuka America Pharmaceutical and Bristol-Myers Squibb: Abilify (Aripiprazole) Package Insert. Rockville, MD, Otsuka America Pharmaceutical and Bristol-Myers Squibb, 2004

Pfizer: Geodon (Ziprasidone HCl) Package Insert. New York, Pfizer, 2004

Pi-Sunyer FX: Medical hazards of obesity. Ann Intern Med 119:655–660, 1993

Pigott TA, Carson WH, Saha AR, et al: Aripiprazole for the prevention of relapse in stabilized patients with chronic schizophrenia: a placebo-controlled 26-week study. J Clin Psychiatry 64:1048–1056, 2003

Reaven G: Syndrome X: 10 years after. Drugs 58 (suppl):19–20, 75–82, 1999

Resnick HE, Valsania P, Halter JB, et al: Differential effects of BMI on diabetes risk among black and white Americans. Diabetes Care 21:1828–1835, 1998

Ryan MC, Collins P, Thakore JH: Impaired fasting glucose tolerance in first-episode, drug-naive patients with schizophrenia. Am J Psychiatry 160:284–289, 2003

Sattar N, Gaw A, Scherbakova R, et al: Metabolic syndrome with and without C-reactive protein as a predictor of coronary heart disease and diabetes in the West of Scotland Coronary Prevention Study. Circulation 108:414–419, 2003

Silverstone T, Smith G, Goodall E: Prevalence of obesity in patients receiving depot antipsychotics. Br J Psychiatry 153:214–217, 1988

Simpson G, Weiden P, Pigott T, et al: Ziprasidone vs olanzapine in schizophrenia: 6-month continuation study. Eur Neuropsychopharmacol 12 (suppl):S310, 2002

Waitzkin L: A survey for unknown diabetics in a mental hospital, I: men under age fifty. Diabetes 15:97–104, 1966a

Waitzkin L: A survey for unknown diabetics in a mental hospital, II: men from age fifty. Diabetes 15:164–172, 1966b

Wilson PW, Kannel WB, Anderson KM: Lipids, glucose intolerance and vascular disease: the Framingham Study. Monogr Atheroscler 13:1–11, 1985

Wilson PW, D'Agostino RB, Levy D, et al: Prediction of coronary heart disease using risk factor categories. Circulation 97:1837–1847, 1998

Wirshing DA, Boyd JA, Meng LR, et al: The effects of novel antipsychotics on glucose and lipid levels. J Clin Psychiatry 63:856–865, 2002

Yang SH, McNeely MJ: Rhabdomyolysis, pancreatitis, and hyperglycemia with ziprasidone. Am J Psychiatry 159:1435, 2002

Yazici KM, Erbas T, Yazici AH: The effect of clozapine on glucose metabolism. Exp Clin Endocrinol Diabetes 106:475–477, 1998

INDEX